D0851116

Oxford American Handbook of
Critical Care

Published and forthcoming Oxford American Handbooks

Oxford American Handbook of Clinical Medicine
Oxford American Handbook of Anesthesia
Oxford American Handbook of Clinical Dentistry
Oxford American Handbook of Clinical Surgery
Oxford American Handbook of Critical Care
Oxford American Handbook of Emergency Medicine
Oxford American Handbook of ENT and Head and Neck Surgery
Oxford American Handbook of Nephrology and Hypertension
Oxford American Handbook of Obstetrics & Gynecology
Oxford American Handbook of Pediatrics
Oxford American Handbook of Psychiatry
Oxford American Handbook of Respiratory Medicine

Oxford American Handbook of Critical Care

Edited by

John A. Kellum, MD

Professor, Department of Critical Care Medicine
University of Pittsburgh
Pittsburgh, Pennsylvania

Scott R. Gunn, MD

Assistant Professor, Department of Critical Care
Medicine, University of Pittsburgh
Pittsburgh, Pennsylvania

with

Mervyn Singer

Professor of Intensive Care Medicine; Director
Bloomsbury Institute of Intensive Care Medicine
University College London, London, UK

Andrew R. Webb

Medical Director and Consultant Physician
Department of Intensive Care
University College London Hospitals
London, UK

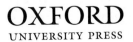

OXFORD
UNIVERSITY PRESS

OXFORD
UNIVERSITY PRESS

Great Clarendon Street, Oxford OX2 6DP

Oxford University Press is a department of the University of Oxford.
It furthers the University's objective of excellence in research, scholarship,
and education by publishing worldwide in

Oxford New York

Auckland Cape Town Dar es Salaam Hong Kong Karachi
Kuala Lumpur Madrid Melbourne Mexico City Nairobi
New Delhi Shanghai Taipei Toronto

With offices in

Argentina Austria Brazil Chile Czech Republic France Greece
Guatemala Hungary Italy Japan Poland Portugal Singapore
South Korea Switzerland Thailand Turkey Ukraine Vietnam

Oxford is a registered trademark of Oxford University Press
in the UK and in certain other countries.

Published in the United States
by Oxford University Press Inc., New York

British Library Cataloguing in Publication Data

Data available

Library of Congress Cataloging in Publication Data
Kellum, John A.

Oxford American handbook of critical care/John A. Kellum, Scott R. Gunn.
p.; cm. – (Oxford American handbooks)

Adapted from: Oxford handbook of critical care/Mervyn Singer, Andrew R. Webb. 2nd ed. 2005.
Includes bibliographical references and index.
ISBN 978-0-19-530528-9 (alk.paper)

1. Critical care medicine–Handbooks, manuals, etc. I. Gunn, Scott R. II. Singer,
Mervyn. Oxford handbook of critical care. III. Title. IV. Series.
[DNLM: 1. Critical Care–Handbooks.
WX 39 K290 2007]
RC86.7.O9448 2007   2007006584
616.02'8–dc22

Typeset by Newgen Imaging Systems (P) Ltd., Chennai, India
Printed in China
on acid-free paper by
Phoenix Offset

ISBN 978–0–19–530528–9 (flexicover: alk.paper)

10 9 8 7 6 5 4 3 2 1

To my beloved wife Nita, and my two wonderful children Brianna and Alston, for understanding my long work hours and time away from home. Their unconditional love and support makes all things possible.

—John A. Kellum

To Sherry, my true companion

—Scott R. Gunn

Preface

Although handbooks abound for virtually every discipline in medicine, critical care largely misses out. Many of us have experience with 'home-grown' notebooks in which trainees try to record all the pearls of wisdom they can catch. Those dog-eared volumes followed many of us through our training and probably still can be found in desk drawers or in the back of closets. But it takes a lot of effort to keep them current and, in our case, legible. We've done our best with this handbook to accomplish both and much more.

The *Oxford Handbook of Critical Care*, by Mervyn Singer and Andrew Webb, is regarded worldwide as a valued 'friend in the pocket' for its practical, clinically relevant content and clear, accessible design for quick access to key information. From the start, we were intrigued by the prospects of adapting this highly successful handbook for an American medical audience. Although the basic principles of management are uniform, critical care is structurally much different in the United States compared with the United Kingdom. Given the much larger population utilizing intensive care units (ICUs) in the United States (roughly five million Americans are admitted to the ICU annually) and severe shortages of full-time critical care specialists on this side of the Atlantic, the need for quick, reliable information on the care of the critically ill is probably even greater.

Consequently, this edition does much more than 'Americanize' the *Handbook*. Several noted developments in critical care have occurred during the last few years; and the practice of critical care medicine is changing rapidly. Much of this change has come from evidence in the medical literature and we have updated the text to reflect these developments. However, the evolution of practice patterns in medicine is as much about centers of excellence and clinical thought leaders as it is about medical literature. As such, we have tried to instill this edition with some of the clinical 'know-how' that has developed during the last quarter of a century at the University of Pittsburgh. In 2001, the University of Pittsburgh became the first medical school in the United States to develop a fully independent department dedicated to critical care medicine. Since its inception under Drs. Peter Safar and Ake Grenvik to the present day, the University of Pittsburgh has been a leading center in the field of critical care medicine around the world. It is our great pleasure to be able to contribute to this project.

John A. Kellum
Scott R. Gunn
2007

Contents

Symbols and abbreviations

↑	increased
↓	decreased
≈	approximately
ACE	angiotensin converting enzyme
ACMV	assisted controlled mechanical ventilation
ACT	activated clotting time
ACTH	adrenocorticotropic hormone
ADQI	Acute Dialysis Quality Initiative
AIDS	acquired immune deficiency syndrome
ALT	alanine aminotransferase
AMI	acute myocardial infarction
APACHE	Acute Physiology and Chronic Health Evaluation
APTT	activated partial thromboplastin time
ARDS	acute respiratory distress syndrome
AST	aspartate aminotransferase
ATP	adenosine triphosphate
ATPase	adenosine triphosphatase
AV	arteriovenous
BBB	bundle branch block
bid	bis in die (twice a day)
BiPAP	bilevel positive airway pressure
BIS	bispectral index
BNP	brain natriuretic peptide
BUN	blood urea nitrogen
cAMP	cyclic adenosine monophosphate
CBF	cerebral blood flow
CBV	cerebral blood volume
CDI	central diabetes insipidus
cGMP	cyclic guanosine monophosphate
CK	creatine kinase
$CMRO_2$	cerebral metabolism of oxygen

CMV	controlled mechanical ventilation
CMV	cytomegalovirus
CNS	central nervous system
CoA	Co-enzyme A
COP	colloid osmotic pressure
COPD	chronic obstructive pulmonary disease
CPAP	continuous positive airway pressure
CPP	cerebral perfusion pressure
CPR	cardiopulmonary resuscitation
CRP	C-reactive protein
CRRT	continuous renal replacement therapy
CSF	cerebrospinal fluid
CT	computed tomography
CVA	cerebrovascular accident
CXR	chest radiograph
DIC	disseminated intravascular coagulation
DS	degree of substitution
DVT	deep vein thrombosis
$ECCO_2R$	extracorporeal CO_2 removal
ECG	electrocardiogram
ECMO	extracorporeal membrane oxygenation
EEG	electroencephalogram
FDP	fibrin degradation product
FEV_1	forced expired volume in 1 s
FFP	fresh frozen plasma
f/V_T	rapid shallow-breathing index
FiO_2	fractional inspired oxygen concentration
FRC	functional residual capacity
FVC	forced vital capacity
γ-GTP	gamma-glutamyl transpeptidase
GCS	Glasgow Coma Scale
GMP	guanosine monophosphate
GVHD	graft versus host disease
Hb	hemoglobin
HELLP	hemolysis, elevated liver enzymes, and low platelets
HFJV	high-frequency jet ventilation

HFOV	high-frequency oscillation ventilation
HITS	heparin-induced thrombocytopenia syndrome
HIV	human immunodeficiency virus
HUS	hemolytic uremic syndrome
ICP	intracranial pressure
ICU	intensive care unit
id	inside diameter
I:E	inspiratory-to-expiratory ratio
IL	interleukin
IM	intramuscularly
IMV	intermittent mandatory ventilation
INR	international normalized ratio
IPPV	intermittent positive-pressure ventilation
ISS	Injury Severity Score
ITP	idiopathic thrombocytopenic purpura
IV	intravenous
kIU	kallikrein inactivation units
LAFB	left anterior fascicular block
LBBB	left bundle branch block
LDH	lactate dehydrogenase
LiDCO	Lithium dilution cardiac output
L-NMMA	L-N-mono-methyl-arginine
LPFB	left posterior fascicular block
LVF	left ventricular failure
MAP	mean arterial pressure
M,C&S	microscopy, culture, and sensitivity
MCA	middle cerebral artery
MCV	mean corpuscular volume
MDMA	3,4-methylenedioxymethamphetamine
MI	myocardial infarction
MIC	minimal inhibitory concentration
MRI	magnetic resonance imaging
MRSA	methicillin-resistant *Staphylococcus aureus*
NIRS	near-infrared spectroscopy
NSAIDS	nonsteroidal anti-inflammatory drugs
PaCO$_2$	arterial partial pressure of carbon dioxide

PAF	platelet activating factor
PaO_2	arterial partial pressure of oxygen
Paw	mean airway pressure
PAWP	pulmonary artery wedge pressure
PCO_2	partial pressure of carbon dioxide
PCR	polymerase chain reaction
PDE	phosphodiesterase
PEEP	positive end expiratory pressure
PEEPi	intrinsic positive end expiratory pressure
PGE_1	prostaglandin E_1
PI	pulsatility index
PImax	maximum inspiratory force
PO	per os (by mouth)
PO_2	partial pressure of oxygen
PR	per rectum
PRN	pro re nata (as needed)
PSV	pressure support ventilation
PT	prothrombin time
PTT	partial thromboplastin time
q	every
qd	quaque die (every day)
qid	quarter in die (four times a day)
Qs/Qt	shunt fraction
RASS	Richmond Agitation Sedation Scale
RBBB	right bundle branch block
REE	resting energy expenditure
RQ	respiratory quotient
RTS	Revised Trauma Score
SaO_2	arterial oxygen saturation
SAPS	Simplified Acute Physiology Score
SAS	Sedation Agitation Scale
SC	subcutaneously
SCUF	slow continuous ultrafiltration
SIADH	syndrome of inappropriate antidiuretic hormone
SIG	strong ion gap
SjO_2	jugular venous bulb saturation

SL	sublingually
SLE	systemic lupus erythematosus
SOFA	Sequential Organ Failure Assessment
SpO_2	pulse oximeter oxygen saturation
SVT	supraventricular tachycardia
TB	tuberculosis
TF	tissue factor
Ti	Inspiratory time
tid	ter in die (three times a day)
TISS	Therapeutic Intervention Scoring System
TMP-SMX	trimethoprim–sulfamethoxazole
TT	thrombin time
TTP	thrombotic thrombocytopenic purpura
VCO_2	carbon dioxide production
Vd	dead space
VF	ventricular fibrillation
VO_2	oxygen consumption
VT	ventricular tachycardia
V_T	tidal volume

Respiratory therapy techniques

Oxygen therapy

All critically ill patients should receive additional inspired oxygen on a 'more not less best' philosophy.

Principles

High-flow, high-concentration oxygen should be given to any acutely dyspneic or hypoxemic patient until accurate titration can be performed using pulse oximetry or arterial blood gas analysis.

In general, maintain arterial oxygen saturation (SaO_2) >90%, although preferably >95%. Compromises may need to be made during acute or chronic hypoxemic respiratory failure, or prolonged, severe acute respiratory distress syndrome (ARDS), when lower values may suffice provided tissue oxygen delivery is maintained.

All patients placed on mechanical ventilation should initially receive a high fractional inspired oxygen concentration (FiO_2) until accurate titration is performed using arterial blood gas analysis or pulse oximetry.

Apart from patients receiving hyperbaric oxygen therapy (e.g., for carbon monoxide poisoning, diving accidents), there is no need to maintain supranormal levels of arterial partial pressure of oxygen (PaO_2).

Cautions

A small proportion of patients with chronic ventilation–perfusion mismatch and hypoxemia will develop an increasing arterial partial pressure of carbon dioxide ($PaCO_2$) and carbon dioxide narcosis when supplemental oxygen is administered. However, this is seldom (if ever) abrupt, and a period of deterioration and increasing drowsiness will alert medical and nursing staff to consider either (1) FiO_2 reduction if overall condition allows, (2) noninvasive or invasive mechanical ventilation if fatiguing, or (3) much less frequently, use of respiratory stimulants such as doxapram. The corollary is that close supervision and monitoring is necessary in all critically ill patients.

A normal pulse oximetry reading may obscure deteriorating gas exchange and progressive hypercapnia.

Oxygen toxicity is described in animal models. Normal volunteers will become symptomatic after several hours of breathing pure oxygen. Furthermore, washout of nitrogen may lead to microatelectasis. However, the relevance and relative importance of oxygen toxicity compared with other forms of ventilator trauma in critically ill patients is still far from clear. Efforts should nevertheless be made to minimize FiO_2 whenever possible. Debate continues regarding whether FiO_2 or airway pressures (e.g., positive end expiratory pressure [PEEP], tidal volume [V_T], inspiratory pressures) should be reduced first. Our current view is to minimize the risks of ventilator trauma by reducing airway pressures.

Monitoring

An oxygen analyzer in the inspiratory limb of the ventilator or continuous positive airway pressure/bilevel positive airway pressure (CPAP/BiPAP) circuit confirms the patient is receiving a known FiO_2. Most modern ventilators have a built-in calibration device.

Adequacy and changes in SaO_2 can be continuously monitored by pulse oximetry and intermittent or continuous invasive blood gas analysis.

Oxygen delivery

- Oxygen delivery via nasal cannula gives an imprecise FiO_2 level and should only be used when hypoxemia is not a major concern.
- Standard face masks allow a slightly higher FiO_2 delivery than nasal cannula. The addition of a reservoir bag and one-way valve significantly increases the delivered FiO_2.
- Masks fitted with a Venturi valve deliver a reasonably accurate FiO_2 (0.24, 0.28, 0.35, 0.40, 0.60) except in patients with very high inspiratory flow rates. These masks do not allow delivery of humidified gas, but are preferable in the short term for dyspneic patients because they enable more precise monitoring of PaO_2-to-FiO_2 ratios.
- A tight-fitting anesthetic mask with a flow-inflating or self-inflating reservoir bag allows 100% oxygen to be delivered.

See also

Ventilatory support—indications, p. 4; Continuous positive airway pressure, p. 26; Basic resuscitation, p. 266; Respiratory failure, p. 278

Ventilatory support—indications

Acute ventilatory insufficiency

Acute ventilatory insufficiency is defined by an acute increase in $PaCO_2$ and a significant respiratory acidosis. $PaCO_2$ is directly proportional to the body's CO_2 production and is inversely proportional to alveolar ventilation (minute ventilation minus dead space ventilation). Causes include

- Respiratory center depression (e.g., depressant drugs or intracranial pathology)
- Peripheral neuromuscular disease (e.g., Guillain–Barré syndrome, myasthenia gravis or spinal cord pathology)
- Therapeutic muscle paralysis (e.g., as part of anesthesia, for management of tetanus or status epilepticus)
- Loss of chest wall integrity (e.g., chest trauma, diaphragm rupture)
- High CO_2 production (e.g., burns, sepsis, or severe agitation)
- Reduced alveolar ventilation (e.g., airway obstruction [asthma, acute bronchitis, foreign body], atelectasis, pneumonia, pulmonary edema [ARDS, cardiac failure], pleural pathology, fibrotic lung disease, obesity)
- Pulmonary vascular disease (e.g., pulmonary embolus, cardiac failure, ARDS)

Oxygenation failure

Hypoxemia is defined by PaO_2 <80 mmHg on FiO_2 ≥0.4. This may be the result of

- Ventilation–perfusion mismatch (reduced ventilation in, or preferential perfusion of, some lung areas), such as that seen in pneumonia, pulmonary edema, pulmonary vascular disease, and extremely high cardiac output
- Shunt (normal perfusion but absent ventilation in some lung zones), such as that seen in pneumonia and pulmonary edema
- Diffusion limitation (reduced alveolar surface area with normal ventilation), such as that seen in emphysema and reduced inspired oxygen tension (e.g., altitude, suffocation)
- Acute ventilatory insufficiency (as mentioned earlier)

To reduce intracranial pressure (ICP)

Reduction of $PaCO_2$ to approximately 30 mmHg causes cerebral vasoconstriction and therefore reduces ICP after brain injury. Recent studies suggest this effect is transient and may impair an already critical cerebral blood flow (CBF).

To reduce work of breathing

Assisted ventilation ± sedation and muscle relaxation reduces respiratory muscle activity and thus the work of breathing. In cardiac failure or noncardiogenic pulmonary edema, the resulting reduction in myocardial oxygen demand is more easily matched to the supply of oxygen.

Indications for ventilatory support

Ventilatory support (invasive or noninvasive) should be considered if
- Respiratory rate, >30 breaths/min
- Vital capacity, <10 to 15 mL/min
- PaO_2 <80 mmHg on FiO_2 ≥0.4
- $PaCO_2$, high with significant respiratory acidosis (e.g., pH <7.2)
- Vd/V_T >60%
- Qs/Qt >15 to 20%
- Exhaustion
- Confusion
- Severe shock
- Severe left ventricular failure (LVF)
- Increased ICP

See also

Intermittent positive-pressure ventilation (IPPV)—description of ventilators

Classification of mechanical ventilators

Mechanical ventilators may be classified by the method of cycling from inspiration to expiration. Volume-cycled ventilation terminates inspiration after the delivery of a preset V_T. Inspiratory pressures vary with lung compliance and airway resistance. Volume cycling is the most common. Pressure-cycled ventilation ends inspiration at a preset inspiratory pressure. Delivered volume varies with lung compliance and airway resistance.

Although the method of cycling is classified according to a single constant, modern ventilators allow a greater degree of control. In volume-cycled mode with pressure limitation, the upper pressure alarm limit is set or the maximum inspiratory pressure controlled. The ventilator delivers a preset V_T unless the lungs are noncompliant or airway resistance is high. This is useful to avoid high peak airway pressures. Newer pressure-cycled modes can vary inspiratory pressure breath by breath until a preset, V_T is reached.

Setting up the mechanical ventilator

V_T

V_T is conventionally set at 8 to 12 mL/kg, although recent data suggest lower values (6 mL/kg) may be better in ARDS, reducing barotrauma and improving outcome. In severe airflow limitation (e.g., asthma, acute bronchitis) a smaller V_T and minute volume may be needed to allow prolonged expiration.

Respiratory rate

The respiratory rate is usually set in accordance with V_T to provide a minute ventilation of 85 to 100 mL/kg/min. In time-cycled or time-limited modes, the set respiratory rate determines the timing of the ventilator cycles.

Inspiratory flow

Inspiratory flow is usually set between 40 to 80 L/min. A higher flow rate is more comfortable for alert patients. This allows for longer expiration in patients with severe airflow limitation, but may be associated with higher peak airway pressures. The flow pattern may be adjusted on most ventilators. A square waveform is often used, but decelerating flow may reduce peak airway pressure.

Inspiratory-to-expiratory (I:E) ratio

The I:E ratio is a function of respiratory rate, V_T, inspiratory flow, and inspiratory time. Prolonged expiration is useful in severe airflow limitation whereas a prolonged inspiratory time is used in ARDS to allow slow-reacting alveoli time to fill. Alert patients are more comfortable with shorter inspiratory times and high inspiratory flow rates.

FiO_2

FiO_2 is set according to arterial blood gases. It is usual to start at 0.6 to 1, then adjust according to arterial blood gases or pulse oximetry.

Airway pressure

In pressure-controlled or pressure-limited modes, the peak airway pressure (circuit rather than alveolar pressure) can be set (usually ≤35–40 cmH_2O). PEEP is usually increased to maintain fractional residual capacity (FRC) when respiratory compliance is low.

Initial ventilator setup

- Check for leaks
- Check oxygen is flowing to
  - FiO_2,   0.6 to 1
  - V_T,   5 to 10 mL/kg
  - Rate,   10 to 15 /min
  - I:E ratio,   1:2
  - Peak pressure,   ≤35 cmH_2O
  - PEEP,   3 to 5 cmH_2O

Key trial

Acute Respiratory Distress Syndrome Network. Ventilation with lower tidal volumes compared with traditional tidal volumes for acute lung injury and the Acute Respiratory Distress Syndrome. *N Engl J Med* 2000; **342**:1301–8.

See also

IPPV—modes of ventilation, p. 8; IPPV—adjusting the ventilator, p. 10; IPPV—failure to tolerate ventilation, p. 12; IPPV—complications of ventilation, p. 14; IPPV—weaning techniques, p. 16; IPPV— assessment of weaning, p. 18; High-frequency ventilation, p. 20; Positive end expiratory pressure (1), p. 22; Positive end expiratory pressure (2), p. 24; Lung recruitment, p. 28; Non-invasive respiratory support, p. 32; CO_2 monitoring, p. 94; Blood gas analysis, p. 102

IPPV—modes of ventilation

Controlled mechanical ventilation (CMV)

A preset number of breaths are delivered to supply all the patient's ventilatory requirements. These breaths may be at a preset V_T (volume controlled) or at a preset inspiratory pressure (pressure controlled).

Assisted controlled mechanical ventilation (ACMV)

Patients can initiate a breath (an assisted breath) and thus determine the respiratory rate. But, as with CMV, a preset number of breaths (controlled breaths) are delivered if the spontaneous respiratory rate decreases to less than the preset level. Assisted and controlled breaths use identical volume or pressure presets.

Intermittent mandatory ventilation (IMV)

A preset mandatory rate is set, but patients are free to breathe spontaneously between set ventilator breaths. Mandatory breaths may be synchronized with patients' spontaneous efforts to avoid mandatory breaths occurring during a spontaneous breath. This effect, known as *stacking*, may lead to excessive tidal volumes, high airway pressure, incomplete exhalation, and air trapping. Pressure support may be added to spontaneous breaths to overcome the work of breathing associated with opening the ventilator demand valve.

Pressure support ventilation (PSV)

With PSV, a preset inspiratory pressure is added to the ventilator circuit during inspiration in spontaneously breathing patients. The preset pressure should be adjusted to ensure adequate V_T.

Choosing the appropriate mode

Volume-cycled ACMV is a standard full-support mode that supplies a guaranteed minute ventilation. Pressure-controlled ventilation may minimize the dangers associated with high peak airway pressures, although it may result in marked changes in V_T if compliance alters. Allowing the patient to make some spontaneous respiratory effort may reduce sedation requirements, retrain respiratory muscles, and reduce mean airway pressures.

Apneic patient

Use of IMV or ACMV in patients who are totally apneic provides the total minute volume requirement if the preset rate is high enough (this is effectively CMV), but allows spontaneous respiratory effort on recovery.

Patient taking limited spontaneous breaths

A guaranteed minimum minute volume is ensured with both ACMV and IMV, depending on the preset rate. The work of spontaneous breathing is reduced by supplying the preset V_T for spontaneously triggered breaths with ACMV, or by adding pressure support to spontaneous breaths with IMV. With ACMV the spontaneous V_T is guaranteed, whereas with IMV and pressure support spontaneous V_T depends on lung compliance and may be less than the preset V_T.

See also

IPPV—adjusting the ventilator

Ventilator adjustments are usually made in response to blood gases, pulse oximetry or capnography, patient agitation or discomfort, or during weaning. 'Migration' of the endotracheal tube, either distally to the carina or beyond, or proximally such that the cuff is at the vocal cord level, may result in agitation, excess coughing, and a deterioration in blood gases. This, and tube obstruction, should be considered and rectified before changing ventilator or sedation dose settings.

The choice of ventilator mode depends on the level of consciousness, the number of spontaneous breaths being taken, and the blood gas values. Volume-cycled ACMV is a common initial ventilatory mode for patients requiring full support. The spontaneously breathing patient can usually cope adequately with pressure support ventilation alone. The paralyzed or heavily sedated patient will require mandatory breaths, either volume or pressure controlled.

The order of change will be dictated by the severity of respiratory failure and individual operator preference. Earlier use of increased PEEP is advocated to recruit collapsed alveoli and thus improve oxygenation in severe respiratory failure.

Low PaO_2 considerations
- Increase FiO_2.
- Review V_T and respiratory rate.
- Increase PEEP (may increase airway pressures).
- Increase I:E ratio.
- Increase pressure support/pressure control.
- In CMV, increase sedation ± muscle relaxants.
- Consider tolerating low level ('permissive hypoxemia') prone ventilation, inhaled nitric oxide.

High PaO_2 considerations
- Decrease level of pressure control/pressure support if V_T adequate.
- Decrease PEEP.
- Decrease FiO_2.
- Decrease I:E ratio.

High $PaCO_2$ considerations
- Increase V_T (if low and peak airway pressure allows).
- Increase respiratory rate.
- Reduce rate if too high (to reduce intrinsic PEEP [PEEPi]).
- Reduce dead space.
- In CMV, increase sedation ± muscle relaxants.
- Consider tolerating high level ('permissive hypercapnia').

Low $PaCO_2$ considerations
- Decrease respiratory rate.
- Decrease V_T.

IPPV—failure to tolerate ventilation

Agitation or 'fighting the ventilator' may occur at any time. Poor tolerance may also be indicated by hypoxemia, hypercapnia, ventilator alarms, or cardiovascular instability.

Poor gas exchange during initial phase of ventilation

- Increase to 1.0 FiO_2 and start manual ventilation.
- Check that the endotracheal tube is correctly positioned and both lungs are being inflated. Consider tube replacement, intratracheal obstruction, or pneumothorax.
- Check that the ventilator circuit is both intact and patent, and the ventilator is functioning correctly. Check ventilator settings, including FiO_2, PEEP, I:E ratio, set V_T, respiratory rate, and/or pressure control. Check pressure limit settings because these may be set too low, causing the ventilator to time-cycle prematurely.

Poor tolerance after previous good tolerance

If agitation occurs in a patient who has previously tolerated mechanical ventilation, either the patient's condition has deteriorated or there is a problem in the ventilator circuit (including the artificial airway) or the ventilator itself.

- The patient should be removed from the ventilator and placed on manual ventilation with 100% oxygen while the problem is resolved. Resorting to increased sedation ± muscle relaxation in this circumstance is dangerous until the cause is resolved.
- Check the patency of the endotracheal tube (e.g., with a suction catheter) and reintubate if in doubt.
- Consider malposition of the endotracheal tube (e.g., cuff above vocal cords, tube tip at carina, tube in main bronchus).
- Seek and treat any changes in the patient's condition, such as tension pneumothorax, sputum plug, or pain.
- When patients are making spontaneous respiratory effort, consider increasing pressure support or adding mandatory breaths.
- If patients fail to synchronize with IMV by stacking spontaneous and mandatory breaths, increasing the pressure support and reducing the mandatory rate may help; alternatively, the use of PSV may be appropriate.

See also

IPPV—complications of ventilation

Hemodynamic complications

Venous return is dependent on passive flow from the central veins to the right atrium. As right atrial pressure increases secondary to the transmitted increase in intrathoracic pressure across compliant lungs, there is a reduction in venous return. This is less of a problem if lungs are stiff (e.g., ARDS), although it will be exacerbated by the use of high airway pressures (inverse I:E ratio and high PEEP). As lung volume is increased by IPPV, the pulmonary vasculature is constricted, thus increasing pulmonary vascular resistance. This will increase diastolic volume of the right ventricle and, by septal shift, impedes filling of the left ventricle. These effects all contribute to a reduced stroke volume. This reduction can be minimized by reducing airway pressures, avoiding prolonged inspiratory times, and maintaining blood volume.

Ventilator trauma

The term *barotrauma* relates to gas escape into cavities and interstitial tissues during IPPV. Barotrauma is a misnomer because it is probably the distending volume and high shear stress that is responsible, rather than pressure. It is most likely to occur with high V_T and high PEEP. It occurs in IPPV and conditions associated with lung overinflation (e.g., asthma). Tension pneumothorax is life threatening and should be suspected in any patient on IPPV who becomes suddenly agitated, tachycardic, or hypotensive, or exhibits sudden deterioration in their blood gases. An immediate chest drainage tube should be inserted if tension pneumothorax develops. Prevention of ventilator trauma relies on avoidance of high V_T and high airway pressures.

Nosocomial infection

Endotracheal intubation bypasses normal defense mechanisms. Ciliary activity and cellular morphology in the tracheobronchial tree are altered. The requirement for endotracheal suction further increases susceptibility to infection. In addition, the normal heat- and moisture-exchanging mechanisms are bypassed, requiring artificial humidification of inspired gases. Failure to provide adequate humidification increases the risk of sputum retention and infection. Maintaining ventilated patients at a 30° upright head tilt has been shown to reduce the incidence of nosocomial pneumonia.

Acid–base disturbance

Ventilating patients with chronic respiratory failure or hyperventilation may, by rapid correction of hypercapnia, cause respiratory alkalosis. This reduces pulmonary blood flow and may contribute to hypoxemia. A respiratory acidosis resulting from hypercapnia may be to the result of inappropriate ventilator settings or may be desired in an attempt to avoid high V_T and ventilator trauma.

Water retention

Vasopressin released from the anterior pituitary is increased as a result of a reduction in intrathoracic blood volume and psychological stress. Reduced urine flow thus contributes to water retention. In addition, the use of PEEP reduces lymphatic flow with consequent peripheral edema, especially affecting the upper body. High airway pressure reduces venous return, again contributing to edema.

Respiratory muscle wasting

Prolonged ventilation may lead to disuse atrophy of the respiratory muscles.

See also

CO_2 monitoring, p. 94; Blood gas analysis, p. 102; Central venous catheter—use, p. 116; Central venous catheter—insertion, p. 118; Bacteriology, p. 158; Acute chest infection (1), p. 286; Acute chest infection (2), p. 288; Acute respiratory distress syndrome (1), p. 290; Acute respiratory distress syndrome (2), p. 292; Pneumothorax, p. 298

IPPV—weaning techniques

Patients may require all or part of their respiratory support to be provided by a mechanical ventilator. Weaning from mechanical ventilation may follow several patterns. In patients ventilated for short periods (no more than a few days) it is common to allow 20 to 30 min of breathing on a T piece or CPAP before removing the endotracheal tube. For patients who have received longer term ventilation, it is less likely that mechanical support can be withdrawn suddenly. Several methods are commonly used to wean these patients from mechanical ventilation. However, daily spontaneous breathing trials with a T piece or CPAP are probably superior in terms of weaning success and rate of weaning.

Intermittent T piece or CPAP

Spontaneous breathing is allowed for increasingly prolonged periods with a rest on mechanical ventilation in between. The use of a T piece for longer than 30 min may lead to basal atelectasis, because the endotracheal tube bypasses the physiological PEEP effect of the larynx. It is therefore common to use 5 cmH$_2$O CPAP as spontaneous breathing periods get longer. During the early stages of weaning, mechanical ventilation is often continued at night to encourage sleep, avoid fatigue, and rest respiratory muscles.

PSV

All respiratory efforts are spontaneous, but positive pressure is added to each breath, the level being chosen to maintain an appropriate V$_T$. Weaning is performed by a gradual reduction of the pressure support level while the respiratory rate is <30 breaths/min. The patient is extubated or allowed to breathe with 5 cmH$_2$O CPAP after pressure support is reduced to minimal settings (<10 cmH$_2$O with modern ventilators).

IMV

The set mandatory rate is gradually reduced as the spontaneous rate increases. Spontaneous breaths are usually pressure supported to overcome circuit and ventilator valve resistance. With this technique, it is important that the patient's required minute ventilation is provided by the combination of mandatory breaths and spontaneous breaths without an excessive spontaneous rate. The reduction in mandatory rate should be slow enough to maintain adequate minute ventilation. It is also important that patients can synchronize their own respiratory efforts with mandatory ventilator breaths; many cannot, particularly when there are frequent spontaneous breaths, some of which may 'stack' with mandatory breaths, causing hyperinflation.

Choice of ventilator

Modern ventilators have enhancements to aid weaning; however, weaning most patients from ventilation is possible with a basic ventilator and the intermittent T-piece technique, provided an adequate fresh gas flow is provided. If IMV and/or pressure support are used, the ventilator should provide the features listed here.

Key features in the choice of ventilator
- Patient triggering allowed by ventilator (i.e., not a minute volume divider)
- Fresh gas flow greater than spontaneous peak inspiratory flow
- Minimum circuit resistance (short, wide-bore, smooth internal lumen)
- Low-resistance ventilator valves
- Sensitive pressure or flow trigger (ideally monitored close to the endotracheal tube)
- Synchronized IMV (avoids stacking mandatory breaths on spontaneous breaths)

Key trial
Esteban A, Frutos F. A comparison of four methods of weaning patients from mechanical ventilation. *N Engl J Med* 1995; **332**:345–50.

See also
IPPV—modes of ventilation, p. 8; IPPV—adjusting the ventilator, p. 10; IPPV—assessment of weaning, p. 18; Continuous positive airway pressure, p. 26; Noninvasive respiratory support, p. 32

IPPV—assessment of weaning

Assessment prior to weaning

Prior to weaning it is important that the cause of respiratory failure and any arising complications have been corrected. Sepsis should be eradicated, as should other factors that increase oxygen demand. Attention is required to nutritional status, and fluid and electrolyte balance. The diaphragm should be allowed to contract unhindered by choosing the optimum position for breathing (sitting up, unless the diaphragm is paralyzed) and ensuring that intra-abdominal pressure is not high. Adequate analgesia must be provided. Sedatives are often withdrawn by this point but may still be needed in specific situations (e.g., residual agitation, increased ICP). Weaning should start after adequate explanation has been given to the patient. Factors predicting weaning success are detailed later in this section. Daily interruption of sedation and spontaneous breathing trials should start as soon as possible to facilitate liberation from mechanical ventilation.

Assessment during weaning

Continuous pulse oximetry and regular clinical review are essential during weaning. After short-term ventilation, extubate if respiratory pattern and arterial gases remain satisfactory, the cough reflex is adeq-uate, and the patient can clear sputum. Patients being weaned from longer term ventilation (>1 week) should generally be allowed to breathe spontaneously with CPAP for at least 8 to 12 h before extubation.

Indications for reventilation

If spontaneous respiration is discoordinate or the patient is exhausted, agitated, or clammy, the ventilator should be reconnected. However, clinical monitoring should avoid exhaustion. Successful weaning is more easily accomplished if excessive fatigue is not allowed to set in. Tachypnea (>30 breaths/min), tachycardia (>110 beats/min), respiratory acidosis (pH, <7.2), increasing $PaCO_2$, and hypoxemia (SaO_2 <90%) should all prompt reconnection of the ventilator.

Factors associated with weaning failure

Failure to wean is associated with
- Increased oxygen cost of breathing
- Muscle fatigue (hypophosphatemia, hypomagnesemia, hypokalemia, malnutrition, peripheral neuropathy, myopathy and drugs [e.g., muscle relaxants, aminoglycosides])
- Inadequate respiratory drive (alkalosis, opiates, sedatives, malnutrition, cerebrovascular accident, coma)
- Inadequate cardiac reserve and heart failure

In the latter case, cardiac function should be monitored during spontaneous breathing periods. Any deterioration in cardiac function should be treated aggressively (e.g., optimal fluid therapy, vasodilators, inotropes).

Factors predicting weaning success

A ratio of respiratory rate to V_T (f/V_T, known as the rapid shallow-breathing index) ≤ 105 breaths/L or f/L has been shown to have a 78% positive predictive value for successful weaning. Other factors are as follows:

- PaO_2 >80 mmHg on FiO_2 = 0.4
- Minute volume <12 L/min
- Vital capacity >10 mL/kg
- Maximum inspiratory force >20 cmH$_2$O
- Qs/Qt <15%
- V_d/V_T <60%
- Hemodynamic stability

Key trial

Yang KL, Tobin MJ. A prospective study of indexes predicting the outcome of trials of weaning from mechanical ventilation. *N Engl J Med* 1991; **324**:1445–50.

See also

IPPV—weaning techniques, p. 16; CO$_2$ monitoring, p. 94; Blood gas analysis, p. 102; Electrolytes (Na$^+$, K$^+$, Cl$^-$, HCO$_3^-$), p. 146; Calcium, magnesium, and phosphate, p. 148; Heart failure—assessment, p. 322; Acute weakness, p. 368; ICU neuromuscular disorders, p. 390

High-frequency ventilation

High-frequency jet ventilation (HFJV)

A high-pressure jet of gas entrains further fresh gas, which is directed by the jet toward the lungs. Respiratory rates of 100 to 300 breaths/min ensure minute volumes of about 20 L/min, although V_T may be lower than dead space. CO_2 elimination is usually more efficient than conventional IPPV. The method of gas exchange is not fully elucidated, but includes turbulent gas mixing and convection. Oxygenation is dependent on mean airway pressure (Paw). Peak airway pressures are lower than with conventional mechanical ventilation, but PEEPi and Paw are maintained. SaO_2 often decreases when starting on HFJV, although usually improves with time. The high gas flow rates used require additional humidification to be provided (30–100 mL/h); this is usually nebulized with the jet.

Indications

Bronchopleural fistula is the only proven intensive care unit (ICU) indication for HFJV. In ARDS, conventional ventilation can lead to ventilator trauma if a high V_T is used. HFJV avoids problems associated with high V_T, but is often unable to provide adequate ventilation in isolation for patients with severe ARDS.

Setting up HFJV

A jet must be provided via a modified endotracheal tube or catheter mount. Entrainment gas is provided via a T piece. The V_T cannot be set directly; rather, it is set by adjusting jet size, I:E ratio, driving pressure, and respiratory rate from a built-in algorithm. The respiratory rate is usually set between 100 to 200 breaths/min. As respiratory rate increases at a constant driving pressure, the $PaCO_2$ may increase as greater PEEPi increases the effective physiological dead space. The I:E ratio is usually set between 1:3 and 1:2. V_T is determined by airway pressure and I:E ratio. Driving pressure is usually set between 1 to 2 bar. These pressures are much higher than the 60 to 100 cmH_2O used in conventional ventilation. PEEPi is related to the driving pressure, I:E ratio, and respiratory rate. External PEEP may be added to increase Paw should this be necessary to improve oxygenation.

Combined HFJV and conventional CMV

Combined HFJV and conventional CMV may be useful in ARDS, when HFJV alone cannot provide adequate gas exchange. Low-frequency pressure-limited ventilation with PEEP provides an adequate Paw to ensure oxygenation while CO_2 clearance is effected by HFJV. Care must be taken to avoid excessive peak airway pressure when HFJV and CMV breaths stack.

Adjusting HFJV according to blood gases

Increasing PaO_2

- Increase FiO_2
- Increase I:E ratio.
- Increase driving pressure.
- Add external PEEP.
- Consider reducing respiratory rate.

Decreasing PaCO₂

- Increase driving pressure.
- Decrease respiratory rate.

High-frequency oscillation ventilation (HFOV)

HFOV effectively uncouples oxygenation and ventilation, allowing changes in flow to determine Paw and oxygenation, while at the same time providing subdead space tidal volumes and smaller pressure amplitudes compared with conventional mechanical ventilation. HFOV can achieve adequate gas exchange in situations when conventional ventilation is not successful. HFOV may be an alternative in patients with ARDS who fail conventional strategies.

Initial settings

1. Ensure adequate venous and arterial access for monitoring and blood gas sampling. Assess airway patency either by bronchoscopy or by passing a suction catheter without resistance. Partially occluded airways attenuate of the HFOV pressure amplitude and impair ventilation.
2. Set FiO₂ at 100%.
3. Set Paw at 5 cmH₂O higher than the measured Paw on the previous conventional settings.
4. Set bias flow at 40 L/min and adjust as needed for airway leaks or the need for increased Paw.
5. Titrate up pressure amplitude until a 'wiggle' is seen from the clavicles to mid thigh.
6. Set frequency at 5 Hz.
7. Set inspiratory time (Ti) at 33%.

Adjusting HFOV according to blood gases

Increasing PaO₂

Increase FiO₂.
Increase Paw (3–5-cmH₂O increments; do not exceed 45 cm).

Decreasing PaCO₂

- Increase pressure amplitude (ΔP) at 10-cm H₂O increments.
- Decrease frequency in 1-Hz decrements. Maximize ΔP first; minimum is 3 Hz.
- Increase Ti to 50% (last resort).
- Monitor chest 'wiggle' to ensure bilateral airflow. Endotrocheal tube repositioning and cuff deflation may also be attempted in refractory hypercarbia.

Weaning from HFOV may be considered when F_iO_2 <60%, Paw is weaned to <20 cmH₂O, and adequate ventilation can be achieved using safe levels of conventional ventilatory support (i.e., plateau pressures of <35 cmH₂O).

See also

Ventilatory support—indications, p. 4; Positive end expiratory pressure (1), p. 22; Positive end expiratory pressure (2), p. 24; Acute respiratory distress syndrome (1), p. 290; Acute respiratory distress syndrome (2), p. 292

Positive end expiratory pressure (1)

PEEP is a modality used in positive-pressure ventilation to prevent the alveoli returning to atmospheric pressure during expiration and collapsing. It is routinely set between 3 to 5 cmH_2O; however, in severe respiratory failure, it will often need to exceed 10 cmH_2O to be more than the lower inflexion point of the pressure–volume curve. This has been suggested as beneficial in patients with severe ARDS. It rarely needs to exceed 20 cmH_2O, to avoid cardiorespiratory complications and alveolar over-distension (discussed later).

Respiratory effects

PEEP improves oxygenation by recruiting collapsed alveoli, redistributing lung water, decreasing arteriovenous (AV) mismatch, and increasing FRC.

Hemodynamics

PEEP usually lowers both left and right ventricular preload and increases right ventricular afterload. Although PEEP may increase cardiac output in left heart failure and fluid overload states by preload reduction, in most other cases cardiac output decreases, even at relatively low PEEP levels. PEEP may also compromise a poorly functioning right ventricle. Improved PaO_2 resulting from a decreased venous admixture may sometimes arise solely from reductions in cardiac output.

Physiological PEEP

A small degree of PEEP (2–3 cmH_2O) is usually provided physiologically by a closed larynx. It is lost when the patient is intubated or is tracheotomized and breathing spontaneously on a T piece with no CPAP valve.

Intrinsic PEEP (auto-PEEP, air trapping, PEEPi)

Increased levels of PEEP resulting from insufficient time for expiration, leading to air trapping, CO_2 retention, increased airway pressures, and increased FRC. Seen in pathological conditions of increased airflow resistance (e.g., asthma, emphysema) and when insufficient expiratory time is set on the ventilator. Used clinically in inverse ratio ventilation to increase oxygenation and decrease peak airway pressures. High levels of PEEPi can, however, slow weaning by an increased work of breathing; use of extrinsic PEEP may overcome this. PEEPi can be measured by temporarily occluding the expiratory outlet of the ventilator at endexpiration for a few seconds to allow equilibration of pressure between the upper and lower airways and then reading the ventilator pressure gauge (or printout).

See also

Positive end expiratory pressure (2)

Adjusting PEEP

- Measure blood gases and monitored hemodynamic variables.
- If indicated, alter level of PEEP in 3 to 5-cmH$_2$O increments.
- Remeasure gases and hemodynamic variables after 15 to 20 min.
- Consider further changes as necessary (including additional changes in PEEP, fluid challenge, or vasoactive drugs).

A number of clinical trials have adjusted PEEP levels according to FiO$_2$ requirements (Table 1.1). Although unlikely to constitute 'optimal PEEP' for an individual patient, this provides a useful approximation and starting point for further titration of therapy.

Table 1.1 PEEP setting recommended for corresponding FiO$_2$

FiO$_2$	0.3	0.4	0.4	0.5	0.5	0.6	0.7	0.7	0.7	0.8	0.9	0.9	0.9	1.0
PEEP (cmH$_2$O)	5	5	8	8	10	10	10	12	14	14	14	16	18	≥18

Indications

- Hypoxemia requiring high FiO$_2$
- Optimization of pressure–volume curve in severe respiratory failure
- Hypoxemia secondary to left heart failure
- Improvement of cardiac output in left heart failure
- Reduced work of breathing during weaning in patients with high PEEPi

Complications

- Reduced cardiac output. May need additional fluid loading or even inotropes. This should generally be avoided unless higher PEEP is necessary to maintain adequate arterial oxygenation. Caution should be exercised in patients with myocardial ischemia.
- Increased airway pressure (and potential risk of ventilator trauma).
- Overinflation leading to air trapping and increased PaCO$_2$. Use with caution in patients with chronic airflow limitation or asthma. In pressure-controlled ventilation, overdistension is suggested when an increase in PEEP produces a significant decrease in V$_T$.
- Decreasing venous return, increasing ICP, and increasing hepatic congestion with high levels.

Continuous positive airway pressure

CPAP is the addition of positive pressure to the expiratory side of the breathing circuit of a spontaneously ventilating patient who may or may not be intubated. This sets the baseline upper airway pressure above atmospheric pressure, prevents alveolar collapse, and possibly recruits already collapsed alveoli. It is usually administered in increments of 2.5 cmH$_2$O to a maximum of 10 cmH$_2$O and is applied via either a tight-fitting face mask (face CPAP), nasal mask (nasal CPAP), or expiratory limb of a T-piece breathing circuit. A high-flow (i.e., more than peak inspiratory flow) inspired air-oxygen supply, or a large reservoir bag in the inspiratory circuit, is necessary to keep the valve open. CPAP improves oxygenation and may reduce the work of breathing by reducing the alveolar-to-mouth pressure gradient in patients with high levels of PEEPi. Transient periods of high CPAP (e.g., 40 cmH$_2$O for 40 s) may be a useful maneuver for recruiting collapsed alveoli and improving oxygenation in ARDS.

Indications
- Hypoxemia requiring high respiratory rate, effort, and FiO$_2$
- Left heart failure to improve hypoxemia and cardiac output
- Weaning modality
- Reducing work of breathing in patients with high PEEPi (e.g., asthma, chronic airflow limitation). NB: Use with caution and monitor closely.

Complications
- With mask CPAP there is an increased risk of aspiration, because gastric dilatation may occur from swallowed air. Insert a nasogastric tube, especially if consciousness is impaired or gastric motility is reduced.
- Reduced cardiac output may result from reduced venous return (increased intrathoracic pressure). May need additional fluid or even inotropes.
- Overinflation leading to air trapping and high PaCO$_2$. Caution is urged in patients with chronic airflow limitation or asthma.
- High levels will reduce venous return and increase ICP.
- Occasionally there is poor patient compliance with a tight-fitting face mask resulting from feelings of claustrophobia and discomfort on the bridge of the nose.
- Inspissated secretions may develop because of high-flow, dry gas.

Management
- Measure blood gases, and monitor hemodynamic variables and respiratory rate.
- Prepare a T-piece circuit with a 5-cmH$_2$O CPAP valve on the expiratory limb. Connect inspiratory limb to flow generator/large-volume reservoir bag. Adjust air–oxygen mix to obtain desired FiO$_2$ (measured by oxygen analyzer in circuit). Use a heat–moisture exchanger to humidify the inhaled gas. If not intubated, consider either nasal or face CPAP. Attach mask to face by appropriate harness and attach T piece to mask. Ensure no air leak around mask. If using a nasal mask, encourage patients to keep their mouth closed.
- Measure gases, respiratory rate, and hemodynamics after 15 to 20 min.
- Consider further changes in CPAP (by 2.5-cmH$_2$O increments).
- Consider need for (1) fluid challenge (or vasoactive drugs) if circulatory compromise and (2) nasogastric tube if gastric atony is present.

See also

Lung recruitment

There has been considerable interest in recent years in the concept of lung recruitment. The rationale is that reopening of collapsed alveoli will result in improved gas exchange, with resulting reductions in airway pressures and FiO_2. Timing is crucial because collapsed alveoli are more likely to be recruitable during the early stages of respiratory failure.

It appears that a benefit is more likely in nonrespiratory causes of ARDS, rather than in cases of direct pulmonary pathology such as pneumonia. Some animal studies suggest that recruitment procedures may even be potentially injurious in the latter situation.

Consideration should be given to lung recruitment soon after intubation in patients with severe respiratory failure, and to procedures causing derecruitment such as endotracheal suction and airway disconnection (e.g., during transport).

Recruitment techniques

A number of techniques are described to recruit collapsed alveoli, such as applying 40 cmH$_2$O PEEP for 40 s with no ventilator breaths; delivering a few large-volume, ventilator-delivered breaths; or using a combination of varying levels of PEEP and increasing pressure-delivered breaths to obtain optimal gas exchange.

Although anecdotal successes are reported, with occasionally dramatic improvements in lung compliance and gas exchange, no comparative trials have been performed, and outcomes have not been assessed prospectively. Hemodynamic compromise may occur during the procedure, although this usually recovers on cessation.

Key trial

Brower RG, et al., for the ARDS Clinical Trials Network. Effects of recruitment maneuvers in patients with acute lung injury and acute respiratory distress syndrome ventilated with high positive end-expiratory pressure. *Crit Care Med* 2003; **31**:2592–7.

Prone positioning

Prone positioning is used to treat patients with ARDS to improve gas exchange. A number of theories have been proposed to explain why the prone position helps. These theories include: reduction in compression atelectasis of dependent lung regions (temporary), reduction in chest wall compliance to increase intrathoracic pressure and alveolar recruitment, better regional diaphragmatic movement, better V/Q (ventilation/perfusion) matching, improved secretion clearance, and less alveolar distension leading to better oxygenation. Although the prone position improves oxygenation in ARDS, it has not been shown to improve survival.

Indications

Prone positioning may be considered when PaO_2 <60 mmHg, FiO_2 ≥6, and PEEP >10 cmH$_2$O despite optimization of other ventilatory support.

Technique

Positioning the patient takes time and preparation. Four staff members are required to turn the patient and one person is needed to secure the head and endotracheal tube. The turn itself is a two-stage procedure via the lateral position. The arm on which the patient is to be rolled is tucked under the hip, with the other arm laid across the chest. Pillows are placed under the abdomen and chest prior to rotation to the lateral position. If stable, the turn may be completed to the prone position. Pillows are placed under the shoulders and pelvis. The head of the bed is raised and one arm is extended at the patient's side while the other is flexed, with the head facing the opposite way.

Frequency of turns

The response to prone ventilation is difficult to predict. Some patients may have no improvement in gas exchange; others may have a temporary benefit, requiring frequent turns, and others may have difficulty returning to a supine position. For compression atelectasis, it is likely that a benefit will last up to 2 h before resumption of a supine position is required. For other conditions, up to 18 h of prone positioning may be required. The head and arms should be repositioned every 2 h.

Complications

There are problems associated with positioning the patient prone, including: facial edema, incorrect positioning of limbs leading to nerve palsy and accidental removal of drains and catheters, pressure necrosis, and myositis ossificans. These problems are preventable, provided there is awareness of their potential.

Contraindications/Cautions

There are two absolute contraindications to prone position: severe head, spinal, or abdominal injury and severe hemodynamic instability. Relative contraindications include
- Recent abdominal surgery
- Large abdomen
- Pregnancy
- Spinal instability (although special beds are available for turning affected patients)
- Frequent seizures
- Multiple trauma
- ↑ICP

Key trial

Gattinoni L, *et al.*, for the Prone–Supine Study Group. Effect of prone positioning on the survival of patients with acute respiratory failure. *N Engl J Med* 2001; **345**:568–73.

See also

Acute respiratory distress syndrome (1), p. 290; Acute respiratory distress syndrome (2), p. 292

Non-invasive respiratory support

Devices of varying sophistication are available to augment spontaneous breathing in the compliant patient by either assisting inspiration (inspiratory support) and/or providing CPAP. Noninvasive support is usually delivered by a tight-fitting face or nasal mask, although a helmet may be used. Some devices allow connection to an endotracheal tube for the intubated but spontaneously breathing patient.

Indications
- Hypoxemia requiring high respiratory rate, effort, and FiO_2
- Hypercapnia in a fatigued patient
- Weaning modality
- To avoid endotracheal intubation when desirable (e.g., severe chronic airflow limitation, immunosuppressed patients)
- To reduce work of breathing in patients with high PEEPi (e.g., asthma, chronic airflow limitation). Use with caution and monitor closely.
- Physiotherapy technique for improving FRC
- Sleep apnea

Inspiratory support

A preset inspiratory pressure is given that is triggered by the patient's breath. This trigger can be adjusted according to the degree of patient effort. Some devices will deliver breaths automatically at adjustable rates and the I:E ratio may also be adjustable. The V_T delivered for a given level of inspiratory support will vary according to the patient's respiratory compliance.

BiPAP

This device delivers adjustable levels of pressure support and PEEP. Delivered breaths can be either patient triggered or mandatory. Some BiPAP devices are driven by air. To increase FiO_2, supplemental oxygen can be given via a circuit connection or through a portal in the mask.

Management
- Select the type and delivery mode of ventilatory support.
- Connect the patient according to device instructions.
- Use an appropriate-size mask that is comfortable and leak free.
- A delivered pressure of 10 to 15 cmH_2O is a usual starting point and can be adjusted according to patient response (e.g., respiratory rate, degree of fatigue, comfort, blood gases).
- Expiratory pressure support levels are usually within the 5 to 12 cmH_2O range.
- Patients in respiratory distress may have initial difficulty in coping with these devices. Constant attention and encouragement help to accustom the patient to the device and/or mask while different levels of support, I:E ratios, and so on, are being tested to find the optimal setting. Cautious administration of low-dose opiates may help to calm the patient without depressing respiratory drive. The tight-fitting mask may be found increasingly claustrophobic after a few days' use. This should be preempted if possible by allowing the patient regular breaks. Pressure areas such as the bridge of the nose should be protected.

Key trials

Antonelli M, *et al.* A comparison of noninvasive positive-pressure ventilation and conventional mechanical ventilation in patients with acute respiratory failure. *N Engl J Med* 1998; **339**:429–35.

Brochard L, *et al.* Noninvasive ventilation for acute exacerbations of chronic obstructive pulmonary disease. *N Engl J Med* 1995; **333**:817–22.

Extracorporeal respiratory support

Extracorporeal respiratory support techniques have declined in popularity during recent years after several trials failed to demonstrate a clear outcome benefit in adults with very severe respiratory failure. Survival rates of 50 to 60% are reported, but clear superiority over conventional vent-ilation has not yet been demonstrated in controlled studies. A large, prospective, randomized study (the CESAR trial) is currently under way in the United Kingdom (www.cesar-trial.org).

Extracorporeal CO_2 removal ($ECCO_2R$)

An extracorporeal venovenous circulation allows CO_2 clearance via a gas exchange membrane. Blood flows of 25 to 33% cardiac output are typically used, which only allow for partial oxygenation support. Low-frequency (4–5 /min) positive-pressure ventilation is usually used with $ECCO_2R$, with continuous oxygenation throughout inspiration and expiration. The lungs are 'held open' with high PEEP (20–25 cmH$_2$O), limited peak airway pressures (35–40 cmH$_2$O), and a continuous fresh gas supply. Thus, oxygenation is effected with lung rest to aid recovery. Anticoagulation of the extracorporeal circuit can be reduced by using heparin-bonded tubing and membranes.

Extracorporeal membrane oxygenation (ECMO)

An extracorporeal venoarterial or venovenous circulation with high blood flows (approaching cardiac output) through a gas exchange membrane enables most, if not all, of the body's gas exchange requirements to be met. The main disadvantage compared with $ECCO_2R$ is the need for high extracorporeal blood flows with the potential for cell damage.

Indications

The primary indication for ECMO is failure of maximum intensive therapy and ventilatory support to sustain adequate gas exchange as evidenced by the criteria below.

Contraindications/Cautions

- Chronic systemic disease involving any major organ system (e.g., irreversible chronic central nervous system [CNS] disease, chronic lung disease with forced expired volume, in 1 s [FEV$_1$] <1 L, FEV$_1$/forced vital capacity [FVC] <0.3 of predicted, chronic PaCO$_2$ >45 mmHg, emphysema or previous admission for chronic respiratory insufficiency, incurable or rapidly fatal malignancy, chronic left heart failure, chronic renal failure, chronic liver failure, human immuno-deficiency virus [HIV]-related disease)
- Lung failure for >7 days (although treatment with extracorporeal respiratory support may persist for longer than 14 days)
- Burns (>40% of body surface)
- More than three organ failures in addition to lung failure

Criteria for ECCO₂R/ECMO

- Rapid failure of ventilatory support. Immediate use of these techniques should be considered in those meeting the following criteria for a period >2 h despite maximum intensive care:
  - PaO_2, <50 mmHg
  - FiO_2, 1.0
  - PEEP, optimally titrated
- Slow failure of ventilatory support. consider use after 48 h maximum of intensive care for those meeting the following gas exchange and mechanical pulmonary function criteria for a period >12 h:
  - PaO_2, <50 mmHg
  - Qs/Qt, >30% on FiO_2 = 1.0
  - PaO_2/FiO_2, <85 mmHg
  - Total static lung compliance, <30 mL/cmH₂O at 10 mL/kg inflation

See also

Anticoagulants, p. 246; Prostaglandins, p. 262; Acute respiratory distress syndrome (1), p. 290; Acute respiratory distress syndrome (2), p. 292

Endotracheal intubation

Indications

An artificial airway is necessary in the following circumstances:

- Apnea—provision of mechanical ventilation (e.g., unconsciousness, severe respiratory muscle weakness, self-poisoning)
- Respiratory failure—provision of mechanical ventilation (e.g., ARDS, pneumonia)
- Airway protection—unconsciousness, trauma, aspiration risk, poisoning
- Airway obstruction—maintenance of airway patency (e.g., trauma, laryngeal edema, tumor, burns)
- Hemodynamic instability—facilitation of mechanical ventilation (e.g., shock, cardiac arrest)

Choice of endotracheal tube

Most adults require a standard high-volume, low-pressure cuffed endotracheal tube. The average-size adult will require a size 8.0 to 9.0-mm inside diameter [id] tube (size 7.5–8.0 mm id for females) at a length of 23 cm (21 cm for females) from the teeth. Particular problems with the upper airway (e.g., trauma, edema) may require a smaller tube. In specific situations nonstandard tubes may be used (e.g., jet ventilation, armored tubes to avoid external compression, and double-lumen tubes to isolate the right or left lung).

Route of intubation

The usual routes of intubation are orotracheal and nasotracheal. Orotracheal intubation is preferred. The nasotracheal route has the advantages of increased patient comfort and the possibility of easier blind placement. It is also easier to secure the tube. However, there are several disadvantages. The tube is usually smaller, there is a risk of sinusitis and otitis media, and the route is contraindicated with concurrent coagulopathy, cerebrospinal fluid [CSF] leak and nasal fractures.

Difficult intubation

If a difficult intubation is predicted, it should not be attempted by an inexperienced operator. Difficulty may be predicted in the patient with a small mouth, high arched palate, large upper incisors, hypognathia, large tongue, anterior larynx, short neck, immobile temporomandibular joints, immobile cervical joints, or morbid obesity. If a difficult intubation presents unexpectedly, the use of a stylet, a straight-blade laryngoscope, or a fiberoptic laryngoscope may help. It is important not to persist for too long; revert to bag and mask ventilation to ensure adequate oxygenation.

Complications of intubation

Early complications

- Trauma (e.g., hemorrhage, mediastinal perforation)
- Hemodynamic collapse (e.g., positive-pressure ventilation, vasodilatation, arrhythmias, or rapid correction of hypercapnia)
- Tube malposition (e.g., failed intubation or endobronchial intubation)

Later complications
- Infection, including maxillary sinusitis if nasally intubated
- Cuff pressure trauma (avoid by maintaining cuff pressure <25 cmH$_2$O)
- Mouth/lip trauma

Equipment required
- Suction (Yankauer tip)
- Oxygen supply, rebreathing bag, and mask
- Laryngoscope (two curved blades and one straight blade)
- Stylet/bougie
- Endotracheal tubes (preferred size and smaller)
- Magill forceps
- Drugs (induction agent, muscle relaxant, sedative)
- Syringe for cuff inflation
- Tape to secure tube
- Capnograph

See also

Tracheotomy

Indications

Tracheotomy provides an artificial airway in place of oro- or nasotracheal intubation. This may provide better patient comfort; avoid vocal cord, mouth, or nasal trauma; or, in an emergency, bypass acute upper airway obstruction. The optimal time to perform a tracheotomy in an intubated patient is not known. Our current practice is 7 to 10 days, or sooner if prolonged intubation is predicted, especially in cases of difficult intubation. Avoiding the risks of vocal cord damage and more rapid weaning of mechanical ventilation are possible advantages for a tracheotomy. The reduced need for sedation; the potential to eat, drink, and speak; and the facilitation of mouth care are all definite advantages.

Percutaneous tracheotomy

Percutaneous tracheotomy is more rapid procedure with less tissue trauma and scarring than the standard open surgical technique. It can be performed in the ICU, avoiding the need to transfer patients to the operating room. Coagulopathy should be excluded or treated first. After a 1 to 1.5-cm midline skin crease incision, the subcutaneous tissue is blunt dissected to the anterior tracheal wall. The endotracheal tube tip is withdrawn to the level of the vocal cords. The trachea is then punctured in the midline with a 14-G needle between the first and second tracheal cartilages (or lower), allowing guide wire insertion. The stoma is created by dilatation to 32 to 36 Fr (Ciaglia technique) or by a guided forceps dilating tool (Schachner–Ovill technique). In the former case, the tracheotomy tube is introduced over an appropriate-size dilator and, in the latter, through the open dilating tool. End-tidal CO_2 monitoring confirms adequate ventilation during the procedure. Fiberoptic bronchoscopy may be used to confirm correct tracheal placement and no trauma to the posterior tracheal wall, although this may compromise ventilation.

Complications

The main early complication is hemorrhage from vessels anterior to the trachea. This is usually controlled with direct pressure or, occasionally, sutures. Bleeding into the trachea may result in clot obstruction of the airway; endotracheal suction is usually effective. Paratracheal placement should be rare, but promptly recognized by inability to ventilate the lungs. Later complications include tracheotomy displacement, stomal infection, and tracheal stenosis. Stenosis is often related to low-grade infection and is claimed to be more common with open tracheotomy. Rare complications include tracheo-esophageal fistula resulting from trauma or pressure necrosis of the posterior tracheal wall, or erosion through the lateral tracheal wall into a blood vessel.

Maintenance of a tracheotomy

Because the upper air passages have been bypassed, artificial humidification is required. Cough is less effective without a functioning larynx, so regular tracheal suction will be necessary. Furthermore, the larynx provides a small amount of natural PEEP that is lost with a tracheotomy. The risk of basal atelectasis can be overcome with CPAP or attention to respiratory exercises that promote deep breathing. A safe fistula forms within 5 to 7 days, allowing replacement of the tracheotomy tube.

Tracheotomy tubes
Standard high-volume, low-pressure cuff
Fenestrated with or without cuff
Useful when airway protection is not a primary concern. May be closed during normal breathing while providing intermittent suction access.

Fenestrated with inner tube
As in previous description but with an inner tube to facilitate closure of the fenestration during intermittent mechanical ventilation.

Fenestrated with speaking valve
Inspiration allowed through the tracheotomy to reduce dead space and inspiratory resistance. Expiration through the larynx, via the fenestration, allowing speech and the advantages of laryngeal PEEP.

Adjustable flange
Accommodates extreme variations in skin-to-trachea depth while ensuring the cuff remains central in the trachea. Should be switched to a fixed flange when possible to avoid dislodgement of the tracheotomy tube.

Pitt speaking tube
A non fenestrated, cuffed tube for continuous mechanical ventilation and airway protection with a port to direct airflow above the cuff to the larynx. When airflow is directed through the larynx, some patients are able to vocalize.

Passy–Muir speaking valve
This is an expiratory occlusive valve placed onto the tracheotomy tube that permits inspiration through the tracheotomy, and expiration through the glottis. The tracheotomy tube cuff must first be deflated. The valve allows phonation, facilitates swallowing, and may reduce aspiration. Small studies have suggested that it may reduce the work of breathing. The potential V_T decrease through cuff deflation makes this valve only suitable in those patients requiring no (or a relatively low level of) invasive ventilatory support.

Silver tube
This is an uncuffed tube used occasionally in ear, nose, and throat practice to maintain a tracheotomy fistula.

See also
Ventilatory support—indications, p. 4; Opioid analgesics, p. 232; Sedatives, p. 236; Muscle relaxants, p. 238; Cardiac arrest, p. 270; Airway obstruction, p. 278; Respiratory failure, p. 280; Acute chest infection (1), p. 286; Acute chest infection (2), p. 288; Acute respiratory distress syndrome (1), p. 290; Acute respiratory distress syndrome (2), p. 292; Asthma—general management, p. 294; Asthma—ventilatory management, p. 296; Poisoning—general principles, p. 454. Postoperative intensive care, p. 536

Minitracheotomy

A minitracheotomy is when a 4-mm-diameter uncuffed plastic tube is inserted through the cricothyroid membrane under local anesthetic.

Indications
- Removal of retained secretions, usually if the patient's cough is weak
- Emergency access to the lower airway if the upper airway is obstructed

Contraindications/Cautions
- Coagulopathy
- Noncompliant, agitated patient (unless sedated)

Technique

Some commercial kits rely on blind insertion of a blunt introducer; others use a Seldinger technique during which a guide wire is inserted via the cricothyroid membrane into the trachea. An introducer passed over the wire dilates the track, allowing easy passage of the tube.

- Use aseptic technique. Clean the site with antiseptic. Locate the cricothyroid membrane (midline 'spongy' area between the cricoid and thyroid cartilages).
- Infiltrate local skin and subcutaneous tissues with 1% lidocaine ± epinephrine. Advance the needle into deeper tissues, aspirating to confirm absence of blood, then infiltrating with lidocaine until the cricothyroid membrane is pierced and air can be easily aspirated.
- (If using the Seldinger technique, insert a guide wire through the membrane into the trachea.) Tether the thyroid cartilage with one hand, incise the skin and tissues vertically in the midline (alongside the wire) with a short-blade guarded scalpel provided with the pack. Insert the scalpel to the blade guard level to make an adequate hole through the cricothyroid membrane. Remove scalpel.
- Insert a blunt introducer through the incision site into the trachea (or over guide wire). Angle caudally. Relatively light resistance will be felt during correct passage. Do not force the introducer if resistance proves excessive.
- Lubricate the plastic tube with gel. Slide the tube over the introducer into the trachea.
- Remove introducer (and the wire), leaving the plastic tube in situ.
- Confirm correct positioning by placing your own hand over the tube and feeling airflow during breathing. Suction down tube to aspirate intratracheal contents (check pH if in doubt). Cap the opening of tube. Suture to skin.
- Acquire chest radiograph (CXR) (unless there is a very smooth insertion and no change in cardiorespiratory variables).
- Oxygen can be entrained through the tube, or an appropriate connector (provided in the pack) can be placed to allow bagging, use of the ventilator, and/or short-term assisted ventilation.

Complications

- Puncture of blood vessel at cricothyroid membrane, causing significant intratracheal or external bleeding. Apply local pressure if this occurs after blade incision. If bleeding continues, insert minitracheotomy tube for a tamponading effect. If bleeding persists, insert deep sutures on either side of the minitracheotomy. If this fails, contact a surgeon for assistance.
- Perforation of esophagus
- Mediastinitis (rare)
- Pneumothorax

See also

Chest physiotherapy, p. 48; Atelectasis and pulmonary collapse, p. 282; Acute chest infection (1), p. 286; Acute chest infection (2), p. 288

Chest drain insertion

Indications

Indications for chest drain insertion include drainage of air (pneumothorax), fluid (effusion), blood (hemothorax), or pus (empyema) from the pleural space.

Insertion technique

- Use a 28-Fr drain (or larger) for a hemothorax or empyema; 20-Fr will suffice for a pure pneumothorax. Seldinger–type drains with an integral guide wire are now also available. The drain is usually inserted through the fifth intercostal space in the midaxillary line, first anesthetizing the skin and pleura with 1% lidocaine. Ensure that air/fluid/blood/pus are aspirated.
- Make a 1 to 1.5-cm skin crease incision, and create a track with a gloved finger (or forceps) to separate the muscle fibers and open pleura.
- Insert the drain through the open pleura with a trochar withdrawn to ensure the tip is blunt to avoid lung damage. Angle and insert the drain to correct position (toward lung apex for a pneumothorax and the lung base for a hemothorax/effusion). Connect the drain to the underwater seal. Computed tomography (CT) or ultrasound may be useful for directing placement for focal/small collections.
- Secure the drain to the chest wall using properly placed sutures.
- Aquire CXR to ensure correct positioning and lung reinflation.
- Place on 20 cmH$_2$O negative pressure (low-pressure wall suction) if lung has not fully expanded.

Subsequent management

- Drains should not be clamped prior to removal or patient transport.
- Drains may be removed when the lung has reexpanded and there is no air leak (no respiratory swing in fluid level or air leak on coughing).
- Unless long-term ventilation is necessary, a drain inserted for a pneumothorax should usually be left in situ during IPPV.
- Remove the drain at end expiration. Cover the hole with thick gauze and Elastoplast; a purse-string suture is not usually necessary. Repeat CXR if indicated by deteriorating clinical signs or blood gas analysis.

Complications

- Morbidity associated with chest drainage may be up to 10%.
- Puncture of intercostal vessel may cause significant bleeding. Consider (1) correcting any coagulopathy, (2) placing deep tension sutures around the drain, or (3) removing the drain, inserting a Foley catheter, inflating the balloon, and applying traction to tamponade the bleeding vessel. If these measures fail, contact a (thoracic) surgeon.
- Puncture of lung tissue may cause a bronchopleural fistula. If chest drain suction (up to 15–20 cmH$_2$O) fails, consider (1) pleurodesis (e.g., with tetracycline), (2) HFJV $\pm$ a double-lumen endobronchial tube, or (3) surgery. Extubate if feasible.

- Perforation of major vessel (often fatal). Clamp but do not remove drain, resuscitate with blood, contact surgeon, consider double-lumen endotracheal tube.
- Infection. Take cultures, administer antibiotics (staphylococcal ± anaerobic coverage), and consider removing/repositioning the drain.
- Local discomfort/pain from pleural irritation may impair cough. Consider simple analgesia, subcutaneous lidocaine, instilling local anesthetic, administering local or regional anesthesia, and so on.
- Drain dislodgement. If needed, replace/reposition a new drain, depending on the cleanliness of the site. Do not advance the old drain (infection risk).
- Lung entrapment/infarction. Avoid milking the drain in the pneumothorax.

See also

IPPV—complications of ventilation, p. 14; High-frequency ventilation, p. 20; Pleural aspiration, p. 44; Basic resuscitation, p. 268; Pneumothorax, p. 298; Hemothorax, p. 300

Pleural aspiration

Pleural aspiration is the drainage of fluid from the pleural space using either a needle, cannula, or flexible small-bore drain. This technique is increasingly being performed under ultrasound guidance. Blood/pus usually require large-bore drain insertion.

Indications
- Improvement of blood gases
- Symptomatic improvement of dyspnea
- Diagnostic 'tap'

Contraindications/Cautions
- Coagulopathy

Complications
- Puncture of lung or subdiaphragmatic viscera
- Bleeding

Fluid protein level
- Protein >30 g/L (this should be viewed in the context of the plasma protein level) exudate. Causes are inflammatory (e.g., pneumonia), pulmonary embolus, neoplasm, and collagen vascular diseases.
- Protein <30 g/L transudate. Causes are increased venous pressure (e.g., heart failure, fluid overload), and decreased colloid osmotic pressure (e.g., critical illness leading to reduced plasma protein from capillary leak and hepatic dysfunction, hepatic failure, nephrotic syndrome).

Technique
- Confirm the presence of an effusion by CXR or ultrasound.
- Select a drainage site either by maximum area of stony dullness under percussion or under ultrasound guidance.
- Use aseptic technique. Clean the area with antiseptic and infiltrate local skin and subcutaneous tissues with 1% lidocaine. Advance into deeper tissues, aspirating to confirm absence of blood, then infiltrating with local anesthetic until the pleura is pierced and the fluid can be aspirated.
- Advance the drainage needle/cannula/drain slowly, applying gentle suction, through the chest wall and intercostal space (above the upper border of the rib to avoid the neurovascular bundle) until fluid can be aspirated.
- Withdraw 50 mL for microbiological (e.g., microscopy, culture, and sensitivity, [M, C&S], tuberclosis, [TB] stain), biochemical (e.g., protein, glucose), and histological/cytological (e.g., pneumocystis, malignant cells) analysis as indicated.
- Either leave the drain in situ, connected to a drainage bag, or connect the needle/cannula by three-way tap to the drainage apparatus.

- Continue aspiration/drainage until no further fluid can be withdrawn or patient becomes symptomatic (pain/dyspneic). Dyspnea or hemodynamic changes may occur as a result of removal of large volumes of fluid (>1–2 L) and subsequent fluid shifts. If this is considered to be a possibility, remove no more than 1 L at a time either by clamping/declamping drain or by repeating needle aspiration after an equilibration interval (e.g., 4–6 h).
- Remove the needle/drain. Cover the puncture site with a firmly applied gauze dressing.

See also

Chest drain insertion, p. 42; Acute chest infection (1), p. 286; Acute chest infection (2), p. 288; Pulmonary embolus, p. 306; Heart failure—assessment, p. 322; Heart failure—management, p. 324; Rheumatic disorders, p. 496; Vasculitides, p. 498

Fiberoptic bronchoscopy

Indications

Diagnostic

- Collection of microbiological ± cytological specimens
  (by bronchoalveolar lavage, protected brush specimen, biopsy)
- Cause of bronchial obstruction (e.g., clot, foreign body, neoplasm)
- Extent of inhalation injury
- Diagnosis of ruptured trachea/bronchus

Therapeutic

- Clearance of secretions, inhaled vomitus, and so on.
- Removal of lumen-obstructing matter (e.g., mucus plug, blood clot, food, tooth). Proximal obstruction rather than consolidation is suggested by the radiological appearance of a collapsed lung/lobe and no air bronchogram.
- Cleaning—removing soot or other toxic materials, irrigation with saline
- Directed physiotherapy ± saline to loosen secretions
- Directed placement of balloon catheter to arrest pulmonary bleeding
- To aid difficult endotracheal intubation

Contraindications/Cautions

- Coagulopathy
- Severe hypoxemia

Complications

- Hypoxemia—from suction, loss of PEEP, partial obstruction of endotracheal tube, and nondelivery of V_T.
- Hemodynamic disturbance including hypertension and tachycardia related to hypoxemia, agitation, tracheal stimulation, and so on).
- Bleeding
- Perforation (unusual, although more common if biopsy taken)

Procedure

It is difficult to perform fiberoptic bronchoscopy in a nasally intubated patient. A narrow-lumen scope can be used, but suction is limited.

- Preoxygenate with $FiO_2 = 1.0$. Monitor with pulse oximetry.
- Increase the pressure alarm limit on the ventilator.
- Lubricate scope with lubricant gel/saline.
- If unintubated, apply lidocaine gel to the nares ± spray to pharynx.
- Consider short-term intravenous (IV) sedation ± paralysis.
- Insert the scope nasally in a nonintubated patient or through a catheter mount port in an intubated patient.
- Inject 2% lidocaine into the trachea to prevent coughing and hemodynamic effects from tracheal/carinal stimulation.
- Perform a thorough inspection and any necessary procedures. If pulse oximeter oxygen, saturation (SpO_2) ≤85% or a hemodynamic disturbance occurs, remove the scope and allow reoxygenation before continuing.

- Bronchoalveolar lavage is performed by instillation of at least 60 mL (preferably warm) isotonic saline into the affected lung area without suction, followed by aspiration into sterile catheter trap. All broncho-scopic samples should be sent promptly to lab.
- Reduction of effective endotracheal tube lumen and suction may affect the V_T, leading to hypoxemia and/or hypercapnia.
- After the procedure, reset the ventilator as appropriate.

See also

Chest physiotherapy

The aim of chest physiotherapy is to expand collapsed alveoli, mobilize chest secretions, or reinflate collapsed lung segments. No scientific validation of effectiveness has been reported. The current view is that routine 'prophylactic' suctioning/bagging should be avoided in the critically ill.

Indications
- Mobilization of secretions
- Reexpansion of collapsed lung/lobes
- Prophylaxis against alveolar collapse and secondary infection

Contraindications/Cautions
- Aggressive hyperinflation in already hyperinflated lungs (e.g., asthma, emphysema), although this can be very useful in removing mucus plugs
- Undrained pneumothorax
- Increased ICP

Techniques
Hyperinflation

Hyperinflation involves hyperinflating to 50% above ventilator-delivered V_T, aiming to expand collapsed alveoli and mobilize secretions. V_T is rarely measured, so either excessive or inadequate hyperinflations may be given depending on lung compliance and operator technique. Pressure-limiting devices ('blow-off valves') or manometers can avoid excessive airway pressures. A recommended technique is slow inspiration, a 1 to 2-s plateau phase, and then rapid release of the bag to simulate a 'huff' and mobilize secretions. Preoxygenation may be needed because PEEP may be lost and the delivered V_T may be inadequate. Cardiac output often decreases with variable blood pressure and heart rate responses. Sedation may blunt the hemodynamic response. Full deflation avoids air trapping.

Suction

Suction is removing secretions from the trachea and main bronchi (usually right). A cough reflex may be stimulated to mobilize secretions further. Tenacious secretions may be loosened by instillation of 2 to 5 mL 0.9% saline. Decreases in SaO_2 and cardiovascular disturbance may be avoided by preoxygenation.

Percussion and vibration

Percussion and vibration are drumming and shaking actions over the chest wall to mobilize secretions.

Inspiratory pressure support

Inspiratory pressure support is used to increase FRC and expand collapsed alveoli.

Postural drainage

Postural drainage is patient positioning to assist drainage (depends on affected lung areas).

Complications
- Hypoxemia—from suction, loss of PEEP, and so on.
- Hemodynamic disturbance affecting cardiac output, heart rate, and blood pressure, which may be related to high V_T, airway pressure, hypoxemia, agitation, tracheal stimulation, and so on.
- Direct trauma from suctioning
- Barotrauma/volutrauma including pneumothorax

General
- Adequate humidification avoids tenacious sputum and mucus plugs.
- Pain relief is important to encourage good chest excursion and cough.
- Mobilization and encouraging deep breathing may avoid infection.

When to request urgent physiotherapy
- Collapsed lung/lobe with no air bronchogram visible, suggesting proximal obstruction rather than consolidation
- Mucus plugging causing subsegmental collapse (e.g., asthma)

When not to request urgent physiotherapy
- Clinical signs of chest infection with no secretions being produced
- Radiological consolidation with air bronchogram but no secretions present

See also

Ventilatory support—indications, p. 4; Endotracheal intubation, p. 36; Tracheotomy, p. 38; Mini-tracheotomy, p. 40; Fiberoptic bronchoscopy, p. 46; Atelectasis and pulmonary collapse, p. 282; Acute chest infection (1), p. 286; Acute chest infection (2), p. 288

Cardiovascular therapy techniques

Defibrillation/cardioversion

Defibrillation/cardioversion is electrical conversion of an arrhythmia to restore normal sinus rhythm. This may be an emergency procedure (when the circulation is absent or severely compromised), semielective (when the circulation is compromised to a lesser degree), or elective (when synchronized cardioversion is performed to restore sinus rhythm for a noncompromising supraventricular tachycardia [SVT]). Synchronization requires initial connection of electrocardiogram (ECG) leads from the patient to the defibrillator so that the shock is delivered on the R wave to minimize the risk of ventricular fibrillation (VF). Newer, biphasic defibrillators require approximately half the energy setting of monophasic defibrillators.

Indications
- Compromised circulation (e.g., VF, VT)
- Restoration of sinus rhythm and more effective cardiac output
- Lower risk of cardiac thrombus formation

Contraindications/Cautions
- Awake/inadequately sedated patient
- Severe coagulopathy
- Caution with recent thrombolysis
- Digoxin levels in toxic range
- Atrial thrombus (risk of embolization)

Complications
- Burns to the chest wall
- Electrocution of bystanders

Technique
(An algorithm is presented in Figure 2.1.)
- The chances of maintaining sinus rhythm are increased in elective cardioversion if K^+ >4.5 mmol/L and plasma Mg^{2+} levels are normal.
- Prior to defibrillation, ensure self and onlookers are not in contact with the patient or bed frame.
- To reduce the risk of superficial burns, replace the gel/gelled pads after every three shocks.
- Consider repositioning the paddle (e.g., anteroposterior) if defibrillation fails.
- The risk of intractable VF after defibrillation in a patient receiving digoxin is small unless the plasma digoxin levels are in the toxic range or the patient is hypovolemic.

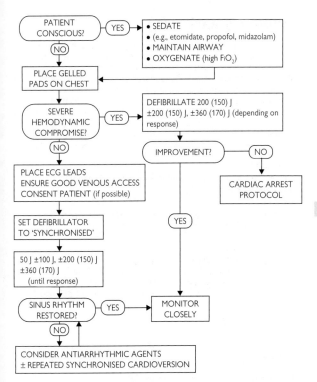

Fig. 2.1 Defibrillation/cardioversion algorithm (Figures in brackets for energy settings refer to biphasic defibrillators.)

See also

Chronotropes, p. 206; Sedatives, p. 236; Cardiac arrest, p. 270; Tachyarrhythmias, p. 314; Hypo-kalemia, p. 424

Temporary pacing (1)

When the heart's intrinsic pacemaking ability fails, temporary internal or external pacing can be instituted. Internal electrodes can be endocardial (inserted via a central vein) or epicardial (placed on the external surface of the heart at thoracotomy). The endocardial wire may be placed under fluoroscopic control or blindly using a balloon flotation catheter. External pacing can be rapidly performed by placement of two electrodes on the front and rear chest wall when asystole or third-degree heart block has produced acute hemodynamic compromise. It is often used as a bridge to temporary internal pacing. It can also be used as a prophylactic measure (e.g., for Mobitz type II second-degree heart block set at a 'backup' rate).

Indications

Placement of transcutaneous patches and active (demand) transcutaneous pacing

Class I

- Sinus bradycardia (rate <50 bpm) with symptoms of hypotension (systolic blood pressure <80 mmHg) unresponsive to drug therapy
- Mobitz type II second-degree AV block
- Third-degree heart block
- Bilateral bundle branch block ([BBB], alternating BBB, or right BBB [RBBB] and alternating left anterior fascicular block [LAFB], left posterior fascicular block [LPFB]; irrespective of time of onset)
- Newly acquired or age-indeterminate left BBB (LBBB), LBBB and LAFB, RBBB, and LPFB
- RBBB or LBBB and first-degree AV block

Class IIa

- Stable bradycardia (systolic blood pressure >90 mmHg, no hemodynamic compromise, or compromise responsive to initial drug therapy)
- Newly acquired or age-indeterminate RBBB

Class IIb

- Newly acquired or age-indeterminate first-degree AV block

Class III

- Uncomplicated acute myocardial infarction (AMI) without evidence of conduction system disease

Temporary transvenous pacing

Class I

- Asystole
- Symptomatic bradycardia (includes sinus bradycardia with hypotension and type I second-degree AV block with hypotension not responsive to atropine)
- Bilateral BBB (alternating BBB or RBBB with alternating LAFB/LPFB; any age)
- New or indeterminate-age bifascicular block (RBBB with LAFB or LPFB, or LBBB) with first-degree AV block

- Mobitz type II second-degree AV block

Class IIa
- RBBB and LAFB or LPFB (new or indeterminate)
- RBBB with first-degree AV block
- LBBB, new or indeterminate
- Incessant VT, for atrial or ventricular overdrive pacing
- Recurrent sinus pauses (>3 s) not responsive to atropine

Class IIb
- Bifascicular block of indeterminate age
- New or age-indeterminate isolated RBBB

Class III
- First-degree heart block
- Type I second-degree AV block with normal hemodynamics
- Accelerated idioventricular rhythm
- BBB or fascicular block known to exist before AMI

Complications
Internal pacing
- As for central venous catheter insertion
- Arrhythmias
- Infection (including endocarditis)
- Myocardial perforation (rare)

External pacing
- Discomfort

Troubleshooting
Failure to pace may be the result of
- No pacemaker spikes seen; check connections, check battery
- No capture (pacing spikes but no QRS complex following); poor posi-
  tioning/dislodgement of wire. Temporarily increase output,
  because this may regain capture. Reposition/replace internal
  pacing wire.

See also
Temporary pacing (2), p. 56; Chronotropes, p. 206; Cardiac arrest, p. 270; Bradyarrhythmias, p. 316

Temporary pacing (2)

General

- Check threshold daily because it will increase slowly over 48 to 96 h, probably because of fibrosis occurring around the electrodes.
- Overpacing is occasionally indicated for a tachycardia not responding to antiarrhythmic therapy or cardioversion. For SVT, pacing is usually attempted with the wire in the right atrium. Pace at rate 20 to 30 bpm above the patient's heart rate for 10 to 15 s, then either decrease the rate immediately to 80 bpm or slowly by 20 bpm every 5 to 10 s.
- If overpacing fails, underpacing may be attempted with the wire situated in either atrium (for SVT) or, usually, ventricle (for either SVT or VT). A paced rate of 80 to 100 bpm may produce a refractory period sufficient to suppress the intrinsic tachycardia.
- Epicardial pacing performed during or after cardiac surgery requires placement of either two epicardial electrodes or one epicardial and one skin electrode (usually a hypodermic needle). The pacing threshold of epicardial wires increases quickly and may become ineffective after 1 to 2 days.
- In asystole, an electrical rhythm produced by pacing does not guarantee an adequate cardiac output is being generated.

Technique (for endocardial electrode placement)

1. If using fluoroscopy, move patient to X-ray suite or place lead shields around bed area. Place patient on 'screening table'. Staff should wear lead aprons.
2. Use aseptic technique throughout. Insert 6-Fr sheath in internal jugular or subclavian vein. Suture in position.
3. Connect pacing wire electrodes to pacing box (black = negative polarity = distal, red = positive polarity = proximal). Set pacemaker to demand. Check box is working and battery charge adequate. Turn pacing rate to ≥30 bpm, above patient's intrinsic rhythm. Set voltage to 4 V.
4. Insert pacing wire through sheath into central vein. If using balloon catheter, insert to 15- to 20-cm depth then inflate balloon. Advance catheter, viewing ECG monitor for change in ECG morphology and capture of pacing rate. If using fluoroscopy, direct wire toward the apex of the right ventricle. Approximate insertion depth from a neck vein is 35 to 40 cm.
5. If pacing impulses not captured, (deflate balloon), withdraw wire to 15-cm insertion depth then repeat step 4.
6. After pacing is captured, decrease voltage by decrements to determine threshold at which pacing is no longer captured. Ideal position determined by a threshold ≤0.6 V. If not achieved, reposition wire.
7. If possible, ask patient to cough to check that wire does not dislodge.
8. Set voltage at three times threshold and set desired heart rate on 'demand' mode. Tape wire securely to patient to prevent dislodgement.

Technique (for external pacing)

1. Connect pacing wire gelled electrodes to pacemaker. Place black (negative polarity) electrode on the anterior chest wall to the left of the lower sternum and red (positive polarity) electrode to the corresponding position on the posterior hemithorax.
2. Connect ECG electrodes from ECG monitor to external pacemaker, and another set of electrodes from pacemaker to patient.
3. Set pacemaker to demand. Turn pacing rate to ≥30 bpm above patient's intrinsic rhythm. Set current to 70 mA.
4. Start pacing. Increase current (by 5-mA increments) until pacing rate captured on monitor.
5. Check pulse to confirm mechanical capture.
6. If pacing rate not captured at current of 120 to 130 mA, reposition electrodes and repeat steps 3 and 4.
7. After pacing is captured, set current at 5 to 10 mA above threshold.

See also

Temporary pacing (1), p. 54; Chronotropes, p. 206; Cardiac arrest, p. 270; Bradyarrhythmias, p. 316

Intra-aortic balloon counterpulsation

Principle

A 30- to 40-mL balloon is placed in the descending aorta. The balloon is inflated with helium during diastole, thus increasing diastolic blood pressure above the balloon. This serves to increase coronary and cerebral perfusion. The balloon is deflated during systole, thus decreasing peripheral resistance and increasing stroke volume. No pharmacological technique exists that can increase coronary blood flow while reducing peripheral resistance. Intra-aortic balloon counterpulsation may improve cardiac performance in situations when drugs are ineffective.

Indications

The most obvious indication is to support the circulation when a structural cardiac defect is to be repaired surgically. However, it may be used in acute circulatory failure in any situation when resolution of the cause of the cardiac dysfunction is expected. In AMI, resolution of peri-infarct edema may allow spontaneous improvement in myocardial function. The use of intra-aortic balloon counterpulsation may provide temporary circulatory support and promote myocardial healing by improving myocardial blood flow. Other indications include acute myocarditis and poisoning with myocardial depressants. Intra-aortic balloon counterpulsation should not be used in aortic regurgitation because the increase in diastolic blood pressure would increase regurgitant flow.

Insertion of the balloon

The usual route is via a femoral artery. Percutaneous Seldinger catheterization (with or without an introducer sheath) provides a rapid and safe technique with minimal arterial trauma and bleeding. Open surgical catheterization may be necessary in patients with atheromatous disease. The balloon position should be checked on a CXR to ensure that the radio-opaque tip is just below the level of the aortic arch in the descending thoracic aorta. Ensure the left radial pulse is not lost.

Anticoagulation

Anticoagulation is often necessary, particularly if the device is to remain in place for more than 24 to 48 h. Risk of thrombus formation is increased significantly if the balloon is left deflated. Therefore, the device is never turned off for longer than 1 min while in situ.

Control of balloon inflation and deflation

Helium is used to inflate the balloon; its low density facilitates rapid transfer from pump to balloon. Inflation is commonly timed to the R wave of the ECG, although timing may be taken from an arterial pressure waveform. Minor adjustment may be made to the timing to ensure that inflation occurs immediately after closure of the aortic valve (after the dicrotic notch of the arterial pressure waveform) and deflation occurs at the end of diastole. The filling volume of the balloon can be varied up to the maximum balloon volume. The greater the filling volume, the greater the circulatory augmentation. The rate at which balloon inflation occurs may coincide with every cardiac beat or every second, third, or fourth cardiac beat. Slower rates are necessary in tachyarrhythmias. Weaning of intra-aortic balloon counterpulsation may be achieved by reducing augmentation or the rate of inflation.

See also

Renal therapy techniques

Continuous renal replacement therapy (1)

Standard hemodialysis requires a pressurized, purified water supply; expensive equipment; and carries a greater risk of hemodynamic instability because of rapid fluid and osmotic shifts. These limitations have prompted the development of techniques that deliver slow continuous renal replacement therapy (CRRT). Modern CRRT machines rely on pumped venovenous circuits and can also operate in a variety of modes from pure hemofiltration (CVVH), which uses replacement fluid and not dialysate, to hemodialysis (CVVHD) to combination therapy (hemodiafiltration, CVVHDF) (see Fig. 3.1). Blood is usually drawn and returned via a standard 10- to 12-Fr double-lumen dialysis catheter.

Indications
- Azotemia (uremia)
- Hyperkalemia
- Metabolic acidosis
- Fluid overload (present or impending)
- Drug/toxin removal

Techniques

In addition to CVVH, CVVHD, and CVVHDF, isolated ultrafiltration, sometimes still referred to as *slow continuous ultrafiltration* (SCUF), can also be performed. With this technique, no replacement fluid or dialysis is used because a small amount of ultrafiltrate (usually 50 to 200 mL) is removed each hour. SCUF does not provide solute clearance. Both CVVH and CVVHD are excellent for small-molecule clearance (e.g., urea), but CVVH has superior larger molecule clearance (e.g., β_2 microglubulin) and can remove substances up to the pore size cutoff of the membrane. In CVVH, filtrate is usually removed at 20 to 35 mL/kg/h and fluid balance is adjusted by varying the fluid replacement rate. High-volume hemofiltration involves much higher ultrafiltration rates (e.g., 50–100 mL/kg/h) in an effort to remove inflammatory mediators (e.g., tumor necrosis factor). Although some studies have suggested improved physiological outcomes, the technique is considered experimental.

Membranes

Membranes are usually hollow fiber polyacrylonitrile, polyamide, or polysulphone. The surface area is usually 0.6 to 1 m^2.

Replacement fluid

A buffered balanced electrolyte solution is given to achieve appropriate electrolyte and acid–base balance. Fluid removal is adjusted to achieve the desired fluid balance. Buffers include lactate, acetate (rarely used), and bicarbonate. Bicarbonate solutions may be more efficient than lactate at reversing severe metabolic acidosis, but outcome benefit has yet to be demonstrated from its use, and care is needed with coadministered calcium because calcium bicarbonate may precipitate. In liver failure and in states of poor tissue perfusion, lactate buffer may not be adequately metabolized.

An increasing metabolic alkalosis may be the result of excessive buffer. In this case, use a 'low-buffer' (i.e., 30 mmol/L) replacement fluid. Potassium can be added, if necessary, to maintain normokalemia. Having 20 mmol KCl in a 4.5 L bag provides a concentration of 4.44 mmol/L. K^+ clearance is increased by decreasing the concentration within the replacement fluid or the dialysate.

Dosage

The optimal amount or 'dose' of CRRT that should be provided is unknown. One trial showed that 35 mL/kg/h of replacement in CVVH was superior to 25 mL/kg/h in terms of hospital mortality. A more recent but smaller study failed to confirm this benefit. Large multicenter studies are underway in the United States and Australia to address this question. Until these data become available, many centers are providing 35 mL/kg/h.

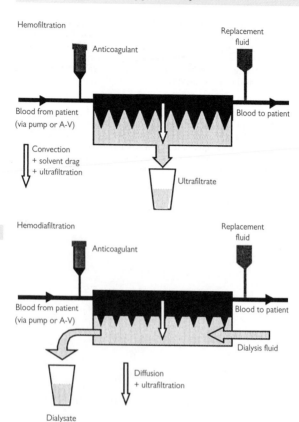

Fig. 3.1 Schematic circuits for hemofiltration and hemodiafiltration.

Key trials

Ronco C, *et al.* Effects of different doses in continuous veno-venous haemofiltration on outcomes of acute renal failure: A prospective randomised trial. *Lancet* 2000; **356**:26–30.

Consensus paper

Kellum JA, Mehta R, Angus DC, Palevsky P, Ronco C, for the ADQI Workgroup. The First International Consensus Conference on Continuous Renal Replacement Therapy. *Kidney Int* 2002; **62**:1855–63.

See also

Continuous renal replacement therapy (2), p. 66; Coagulation monitoring, p. 156; Anticoagulants, p. 246; Oliguria, p. 328; Acute renal failure—diagnosis, p. 330; Acute renal failure—management, p. 332; Metabolic acidosis, p. 436; Metabolic alkalosis, p. 438; Poisoning—general principles p. 322; Metabolic acidosis, p. 436; Metabolic alkalosis, p. 438; Poisoning—general principles, p. 454; Rhabdomyolysis, p. 530

Continuous renal replacement therapy (2)

Anticoagulation

- Anticoagulation of the circuit is usually done with unfractionated heparin (200–2000 IU/h), citrate, or a prostanoid (prostacyclin or prostaglandon E_1 [PGE_1]) at 2 to 10 ng/kg/min, or (rarely) a combination of the two. Little experience is available on the use of low-molecular weight heparin, or other anticoagulants such as hirudin.
- No anticoagulant may be needed if the patient is autoanticoagulated.
- Premature clotting may be the result of mechanical kinking/obstruction of the circuit, insufficient anticoagulation, or inadequate blood flow rates, or the result of a lack of endogenous anticoagulants (antithrombin III, heparin cofactor II).
- Filters should usually be changed every 2 to 3 days. Usual filter life span should be at least 2 days, but is often decreased in septic patients because of decreased endogenous anticoagulant levels. In this situation, consider the use of fresh frozen plasma (FFP), a synthetic protease inhibitor such as aprotinin, or antithrombin III replacement (costly).

Filter blood flow

Flow through the filter is usually 100 to 200 mL/min. Too slow a flow rate promotes clotting. Too high a flow rate will increase transmembrane pressures and decrease filter life span without significant improvement in clearance of 'middle molecules' (e.g., urea).

Complications

- Disconnection leading to hemorrhage
- Infection risk (sterile technique must be used)
- Electrolyte, acid–base, or fluid imbalance (excess input or removal)
- Hemorrhage (vascular access sites, peptic ulcers) related to anticoagulation therapy. Heparin-induced thrombocytopenia may rarely occur
- Hypocalcemia and metabolic alkalosis with citrate anticoagulation

Cautions

- Hemodynamic instability related to hypovolemia (especially at start)
- Membrane–drug interaction; sporadic case reports on hypersensitivity when AN69 membranes are used in patients receiving angiotension converting enzyme (ACE) inhibitors
- Possible revision of drug dosages (consult pharmacist)
- Amino acid losses through the filter
- Heat loss leading to hypothermia and masking of pyrexia
- Hypophosphatemia

See also

Oliguria p. 328; Acute renal failure—diagnosis p. 330; Acute renal failure—management p. 332

Peritoneal dialysis

Peritoneal dialysis is a slow form of dialysis utilizing the peritoneum as the dialysis membrane. Slow correction of fluid and electrolyte disturbance may be better tolerated by critically ill patients, and the technique does not require complex equipment. However, treatment is labor intensive and there is considerable risk of peritoneal infection. In addition, the dose of dialysis provided by this form of therapy may be inadequate for many critically ill patients. It has been largely superseded by hemofiltration in most ICUs.

Peritoneal access

For acute peritoneal dialysis, a trocar and cannula are inserted through a small skin incision under local anesthetic. The skin is prepared and draped as for any sterile procedure. The most common approach is through a small midline incision 1 cm below the umbilicus. The subcutaneous tissues and peritoneum are punctured by the trocar, which is withdrawn slightly before the cannula is advanced toward the pouch of Douglas. To avoid damage to intra-abdominal structures, 1 to 2 L warmed peritoneal dialysate may be infused into the peritoneum by a standard, short intravascular cannula prior to placement of the trocar and cannula system. If the midline access site is not available, an alternative is to use a lateral approach, lateral to a line joining the umbilicus and the anterior superior iliac spine (avoiding the inferior epigastric vessels).

Dialysis technique

Warmed peritoneal dialysate is infused into the peritoneum in a volume of 1 to 2 L at a time. During the acute phase, fluid is flushed in and drained continuously (i.e., with no dwell time). After biochemical control is achieved, it is usual to leave fluid in the peritoneal cavity for 4 to 6 h before draining. Heparin (500 IU/L) may be added to the first six cycles to prevent fibrin catheter blockage. Thereafter, it is only necessary if there is blood or cloudiness in the drainage fluid.

Peritoneal dialysate

The dialysate is a sterile, balanced electrolyte solution with glucose at 75 mmol/L for a standard fluid or 311 mmol/L for a hypertonic fluid (used for greater fluid removal). The fluid is usually potassium free, because potassium exchanges slowly in peritoneal dialysis, although potassium may be added if necessary.

Complications

- Fluid leak—caused by poor drainage, steroid therapy, obese or elderly patient
- Catheter blockage—caused by bleeding, omental encasement
- Infection—caused by white cells >50 cells/mL, cloudy drainage fluid
- Hyperglycemia—caused by absorption of hyperosmotic glucose
- Diaphragm splinting

Treatment of infection

It is often possible to sterilize the peritoneum and catheter by adding appropriate antibiotics to the dialysate. Suitable regimens include
- Cefuroxime 500 mg/L for two cycles then 200 mg/L for 10 days
- Gentamicin 8 mg/L for one cycle daily

See also

Oliguria, p. 328; Acute renal failure—diagnosis, p. 330; Acute renal failure—management, p. 332

Plasma exchange

Indications

Plasma exchange may be used to remove circulating toxins or to replace missing plasma factors. It has also been used in fulminant forms of sepsis (e.g., meningococcemia). In patients with immune-mediated disease, plasma exchange is usually a temporary measure while systemic immunosuppression takes effect. There are some immune-mediated diseases (e.g., Guillain–Barré syndrome, thrombotic thrombocytopenic purpura (TTP), hemolytic uremic syndrome) when an isolated rather than a continuous antibody–antigen reaction can be treated with early plasma exchange and no follow-up immunosuppression. Most diseases require a daily 3- to 4-L plasma exchange, repeated for at least four additional occasions over 5 to 10 days.

Techniques

Cell separation by centrifugation

Blood is separated into components in a centrifuge. Plasma (or other specific blood components) is discarded and a plasma replacement fluid is infused in equal volume. Centrifugation may be continuous, when blood is withdrawn and returned by separate needles, or intermittent, when blood is withdrawn, separated, and then returned via the same needle.

Membrane filtration

Plasma is continuously filtered through a large-pore filter (molecular weight cutoff typically 1,000,000 Da). The plasma is discarded and replaced by infusion of an equal volume of replacement fluid. The technique is similar to hemofiltration and uses the same equipment.

Replacement fluid

Most patients will tolerate replacement with a plasma substitute. Our preference is to replace plasma loss with equal volumes of 6% hydroxy-ethyl starch and 5% albumin. However, some use partial crystalloid replacement and others use all-albumin replacement. Some FFP will be necessary after the exchange to replace coagulation factors. The only indication to replace plasma loss with all FFP is when plasma exchange is being performed to replace missing plasma factors (e.g., thrombotic thrombocytopenic purpura).

Complications

- Circulatory instability—intravascular volume changes, removal of circulating catecholamines, hypocalcemia
- Reduced intravascular COP (colloid osmotic pressure)—if replacement with crystalloid
- Infection—reduced plasma opsonization
- Bleeding—removal of coagulation factor

Indications

Autoimmune disease
- Goodpasture's syndrome
- Guillain–Barré syndrome
- Myasthenia gravis
- Pemphigus
- Rapidly progressive glomerulonephritis
- Systemic lupus erythematosus (SLE)
- TTP
- HUS

Immunoproliferative disease
- Cryoglobulinemia
- Multiple myeloma
- Waldenström's macroglobulinemia

Poisoning
- Paraquat

Others
- Meningococcal septicemia (possible benefit)
- Sepsis (possible benefit, especially when there is a consumptive thrombocytopenia)
- Reye's syndrome

See also

Coagulation monitoring, p. 156; Anticoagulants, p. 246; Guillain–Barré syndrome, p. 386; Myasthenia gravis, p. 388; Platelet disorders, p. 408; Poisoning—general principles, p. 454; Vasculitides, p. 498

Gastrointestinal therapy techniques

Balloon tamponade tube

A balloon tamponade tube is used to manage esophageal variceal hemorrhage that continues despite pharmacological ± endoscopic therapy. The Sengstaken–Blakemore is a large-bore rubber tube that contains gastric and esophageal balloons with a single gastric aspiration port. The Minnesota tube contains gastric and esophageal balloons as well as gastric and esophageal aspiration ports. Either device is usually effective, with the gastric balloon alone inflated and compressing the varices at the cardia. Inflation of the esophageal balloon is rarely necessary and is associated with more complications compared with the gastric balloon alone.

Insertion technique

The tubes may be cooled by placing them in the refrigerator or by flushing them with iced saline to provide added stiffness for easier insertion.

- The patient usually requires sedation and mechanical ventilation (as warranted by state of consciousness/level of agitation) prior to insertion.
- Check balloons inflate properly beforehand. Lubricate end of tube.
- Insert via mouth.
- Place to depth of 55 to 60 cm (i.e., to ensure gastric balloon is in stomach prior to inflation).
- Inflate gastric balloon with 50 mL air and confirm placement radiographically prior to full inflation of gastric balloon. There is a high risk of esophageal rupture if gastric balloon is fully inflated while in the esophagus.
- Inflate gastric balloon to volume instructed by manufacturer (usually, ≈200 mL). Negligible resistance to inflation should be felt. Clamp gastric balloon lumen.
- Pull tube back until resistance is felt (i.e., gastric balloon is at cardia). Fix tube in place by applying countertraction at the mouth or attaching tube to free-hanging traction weights.
- Perform radiography to check satisfactory position of gastric balloon.
- If bleeding continues (continued large aspirates from gastric or esophageal lumens), inflate esophageal balloon (approximately 50 mL).

Subsequent management

- The gastric balloon is usually kept inflated for 12 to 24 h and is deflated prior to endoscopy ± sclerotherapy. The traction on the tube should be tested hourly by the nursing staff. The esophageal lumen should be placed on continuous drainage whereas enteral nutrition and administration of drugs can be given via the gastric lumen.
- If the esophageal balloon is used, deflate for 5 to 10 min every 1 to 2 h to reduce the risk of esophageal pressure necrosis. Do not leave esophageal balloon inflated for longer than 12 h after sclerotherapy.
- The tube may need to stay in situ for 2 to 3 days, although periods of deflation should then be allowed.

Complications
- Aspiration
- Perforation
- Ulceration
- Esophageal necrosis

See also
Upper gastrointestinal hemorrhage, p. 342; Bleeding varices, p. 344

Upper gastrointestinal endoscopy

Upper gastrointestinal endoscopy is identical in ventilated and nonventilated patients, although a protected airway ± sedation usually facilitates the procedure.

Indications
- Investigation of upper gastrointestinal signs/symptoms (e.g., bleeding, pain, mass, obstruction)
- Therapeutic (e.g., sclerotherapy for varices, local epinephrine [adrenaline] injection for discrete bleeding points such as in ulcer base)
- Placement of nasojejunal tube (when gastric atony prevents enteral feeding) or percutaneous gastrostomy
- Endoscopic retrograde cholangiopancreatography—unusual in the ICU patient

Complications
- Local trauma causing hemorrhage or perforation
- Abdominal distension compromising respiratory function

Contraindications/Cautions
- Severe coagulopathy (should ideally be corrected)

Procedure
Upper gastrointestinal endoscopy should be performed by an experienced operator to minimize the duration and trauma of the procedure, and to minimize gaseous distension of the gut.
- The patient is usually placed in a lateral position, although can be supine if intubated.
- Increase FiO_2 and ventilator pressure alarm settings. Consider increasing sedation and adjusting ventilator mode.
- Monitor ECG, SpO_2, airway pressures, and hemodynamic variables throughout. If patient is on pressure support or pressure control ventilatory modes, also monitor tidal volumes. Operator should cease procedure, at least temporarily, if patient becomes compromised.
- At end of procedure, operator should aspirate as much air as possible out of gastrointestinal tract to decompress the abdomen.

See also

Pulse oximetry, p. 92; Upper gastrointestinal hemorrhage, p. 342; Bleeding varices, p. 344

Nutrition

Nutrition—use and indications

Malnutrition leads to poor wound healing, postoperative complications, and sepsis. Adequate nutritional support is important for critically ill patients and should be provided early during the illness. Evidence for improved outcome from early nutritional support exists for patients with trauma and burns. Enteral nutrition is indicated when swallowing is inadequate or impossible, but gastrointestinal function is otherwise intact. Parenteral nutrition is indicated when the gastrointestinal tract cannot be used to provide adequate nutritional support (e.g., obstruction, ileus, high small bowel fistula, or malabsorption). Parenteral nutrition may be used to supplement enteral nutrition when gastrointestinal function allows partial nutritional support.

Consequences of malnutrition

Underfeeding	*Overfeeding*
Loss of muscle mass	Increased oxygen consumption (VO_2)
Reduced respiratory function	Increased CO_2 production (VCO_2)
Reduced immune function	Hyperglycemia
Poor wound healing	Fatty infiltration of liver
Gut mucosal atrophy	
Reduced protein synthesis	

Calorie requirements

Various formulas exist to calculate the patient's basal metabolic rate, but, they can be misleading in critical illness. Metabolic rate can be measured by indirect calorimetry, but most patients are assumed to require 2000 to 2700 KCal/day, or less if starved or underweight.

Protein requirements

Nitrogen balance can be used to assess the adequacy of protein intake. Nitrogen balance can be calculated in the absence of renal failure using 24-h urea excretion:

Nitrogen balance = Protein intake (g/24 h) − 2 + [Urinary urea nitrogen (g/24 h) × 6.25]

However, as with most formulas, this method lacks accuracy. Most patients require 1 to 1.5 g/kg of protein daily.

Other requirements

The normal requirements of substrates, vitamins, and trace elements are presented in Table 5.1. Most long-term critically ill patients require folic acid and vitamin supplementation during nutritional support. Trace elements are usually supplemented in parenteral formulas, but should not be required during enteral nutrition.

Table 5.1 Normal daily nutritional requirements

Normal daily requirements (for a 70-kg adult)	
Water	2100 mL
Energy	2000–2700 KCal
Protein	70–105 g
Glucose	210 g
Lipid	140 g
Sodium	70–140 mmol
Potassium	50–120 mmol
Calcium	5–10 mmol
Magnesium	5–10 mmol
Phosphate	10–20 mmol
Vitamins	
Thiamine	16–19 mg
Riboflavin	3–8 mg
Niacin	33–34 mg
Pyridoxine	5–10 mg
Folate	0.3–0.5 mg
Vitamin C	250–450 mg
Vitamin A	2800–3300 IU
Vitamin D	280–330 IU
Vitamin E	1.4–1.7 IU
Vitamin K	0.7 mg
Trace elements	
Iron	1–2 mg
Copper	0.5–1.0 mg
Manganese	1–2 µg
Zinc	2–4 mg
Iodide	70–140 µg
Fluoride	1–2 mg

Additional requirements are needed to satisfy excess loss or increased metabolic activity.

See also

Electrolytes (Na^+, K^+, Cl^-, HCO_3^-) p. 146; Calcium, magnesium, and phosphate, p. 148; Gut motility agents, p. 224; Vomiting/gastric stasis, p. 336; Diarrhea, p. 338; Bowel perforation and obstruction, p. 346; Hypernatremia, p. 418; Hyponatremia, p. 420; Hyperkalemia, p. 422; Hypokalemia, p. 424; Hypomagnesemia, p. 426; Hypocalcemia, p. 430; Hypophosphatemia, p. 432

Enteral nutrition

Enteral nutrition routes include nasogastric and nasoduodenal/jejunal, and gastrostomy, gastrojejunostomy, and jejunostomy. Nasal tube feeding should be via a soft, fine-bore tube to aid patient comfort and avoid ulceration of the nose or esophagus. Prolonged enteral feeding may be accomplished via a percutaneous/surgical gastrostomy/gastrojejunostomy or surgical jejunostomy. Enteral feeding provides a more complete diet than parenteral nutrition, maintains structural integrity of the gut, improves bowel adaptation after resection, and reduces infection risk.

Feed composition

Most patients tolerate iso-osmolar, nonlactose feed. Carbohydrates are provided as sucrose or glucose polymers, protein as whole protein or oligopeptides (may be better absorbed than free amino acids in 'elemental' feeds), and fats as medium-chain or long-chain triglycerides. Medium-chain triglycerides are better absorbed. Standard feed is formulated at 1 KCal/mL. Special feeds are available (e.g., high fiber, high protein–calorie, restricted salt, high fat, or concentrated [1.5 or 2 KCal/mL] for fluid restriction). Immune-enhanced feeds contain various mixtures of essential amino acids such as glutamine and arginine, nucleotides, and omega-3 fatty acids. Several studies have shown a reduced incidence of nosocomial infection, but no evidence of outcome benefit has been shown from large, prospective studies. A large-scale randomized trial run by the Canadian Critical Care Trialists is currently in process.

Management of enteral nutrition

After a decision is made to start enteral nutrition, 20 mL/h full-strength standard feed may be started immediately. Starter regimens incorporating dilute feed are not necessary. After 6 h at 20 mL/h, the feed should be stopped for 30 min prior to aspiration of the stomach. Because gastric juice production is increased by the presence of a nasogastric tube, it is reasonable to accept an aspirate of <200 mL as evidence of gastric emptying, and therefore to increase the infusion rate in 20-mL/h increments. This process is repeated every 6 h until the target feed rate is achieved. Thereafter, aspiration of the stomach can be reduced to every 8 h. If the gastric aspirate volume is >200 mL, the infusion rate is not increased but the feed is continued. If aspirates remain at high volume despite measures to promote gastric emptying (e.g., metoclopramide or erythromycin), then either bowel rest or nasoduodenal/nasojejunal feeding should be considered. Parenteral nutrition may be considered after all options for enteral feeding are exhausted.

Complications

- Tube placement—tracheobronchial intubation, nasopharyngeal perforation, intracranial penetration (basal skull fracture), esophageal perforation
- Reflux
- Pulmonary aspiration
- Nausea and vomiting
- Abdominal distension

- Diarrhea—large volume, bolus feeding, high osmolality, infection, lactose intolerance, antibiotic therapy, high fat content
- Constipation
- Metabolic—dehydration, hyperglycemia, electrolyte imbalance

Key trial

Atkinson S, et al. A prospective, randomized, double-blind, controlled clinical trial of enteral immunonutrition in the critically ill. *Crit Care Med* 1998; **26**:1164–72.

See also

Nutrition—use and indications, p. 80; Electrolytes (Na^+, K^+, Cl^-, HCO_3^-) p. 146; Calcium, magnesium, and phosphate, p. 148; Gut motility agents, p. 224; Vomiting/gastric stasis, p. 336; Diarrhea, p. 338; Bowel perforation and obstruction, p. 346; Hypernatremia, p. 418; Hyponatremia, p. 420; Hyperkalemia, p. 422; Hypokalemia, p. 424; Hypomagnesemia, p. 426; Hypocalcemia, p. 430; Hypophosphatemia, p. 432

Parenteral nutrition

Feed composition

Carbohydrate is normally provided as concentrated glucose. 30 to 40% of total calories are usually given as lipid (e.g., soy bean emulsion). The protein source is synthetic, crystalline L-amino acids, which should contain appropriate quantities of all essential and most nonessential amino acids. Carbohydrate, lipid, and protein sources are usually mixed into a large bag in a sterile pharmacy unit. Vitamins, trace elements, and appropriate electrolyte concentrations can be achieved in a single infusion, thus avoiding multiple connections. Volume, protein, and calorie content of the feed should be determined on a daily basis in conjunction with the dietitian.

Choice of parenteral feeding route

Central venous

A dedicated catheter (or lumen of a multilumen catheter) is placed under sterile conditions. For long-term feeding, a subcutaneous tunnel is often used to separate skin and vein entry sites. This may reduce the risk of infection and clearly identifies the special purpose of the catheter. Ideally, blood samples should not be taken nor other injections or infusions given via the feeding lumen. The central venous route allows infusion of hyperosmolar solutions, providing adequate energy intake in reduced volume.

Peripheral venous

Parenteral nutrition via the peripheral route requires a solution with osmolality <800 mOsmol/kg. Either the volume must be increased or the energy content (particularly from carbohydrate) reduced. Peripheral cannula sites must be changed frequently.

Complications

- Catheter related—misplacement, infection, thromboembolism
- Fluid excess
- Hyperosmolar, hyperglycemic state
- Electrolyte imbalance
- Hypophosphatemia
- Metabolic acidosis—hyperchloremia, metabolism of cationic amino acids
- Rebound hypoglycemia—high endogenous insulin levels
- Vitamin deficiency—folate – pancytopenia; thiamine – encephalopathy; vitamin K – hypoprothrombinemia;
- Vitamin excess—vitamin A – dermatitis; vitamin D – hypercalcemia
- Fatty liver

.

See also

Special support surfaces

Special support surfaces

Pressure sores

Pressure sores occur as a result of compression of tissue between bone and the support surface and as a result of shearing forces, friction, and maceration of tissues against the support surface. The use of special beds attempts to reduce the pressure at the contacting skin surface to a level lower than the capillary occlusion pressure. In the majority of cases, it is sufficient to minimize the time that the support surface contacts any one area of skin by position changes.

Factors suggesting the need for a special bed

- Patients with severely restricted mobility resulting from traction or cardiorespiratory instability. These patients cannot be turned frequently, if at all.
- Patients with decreased skin integrity (e.g., burns, pressure sores already present, chronic steroid use, diabetes mellitus)
- Patients on vasoactive drug infusions

Types of special support surfaces

Air mattress

An air mattress either replaces or is placed on top of a standard hospital bed mattress. It provides minimum reduction in contact pressure, but should be considered as minimum support for any patient with the previously listed factors.

Low-air loss bed

These purpose-built, pressure-relieving beds allow easier patient mobility than other support surfaces. Contact pressure may still be higher than capillary occlusion pressure, so positioning is still required. The presence of pressure sores with intact skin is an indication for a low-air loss bed. Rotational low-air loss beds allow automated lateral rotation at variable time intervals to facilitate chest drainage. These may also be useful when manual positioning is impractical.

Air-'fluidized' bed

This is the only support surface that consistently lowers contact pressure to below capillary occlusion pressure. Consequently, patients with severe cardiorespiratory instability, who cannot be turned, and patients with pressure sores with broken skin benefit most. The additional ability to control the temperature of the immediate environment is an advantage in hypothermic patients and in those with large surface area burns. Any exudate from the skin is adsorbed into the silicone beads on which the patient floats. This drying effect is particularly useful in major burns (although it must be taken into account for fluid replacement therapy). The air-fluidized bed also has a role in pain relief.

Respiratory monitoring

Pulse oximetry

Pulse oximetry is continuous, noninvasive monitoring of arterial oxygen saturation by a probe emitting red and near-infrared light over the pulse on a digit, earlobe, cheek, or bridge of the nose. It is unaffected by skin pigmentation, hyperbilirubinemia, or anemia (unless profound).

Physics

The color of blood varies with oxygen saturation as a result of the optical properties of the hemoglobin (Hb) moiety. As Hb gives up oxygen, it becomes less permeable to red light and takes on a blue tint. Saturation is determined spectrophotometrically by measuring the 'blueness', utilizing the ability of compounds to absorb light at a specific wavelength. The use of two wavelengths (650 nm and 940 nm) permits the relative quantities of reduced and oxyhemoglobin to be calculated, thereby determining saturation. The arterial pulse is used to provide time points to allow subtraction of the constant absorption of light by tissue and venous blood. The accuracy of pulse oximetry is within 2% when above 70% SaO_2.

Indications

- Continuous monitoring of SaO_2

Cautions

- Because only two wavelengths are used, pulse oximetry measures functional rather than fractional oxyhemoglobin saturation. Erroneously high readings are given with carboxyhemoglobin and methemoglobin.
- With poor peripheral perfusion or intense vasoconstriction the reading may be inaccurate ('fail soft') or, in newer models, absent ('fail hard').
- Motion artifacts and high levels of ambient lighting may affect readings.
- An erroneous signal may be produced by significant venous pulsation from tricuspid regurgitation or venous congestion. Venous pulsatility accounts for differences between ear and finger SpO_2 in the same subject.
- Ensure a good LED signal indicator or a pulse waveform (if available) is seen on the monitor.
- Vital dyes (e.g., methylthionine chloride [methylene blue], indocyanine green) may affect SpO_2 readings.

See also

CO_2 monitoring

Capnography

For capnography, respiratory gases must be sampled continuously and measured by a rapid response device. Because CO_2 has an absorption band in the infrared spectrum, measurement is facilitated in gas mixtures. Other gases can interfere with infrared absorption by CO_2. This may be overcome by calibrating the instrument with known concentrations of CO_2 in the required measurement range, diluted with a gas mixture similar to exhaled gas.

The capnogram

The CO_2 concentration of exhaled gas consists of four phases (Fig. 7.1). The presence of significant concentrations of CO_2 in phase 1 implies rebreathing of exhaled gas. Failure of an expiratory valve to open is the most likely cause of rebreathing during manual ventilation, although an inadequate flow of fresh gas into a rebreathing bag is a common cause. The slope of phase 3 is dependent on the rate of alveolar gas exchange. A steep slope may indicate ventilation–perfusion mismatch, because alveoli that are poorly ventilated but well perfused discharge late in the respiratory cycle. A steep slope is seen in patients with significant auto-PEEP.

Phase 1

During the early part of the exhaled breath, anatomic dead space and sampling device dead space gas are sampled. There is negligible CO_2 in phase 1.

Phase 2

As alveolar gas begins to be sampled, there is a rapid increase in CO_2 concentration.

Phase 3

Phase 3 is known as the *alveolar plateau* and represents the CO_2 concentration in mixed, expired alveolar gas. There is normally a slight increase in the partial pressure of CO_2 (PCO_2) during phase 3 as alveolar gas exchange continues during expiration. Airway obstruction or a high rate of VCO_2 will increase the slope. End-tidal PCO_2 will be less than the PCO_2 of ideal alveolar gas because the sampled exhaled gas is mixed with alveolar dead space gas.

Phase 4

As inspiration begins, there is a rapid decrease in sample PCO_2.

Colorimetric devices

The underlying principle is that the change in pH produced by different CO_2 concentrations in solution will change the color of an indicator. Colorimetric devices are small devices that fit onto an endotracheal tube or the ventilator circuit and respond rapidly (up to 60 breaths/min). They can be affected by excessive humidity and generally only work in the range of 0 to 4% CO_2. They are useful to confirm tracheal intubation during patient transfer and in a cardiac arrest situation.

PCO₂

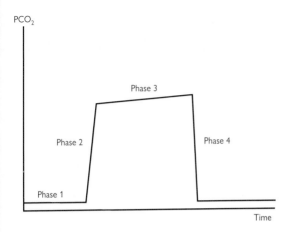

Fig. 7.1 The components of a normal capnogram.

End-tidal partial pressure of CO₂ (PCO₂)

End-tidal PCO_2 approximates $PaCO_2$ in patients with normal lung function. In ICU patients, pulmonary function is rarely normal; thus, end-tidal PCO_2 is a poor approximation of $PaCO_2$. Large differences may represent an increased Vd-to-V_T ratio, poor pulmonary perfusion, or intrapulmonary shunting. A progressive increase in end-tidal PCO_2 may represent hypoventilation, airway obstruction, or increased CO_2 production resulting from an increased metabolic rate. End-tidal PCO_2 decreases with hyperventilation and in low cardiac output states. It is absent with ventilator disconnection and during cardiac arrest, but increases with effective cardiopulmonary resuscitation (CPR) or restoration of a spontaneous circulation.

Vd-to-V_T ratio

The arterial to end-tidal PCO_2 difference may be used to calculate the physiological Vd-to-V_T ratio via the Bohr equation:

$$Vd/V_T = (PaCO_2 - \text{end-tidal } PCO_2)/PaCO_2$$

In a healthy person, a value between 30% and 45% should be expected.

See also

Ventilatory support—indications, p. 4; IPPV—adjusting the ventilator, p. 10; Endotracheal intubation, p. 36; Tracheotomy, p. 38; Fiberoptic bronchoscopy, p. 46; Blood gas analysis, p. 102; Basic resuscitation, p. 268

Pulmonary function tests

Few of the numerous pulmonary function tests currently available affect clinical management of the critically ill (Table 7.1), particularly if the patient has to be moved to a laboratory. A number of other tests require highly specialized equipment and fulfill a predominant research role (Table 7.2).

Table 7.1 Clinically relevant tests

Measurement	Test	Common clinical use
PaO_2, SaO_2, $PaCO_2$	Arterial blood gases	
SpO_2	Pulse oximetry	
End-tidal PCO_2	Capnography	
VC, V_T	Spirometry, electronic flowmetry	Serial measurement of borderline function (VC <10–15 mL/kg); (e.g., Guillain–Barré syndrome)
Peak expiratory flow rate FEV_1, FVC	Wright peak flow meter, spirometry, electronic flowmetry	(Spontaneous ventilation) asthma, (Spontaneous ventilation) asthma, obstructive/restrictive disease
Lung/chest wall compliance (see 'Equations')	Pressure–volume curve	Ventilator adjustments monitoring disease progression
Flow–volume loop, pressure–volume loop	Pneumotachograph manometry	Ventilator adjustments

Table 7.2 Research tests (examples)

Measurement	Test	Research use
Diaphragmatic strength (transdiaphragmatic pressure)	Gastric and esophageal manometry	Respiratory muscle function, weaning
Pleural (intrathoracic) pressure	Esophageal manometry	Ventilator trauma, work of breathing, weaning
FRC	Closed-circuit helium dilution (bag-in-a-box), open circuit N_2 washout	Lung volumes, compliance
Ventilation–perfusion relationship	Multiple inert gas elimination technique, isotope techniques	Regional lung ventilation–perfusion, pulmonary gas exchange
Pulmonary diffusing capacity	Carbon monoxide uptake	Pulmonary gas exchange

Notes

- Compliance equals the change in pressure during a linear increase of 1 L in volume above FRC.
- The alveolar–arterial oxygen difference is <15 mmHg in youth and <25 mmHg in older patients.

- The Bohr equation calculates physiological dead space. The normal value is >30%.
- The shunt equation estimates the proportion of blood shunted past poorly ventilated alveoli (Q_S) compared with total lung blood flow (Q_T).

These equations allow estimation of ventilation/perfusion mismatch:
- V/Q = 1, ventilation and perfusion are wellmatched
- V/Q >1, increased dead space (when alveoli are poorly perfused but well ventilated)
- V/Q <1, increased venous admixture or shunt (when alveoli are perfused but poorly ventilated)

The normal range is <15%.

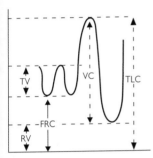

TLC = total lung capacity
VC = vital capacity
FRC = functional residual capacity
TV = tidal volume
RV = residual volume

Fig. 7.2 Lung volumes and capacity

Equations

Alveolar gas equation

$$P_AO_2 = FiO_2 - (PaCO_2/\text{respiratory quotient (RQ)})$$

[RQ often approximated to 0.8]

Alveolar–arterial oxygen difference

$$(A - a) \text{ difference} = FiO_2 \times 94.8 - PaCO_2 - PaO_2$$

Bohr equation

$$Vd/V_T = (PaCO_2 - \text{expired } PCO_2)/PaCO_2$$

Shunt equation

$$Q_S/Q_T = (CcO_2 - CaO_2)/(CcO_2 - CvO_2)$$

where CcO_2 is end-capillary O_2 content, a is arterial, and v is mixed venous.

See also

Ventilatory support—indications, p. 4; IPPV—adjusting the ventilator, p. 10; IPPV—weaning techniques, p. 16; IPPV—assessment of weaning, p. 18; Pulse oximetry, p. 92; CO₂ monitoring, p. 98; Blood gas analysis, p. 102; Chronic airflow limitation, p. 284; Asthma—general management, p. 294; Asthma—ventilatory management, p. 296; Acute weakness, p. 368; Guillain–Barré syndrome, p. 386; Myasthenia gravis, p. 388; Rheumatic disorders, p. 496; Vasculitides, p. 498

Pressure–volume relationship

The pressure–volume relationship is determined by the compliance of the lungs and chest wall. The inspiratory pressure–volume relationship contains three components: an initial increase in pressure with no significant volume change, a linear increase in volume as pressure increases (the slope of which represents respiratory system compliance), and a further period of pressure increase with no volume increase. These three phases are separated by two inflection zones, the lower representing the opening pressure of the system after flow resistance has been overcome in smaller airways and the upper approximating to total lung capacity. The normal expiratory pressure–volume relationship is slightly left shifted from the inspiratory relationship, indicating a higher volume per given distending pressure. This shift, or *hysteresis*, is probably related to differences in surface tension (see Fig. 7.3).

Dynamic measurement

A pressure–volume loop may be viewed on most modern mechanical ventilators. A square wave inspiratory waveform (constant flow) and no inspiratory pause are necessary for waveform interpretation.

Static measurement

Small incremental lung volumes (200 mL) are delivered with a calibrated syringe. The pressure measurement after each increment is taken under zero-flow conditions, allowing construction of a pressure–volume curve. A quasi-static curve can be constructed by setting incremental tidal volumes (e.g., between 100 mL and 1000 mL) for successive ventilator breaths and measuring the pressure during an inspiratory pause.

Use of pressure–volume curves

Because respiratory muscle activity can alter intrathoracic pressure, the pressure–volume curve is more easily obtained in the relaxed, fully ventilated patient. Both static and dynamic respiratory system compliance can be determined as the slope of the linear portion of the curve (i.e., where incremental pressure inflates the lungs). Below the lower inflexion zone, the small airways are closed and expiration does not reach FRC. The lower inflexion zone therefore represents the appropriate setting for external PEEP to avoid gas trapping. Above the upper inflexion zone, the lungs cannot inflate further. The upper inflexion zone therefore represents the maximum setting for peak airway pressure.

Compliance: calculations

- Lung compliance = V_L/P_L

where L, the liter above FRC, is the slope of the linear portion of the curve and lung compliance is measured in liters per centimeter water.

- Total respiratory system compliance is derived from the equation

    (1/Total compliance) = (1/Lung compliance) + (1/Chest wall compliance)

- Total compliance can be calculated in well-sedated, ventilated patients as

    V_T/(End-inspiratory pause pressure − PEEP)

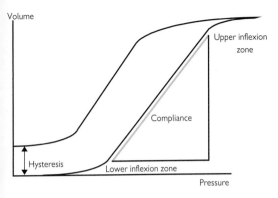

Fig. 7.3

See also

Ventilatory support—indications, p. 4; IPPV—adjusting the ventilator, p. 10; Positive end expiratory pressure (1), p. 22; Positive end expiratory pressure (2), p. 24; Chronic airflow limitation,
p. 284; Asthma—general management, p. 284; Asthma—ventilatory management, p. 296

Blood gas machine

A small amount of heparinized blood is either injected from a syringe or aspirated from a capillary tube into the machine. The blood comes into contact with three electrodes that measure pH, partial pressure of oxygen (PO_2), and PCO_2.

- pH—measured by the potential across a pH-sensitive glass membrane separating a sample of known pH and the test sample.
- PO_2—measured by applying a polarizing voltage between a platinum cathode and a silver anode (Clark electrode), O_2 is reduced, generating a current proportional to PO_2.
- PCO_2—utilizes a pH electrode with a Teflon membrane (Severinghaus electrode) that allows through uncharged molecules (CO_2) but not charged ions (H^+). CO_2 alone thus changes the pH of a bicarbonate electrolyte solution, the change being linearly related to PCO_2.
- Hb—estimated photometrically, not as accurate as co-oximetry (discussed later).
- Bicarbonate—calculated by the Henderson–Hasselbach equation:

$$pH = 6.1 + Log_{10}\frac{arterial\ [HCO_3^-]}{PaCO_2 \times 0.03}$$

Actual HCO_3^- includes bicarbonate, carbonate, and carbamate.

- Actual base excess (deficit)—the difference in concentration of strong base (acid) in whole blood and that titrated to pH 7.4 at a PCO_2 of 40 mmHg and 37°C.
- Standard base excess (deficit)—a calculated *in vivo* base excess (deficit).

Blood gas values can be given either as 'pH-stat' or 'alpha-stat', the former correcting for body temperature by shifting the calculated Bohr oxyhe-moglobin dissociation curve (hyperthermia to the right, hypothermia to the left). The alpha-stat method is generally considered the standard and measures actual blood gas levels in the sample.

Co-oximeter

This differs from a blood gas machine in that the blood is hemolyzed to calculate (1) total Hb and fetal Hb, and; (2) oxyhemoglobin, carboxy-hemoglobin, methemoglobin, and sulfhemoglobin by utilizing absorbance at six wavelengths (535, 560, 577, 622, 636, and 670 nm).

Taking a good blood gas sample

Use a 1 mL syringe containing preferably a dry heparin salt (if not, liquid sodium heparin 1000 IU/mL solution just filling the hub). Take sample, expel air, mix sample thoroughly, and insert without delay.

Cautions

- Too much heparin causes dilution errors and is acidic.
- Nitrous oxide or halothane anesthesia may give unreliable PO_2 values.
- IV lipid administration may affect pH values.
- Abnormal (high/low) plasma protein concentrations affect base deficit.

See also

Blood gas analysis, p. 102; Invasive blood gas monitoring, p. 104

Blood gas analysis

A heparinized (arterial, venous, capillary) blood sample can be inserted into a blood gas machine and/or co-oximeter for measurement of gas tensions and saturations, and acid–base status.

Measurements

- Identification of arterial hypoxemia and hyperoxia, and hypercapnia and hypocapnia enables monitoring of disease progression and efficacy of treatment. Ventilator and FiO_2 adjustments can be made precisely.
- pH, $PaCO_2$, and base deficit (or bicarbonate) values can be reviewed in parallel for diagnosis of acidosis and alkalosis, whether they be respiratory or metabolic in origin, and whether any compensation has occurred (Fig. 7.4).
- Using a co-oximeter, accurate measurement can be made of Hb oxygen saturation and also the total Hb level. The more sophisticated co-oximeters permit measurement of the fraction of methemoglobin, carboxyhemoglobin, deoxyhemoglobin, and fetal Hb.
- Measure mixed venous oxygen saturation to calculate oxygen consumption and monitor oxygen supply–demand balance.

Causes of acid–base disturbances

- Respiratory acidosis—excess CO_2 production and/or inadequate excretion (e.g., hypoventilation, excess narcotic)
- Respiratory alkalosis—reduction in $PaCO_2$ resulting from hyperventilation
- Metabolic acidosis—usually lactic, keto, or hyperchloremic; consider tissue hypoperfusion, ingestion of acids (e.g., aspirin), loss of alkali (e.g., diarrhea, renal tubular acidosis), diabetic ketoacidosis, and hyperchloremia (e.g., from excess normal saline administration)
- Metabolic alkalosis—consider excess alkali (e.g., bicarbonate or buffer infusion), loss of acid (e.g., large gastric aspirates), hypokalemia, drugs (e.g., diuretics)

Normal values

Arterial pH, 7.35 to 7.45
$PaCO_2$, 35 to 45 mmHg
PaO_2, 80 to 100 mmHg
Arterial HCO_3^-, 22 to 26 mmol/L
SBE (standard base excess), −2 to +2 mEq/L
SaO_2, 95% to 98%
Mixed venous oxygen saturation, 70% to 75%

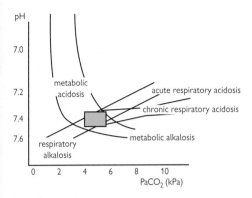

Fig. 7.4 Acid–base map.

Invasive blood gas monitoring

Continuous blood gas monitoring can be achieved via an intra-arterial heparin-bonded catheter with online display of directly measured and computed blood gas variables. Results are updated every 20 to 30 s. Recalibration is generally recommended at 12-h intervals.

Technology

- Systems use either electrode, tonometric, or optode technology.
- Electrode technology is similar to that described for blood gas machine measurement. Optical sensors use either absorbance or fluorescence spectrophotometry to measure the signal from the chemical interaction between the analyte (O_2, CO_2, and H^+) and an indicator phase.

Problems

- Damping of the arterial pressure waveform can occur through the presence of the catheter within the arterial cannula. A dedicated, nontapering 20-G cannula reduces this damping effect.
- An increasing drift in accuracy is recognized after several days.

See also

Blood gas analysis, p. 102

Cardiovascular monitoring

ECG monitoring

Continuous ECG monitoring is routine in every ICU. The standard technique is to display a three-lead ECG (commonly lead II). Other limb leads may be used, although the electrodes are placed at the shoulders and left side of the abdomen. Other lead configurations can be used for specific purposes:
- Chest–shoulder–V5, early detection of left ventricular strain
- Chest–manubrium–V5, early detection of left ventricular strain
- Chest–back–V5, P-wave monitoring

Modern, continuous monitors include alarm functions for bradycardia and tachycardia monitoring, and software routines for arrhythmia detection or ST segment analysis.

Causes of changes in heart rate or rhythm

Changes in heart rate or rhythm may be an indication of
- Sympathetic activity
  - Circulatory insufficiency
  - Pain
  - Anxiety
  - Hypoxemia
  - Hypercapnia
- Adverse drug effects
  - Antiarrhythmics
  - Sedatives
- Electrolyte imbalance
- Fever

See also

Blood pressure monitoring

Noninvasive techniques

Noninvasive techniques are intermittent but automated. They include oscillotonometry (detection of cuff pulsation as the systolic pressure), detection of arterial turbulence under the cuff, ultrasonic detection of arterial wall motion under the cuff, and detection of blood flow distal to the cuff. Any cuff system should use a cuff large enough to cover two thirds of the surface of the upper arm.

Invasive (direct) arterial monitoring

Blood pressure is most accurately monitored from larger limb arteries (e.g., femoral or brachial). However, the potential for damage to these arteries is considerable, and most consider it safer to use the radial artery, the pressure in which is slightly higher. The arterial cannula is connected to an appropriate transducer system via a short length of noncompliant manometer tubing. The transducer should be matched to the monitor as recommended by the manufacturer of the monitor. The transducer must be zeroed to atmospheric pressure. The transducer should be positioned at the level of the fourth intercostal space in the midaxillary line. The transducer, manometer tubing, and cannula should be flushed with saline.

Damping errors

It is important that the monitoring system is correctly damped. An under-damped system will overestimate systolic blood pressure and underestimate diastolic blood pressure. The converse is true for an overdamped system. Moreover, it is not possible to interpret waveform shape correctly if damping is not correct. A correctly damped system will return immediately to the pressure waveform after flushing. Return is slow in an overdamped system and there is often resonance around the baseline before return to the pressure waveform in an underdamped system.

Interpretation of waveform

The shape of the arterial pressure waveform gives useful qualitative information about the state of the heart and circulation (see Fig. 8.1):
- Short systolic time
  - Hypovolemia
  - High peripheral resistance
- Marked respiratory swing
  - Hypovolemia
  - Pericardial effusion
  - Airways obstruction
  - High intrathoracic pressure
- Slow systolic upstroke
  - Poor myocardial contractility
  - High peripheral resistance

Limitations of blood pressure monitoring

It is important not to rely on arterial blood pressure monitoring alone in the critically ill. A normal blood pressure does not guarantee adequate organ blood flow. Conversely, a low blood pressure may be acceptable if perfusion pressure and blood flow is adequate for all organs. Measurement of cardiac output, in addition to blood pressure, is necessary when there is doubt about the adequacy of the circulation.

Normal arterial waveform

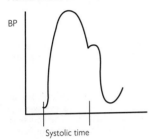

Short systolic time

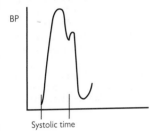

Slow systolic upstroke

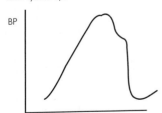

Fig. 8.1 Examples of arterial wavefom shape.

See also

Arterial cannulation, p. 114; Hypotension, p. 310; Hypertension, p. 312

Arterial cannulation

Indications
Performed correctly, arterial cannulation is a safe technique that allows continuous monitoring of blood pressure and frequent sampling of blood. It is indicated in any patient with unstable or potentially unstable hemodynamic or respiratory status.

Radial artery cannulation
The radial artery is most frequently chosen because it is accessible and has good collateral blood flow. Allen's test, used to confirm ulnar arterial blood supply, is not reliable.

Technique of cannulation
The wrist is hyperextended and the thumb abducted. After cleaning the skin, local anesthetic (1% plain lidocaine) is injected into the skin and subcutaneous tissue over the most prominent pulsation. The course of the artery is noted and a 20-G Teflon cannula is inserted along the line of the vessel. The usual technique is to enter the vessel in the same way as an IV cannula would be inserted. There is usually some resistance to skin puncture. To avoid accidentally puncturing the posterior wall of the artery, the skin and artery should be punctured as two distinct maneuvers. Alternatively, a small skin nick may be made to facilitate skin entry.

Seldinger–type kits are also available for arterial cannulation. A guide wire is first inserted through a rigid steel needle. The indwelling plastic cannula is then placed over the guide wire.

The cannula should be connected to a continuous flushing device after successful puncture. Flushing with a syringe should be avoided because the high pressures generated may lead to a retrograde cerebral embolus.

Alternative sites for cannulation
Brachial artery
Thus end artery supplies a large volume of tissue, thus thrombosis has potentially severe consequences.

Ulnar artery
The ulnar artery should be avoided if the radial artery is occluded.

Femoral artery
The femoral artery may be difficult to keep clean. It also supplies a large volume of tissue. A longer catheter should be used to avoid displacement.

Dorsalis pedis artery
The dorsalis pedis artery is notoriously technically difficult both for monitoring (blood pressure will be at least 10–20 mmHg higher than in the central circulation) and in terms of maintaining patency.

Axiliary artery
Use of the axilary artery increases risk of injury to the brachial plexus. This should only be performed by an experienced clinician.

Complications
- Digital ischemia resulting from arterial spasm, thrombosis, or embolus
- Bleeding in cases with altered coagulation status
- Risk of infection in prolonged cannulation
- False aneurysm

See also
Blood gas analysis, p. 102; Invasive blood gas monitoring, p. 104; Blood pressure monitoring, p. 112; Routine changes of disposables, p. 480

Central venous catheter—use

Types of catheter

- Single-, double-, triple-, or quadruple-lumen
- Antimicrobial coating (available for some catheters)
- Sheaths for insertion of pulmonary artery catheter or pacing wire
- Tunneled catheter for long-term use
- Multilumen catheters, which allow multiple infusions to be given separately ± continuous pressure monitoring; minimizes accidental bolus risk
- Large-bore double-lumen catheters for venovenous dialysis/filtration
- Common routes—internal jugular, subclavian, and femoral
- 'Long' catheters for insertion via brachial or axillary veins; generally not used because of the risk of thrombosis

Uses

- Invasive hemodynamic monitoring
- Infusion of drugs that can cause peripheral phlebitis or tissue necrosis if tissue extravasation occurs (e.g., TPN (total parenteral nutrition), epinephrine, amiodarone)
- Rapid-volume infusion (Note: The rate of flow is inversely proportional to the length of the cannula and directly proportional to the diameter.)
- Access (e.g., for pacing wire insertion)
- Emergency access when peripheral circulation is 'shut down'
- Renal replacement therapy, plasmapheresis, exchange transfusion

Contraindications/Cautions

- Coagulopathy
- Undrained pneumothorax on contralateral side
- Agitated, restless patient

Complications

- Arterial puncture
- Hemorrhage
- Arrhythmias
- Infection (usually skin, occasionally sepsis or endocarditis)
- Pneumothorax
- Air embolism, venous thrombosis, hemothorax, chylothorax (rare)

Central venous pressure measurement

Use of an electronic pressure transducer is preferable to manometry. The pressure transducer should be placed and 'zeroed' at the level of the left atrium (approximately, midaxillary line) rather than the sternum, which is more affected by patient position (supine/semierect/prone). Venous pulsation and some respiratory swing should be seen in the trace, but not an RV pressure waveform (i.e., catheter inserted too far).

Troubleshooting

Excessive bleeding at the insertion site is usually controlled by direct compression. If not controlled, correct any coagulopathy. If postthrombolysis, consider tranexamic acid.

The incidence of local infection (usually coagulase-negative staphylococci or *Staphylococcus aureus*) increases after 5 days. Routine change of catheter at 5 to 7 days is not necessary although change over a wire may be sufficient if the patient develops an unexplained fever or leukocytosis. However, removal ± change of site is needed if the site is cellulitic or blood cultures taken through the catheter are positive, or in high-risk patients with unexplained fever or leukocytosis.

See also

Continuous renal replacement therapy, (1), p. 62; Continuous renal replacement therapy, (2), p. 66; Parenteral nutrition, p. 84; Temporary pacing (1), p. 54; Temporary pacing (2), p. 56; Central venous catheter—insertion, p. 118; Pulmonary artery catheter—insertion, p. 122; Fluid challenge, p. 272; Routine changes of disposables, p. 480

Central venous catheter—insertion

Ultrasound-guided placement should be considered, especially for difficult placements. The technique with ultrasound guidance is different from the landmark technique; operators should to be able to identify a patent vein and manipulate both probe and cannula simultaneously. There will be many situations when an ultrasound device may be unavailable, so placement using anatomic landmarks alone should still be learned.

Landmarks

Various landmarks have been described. For example,

- Internal jugular—halfway between mastoid process and sternal notch, lateral to carotid pulsation and medial to medial border of sternocleidomastoid. Aim toward ipsilateral nipple, advancing under body of sternocleidomastoid until vein entered.
- Subclavian—3 cm below junction of lateral third and medial two thirds of clavicle. Turn head to contralateral side. Aim for point between jaw and contralateral shoulder tip. Advance needle subcutaneously (SC) to hit clavicle. Scrape needle under clavicle and advance farther until vein entered.
- Femoral—locate femoral artery in groin. Insert needle 3 cm medially and angled rostrally. Advance until vein entered.

Insertion technique

The Seldinger technique (described here) is safer than the 'catheter-over-needle' technique and should generally be used in ICU patients.

- Use aseptic technique throughout. Clean area with antiseptic and surround with sterile drapes. Anesthetize local area with 1% lidocaine. Flush lumens catheter with saline.
- Use metal needle to locate central vein.
- Pass wire (with 'J' or floppy end leading) through needle into vein. Only minimal resistance at most should be felt. If not, remove wire and confirm needle tip is still located within vein lumen. Monitor for arrhythmias. If these occur, wire is probably at tricuspid valve. Usually responds to retracting wire a few centimeters.
- Remove needle, leaving wire extruding from skin puncture site.
- Depending on size/type of catheter to be inserted, a rigid dilator (± preceded by a scalpel incision to enlarge puncture site) may be passed over the wire to form a track through SC tissues to the vein. Remove dilator.
- Thread catheter over wire. Ensure end of wire extrudes from catheter to prevent accidental loss of wire in vein. Insert catheter into vein to a depth of 15 to 20 cm. Remove wire.
- Check for flashback of blood down each lumen and respiratory swing, then flush with saline.
- Suture catheter to skin. Clean and dry area. Cover with sterile transparent semipermeable dressing.
- A CXR is usually acquired to verify correct position of tip (junction of superior vena cava and right atrium) and to exclude a pneumothorax. Unless in an emergency situation, a satisfactory position should generally be confirmed before use of the catheter.

Pulmonary artery catheter—use

Although in clinical use for 30 years, evidence from large trials does not suggest a mortality benefit associated with pulmonary artery catheter use. Studies have also found an inadequate knowledge base regarding insertion and data interpretation, so proper training in its use is mandated.

Uses

- Pressure monitoring—RA, RV, PA pulmonary artery wedge pressure (PAWP)
- Flow monitoring—(right ventricular) cardiac output
- Oxygen saturation—mixed venous (i.e., in RV outflow tract/PA), determination of left to right shunts (ASD, VSD)
- Derived variables—SVR, PVR, LVSW, RVSW, DO_2, VO_2, O_2ER
- Temporary pacing
- Right ventricular ejection fraction and end-diastolic volume

Specialized catheters

- Continuous mixed venous oxygen saturation measurement
- Continuous cardiac output measurement
- RV end-diastolic volume, RV ejection fraction calculation
- Ventricular (± atrial) pacing

Management

Monitor PA pressure continuously to recognize forward catheter migration and pulmonary arterial occlusion. If so, correct immediately by partial catheter withdrawal to prevent infarction.

The risk of local infection (usually *S. aureus* or coagulase-negative staphylococci) increases after 5 days. A catheter change over a guide wire may be sufficient if unexplained fever or leukocytosis develops. Removal ± change of site is needed if the site is cellulitic, or positive cultures are grown from either the line tip or blood, or in high-risk patients with unexplained fever or leukocytosis.

Withdraw samples of pulmonary artery blood slowly from the distal lumen to prevent 'arterialization' (i.e., pulmonary venous sampling).

Wedge pressure measurements

Inflate balloon slowly, monitoring the waveform to avoid overwedging and potential vessel rupture, especially if the patient is elderly and/or pulmonary hypertensive. The trace should only 'wedge' after ≥1.3 mL air has been injected.

Measure at end-expiration when intrathoracic pressure is closest to atmospheric pressure. The highest reading is seen during spontaneous breathing end expiration. For ventilated patients end expiration typically corresponds to the lowest wedge reading, although significant spontaneous breathing effort may alter the appearance. Measurement is difficult in the dyspneic patient; a 'mean' wedge reading is sometimes used in this instance.

- The PAWP cannot be higher than the PA diastolic pressure.
- Central venous pressure, PAWP, and Cardiac output should not be measured during rapid-volume infusion, but after a period of equilibration (5–10 min).

- The PAWP does not equal the LVEDP in mitral stenosis.
- In mitral regurgitation, measure PAWP at the end of the 'A' wave.

West's zones

- The catheter tip should lie in a zone III region where PA pressure >PV pressure >alveolar pressure, and is below the left atrial level on a lateral CXR.
- Suspect a nonzone III position if (1) after an increase in PEEP, the PAWP increases by >50% of the increment; or (2) the wedge trace shows no detectable cardiac pulsation and/or excess respiratory variation.
- A nonzone III position is more likely with PEEP and/or hypovolemia.

Normal values

Stroke volume, 70 to 100 mL
Cardiac output, 4 to 6 L/min
Right atrial pressure, 0 to 5 mmHg
Right ventricular pressure, 20 to 25/0 to 5 mmHg
Pulmonary artery pressure, 20 to 25/10 to 15 mmHg
Pulmonary artery wedge pressure, 6 to 12 mmHg
Mixed venous oxygen saturation, 70 to 75%

Table 8.1 Derived variables

Variable	Calculation	Normal range
Cardiac index	$\dfrac{CO}{\text{Body surface area } (m^2)}$	2.5–3.5 L/min/m^2
Stroke index	$\dfrac{SV}{\text{Body surface area } (m^2)}$	40–60 mL/m^2
Systemic vascular resistance	$\dfrac{MAP - RAP \times 79.9}{CO}$	960–1400 dyns/cm^5
Pulmonary vascular resistance	$\dfrac{PAP - PAWP \times 79.9}{CO}$	25–125 dyns/cm^5
Left ventricular stroke work index	$(MAP - PAWP) \times SI \times 0.0136$	44–68 gm × m/m^2/beat
Right ventricular stroke work index	$(MPAP - RAP) \times SI \times 0.0136$	4–8 gm × m/m^2/beat
Oxygen delivery	$0.134 \times CO \times Hb_a \times SaO_2$	950–1300 mL/min
Oxygen consumption	$0.134 \times CO \times (Hb_a \times SaO_2 - Hb_v \times SvO_2)$	180–320 mL/min
Oxygen extraction ratio	$1 - \dfrac{SaO_2 - SvO_2}{SaO_2}$	0.25–0.30

CO, Cardiac output.

Key trials

Harvey S, *et al.* Assessment of the clinical effectiveness of pulmonary artery catheters in management of patients in intensive care (PAC-Man): A randomised controlled trial. *Lancet.* 2005; **366**(9484):472–7.

Iberti TJ *et al.* A multicenter study of physicians' knowledge of the pulmonary artery catheter. JAMA 1990; **264**:2928–32.

Richard C, *et al.* Early use of the pulmonary artery catheter and outcomes in patients with shock and acute respiratory distress syndrome: A randomized controlled trial. JAMA 2003; **290**:2713–20.

See also

Positive end expiratory pressure (1), p. 22; Positive end expiratory pressure (2), p. 24; Blood gas analysis, p. 102; Central venous catheter—use, p. 116; Central venous catheter—insertion, p. 118; Pulmonary artery catheter—insertion, p. 122; Cardiac output—thermodilution, p. 124; Cardiac output—other invasive, p. 126; Fluid challenge, p. 272; Heart failure—assessment, p. 322; Routine changes of disposables, p. 480

Pulmonary artery catheter—insertion

Insertion

- Insert 8-Fr central venous introducer sheath under strict aseptic technique. Pulmonary artery catheterization is easier via internal jugular or subclavian veins.
- Prepare catheter preinsertion—three-way stopcocks on all lumens; flush lumens with crystalloid; inflate balloon with 1.6 mL air, and check for concentric inflation and leaks; place transparent sleeve over catheter to maintain future sterility; 'pressure transduce' distal lumen and zero to a reference point (usually midaxillary line). Depending on catheter type, other preinsertion calibration steps may be required (e.g., oxygen saturation).
- Insert catheter 15 cm (i.e., beyond the length of the introducer sheath) before inflating balloon. Advance catheter smoothly through the right heart chambers. Pause to record pressures and note waveform shape in RA, RV, and PA. When a characteristic PAWP waveform is obtained (see Fig. 8.2), stop advancing catheter, deflate balloon, and ensure that PA waveform reappears. If not, withdraw catheter by a few centimeters.
- Slowly reinflate balloon, observing waveform trace. The wedge recording should not be obtained until at least 1.3 mL air has been injected into the balloon. If not, withdraw catheter 1 to 2 cm and repeat. If 'overwedged' (pressure continues to increase on inflation), catheter is inserted too far and balloon has inflated forward over the distal lumen. Immediately deflate, withdraw catheter 1 to 2 cm, and repeat.
- After insertion, a CXR is usually acquired to verify catheter position and to exclude pneumothorax.

Contraindications/Cautions

- Coagulopathy
- Tricuspid valve prosthesis or disease

Complications

- Problems of central venous catheterization
- Arrhythmias (especially when traversing tricuspid valve)
- Infection (including endocarditis)
- Pulmonary artery rupture
- Pulmonary infarction
- Knotting of catheter
- Valve damage (do not withdraw catheter unless balloon deflated)

Troubleshooting

Excessive catheter length in a heart chamber causes coiling and a risk of knotting. No more than 15 to 20 cm should be passed before the waveform changes. If not, deflate balloon, withdraw catheter, and repeat. A knot can be managed by (1) 'unknotting' with an intraluminal wire, (2) pulling taut and removing catheter and introducer sheath together, or (3) surgical or angiographic intervention.

If the catheter fails to advance to next chamber, consider 'stiffening' catheter by injecting iced crystalloid through the distal lumen, rolling the patient to the left lateral position, or advancing the catheter slowly with the balloon deflated. The catheter should never be withdrawn with the balloon inflated.

Arrhythmias on insertion usually occur when the catheter tip is at the tricuspid valve. These usually resolve on withdrawing the catheter or, occasionally, after a slow bolus of 1.5 mg/kg lidocaine is administered.

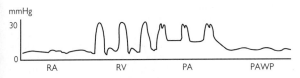

Fig. 8.2 Typical waveforms associated with a PA catheter as it is inserted.

See also

Central venous catheter—insertion, p. 118; Pulmonary artery catheter—use, p. 120; Pneumothorax, p. 298; Hemothorax, p. 300; Tachyarrhythmias, p. 314

Cardiac output—thermodilution

Thermodilution is the technique used by the pulmonary artery catheter to measure right ventricular cardiac output. The principle is a modification of the Fick principle whereby a bolus of cooled 5% glucose is injected through the proximal lumen into the central circulation (right atrium) and the temperature change is detected by a thermistor at the catheter tip, some 30 cm distal. A modification of the Hamilton–Stewart equation, using the volume, temperature, and specific heat of the injectate, enables cardiac output to be calculated by an online computer from a curve measuring temperature change in the pulmonary artery.

Continuous thermodilution measurement uses a modified catheter that emits heat pulses from a thermal filament lying within the right ventricle and right atrium, 14 to 25 cm from the tip. A total of 7.5 W of heat are added to the blood intermittently every 30 to 60 s, and these temperature changes are measured by a thermistor 4 cm from the tip. Although updated frequently, the cardiac output displayed is usually an average of the previous 3 to 6 min.

Thermodilution injection technique

The computer constant must be set for the volume and temperature of the 5% glucose used. Ten milliliters of ice-cold glucose provides the most accurate measure. Five milliliters of room-temperature injectate is sufficiently precise for normal and high output states, however, its accuracy does worsen at low output values.

- Press start button on computer.
- Inject fluid smoothly over 2 to 3 s.
- Repeat at least twice more at random points in the respiratory cycle.
- Average three measurements falling within 10% of each other. Reject outputs gained from curves that are irregular/nonsmooth.

Erroneous readings

- Valve lesions—Tricuspid regurgitation will allow some of the injectate to reflux back into the right atrium. Aortic incompetence produces a higher left ventricular output because a proportion will regurgitate back into the left ventricle.
- Septal defects
- Loss of injectate—check that connections are tight and do not leak.

Advantages

- Most commonly used and familiar ICU technique, computer warnings of poor curves

Disadvantages

- Noncontinuous (by injection technique)
- 5% to 10% inter- and intraobserver variability
- Erroneous readings with tricuspid regurgitation, intracardiac shunts
- Considerable volumes of 5% glucose being injected from frequently repeated measurements

See also

Cardiac output—other invasive

Dye dilution

Mixing of a given volume of indicator with an unknown volume of fluid allows calculation of this volume from the degree of indicator dilution. The time elapsed for the indicator to pass some distance in the cardiovascular system yields a cardiac output value, calculated as

$$\frac{60 \times I}{C_m \times t}$$

where I is the amount of indicator injected, C_m is the mean concentration of the indicator, and t is the total duration of the curve. The traditional dye dilution technique is to inject indocyanine green into a central vein followed by repeated sampling of arterial blood to enable construction of a time–concentration curve with a rapid upstroke and an exponential decay. Plotting the dye decay curve semilogarithmically and extrapolating values to the origin produces the cardiac output. The COLD-Pulsion device measures the concentration decay directly from an indwelling arterial probe, thus computing cardiac output. Alternatively, this device may use the thermodilution approach, avoiding pulmonary artery catheterization. The lithium dilution cardiac output (LiDCO) device is based on a similar principle using lithium as the 'dye'.

Advantages

- Is reasonably accurate and less invasive than pulmonary artery catheter placement.
- Some techniques (e.g., LiDCO) can measure cardiac output 'beat to beat' and thus provide rapid assessment during clinical changes.
- Can also be used to estimate preload responsiveness and thus guide fluid resuscitation

Disadvantages

- Recirculation of dye prevents multiple repeated measurements.
- This is a lengthy procedure and it may underestimate low output values.
- It may be inaccurate with moderate/severe valvular regurgitation.
- The use of some neuromuscular blocking agents may interfere with lithium measurement.

Direct Fick

The amount of substance passing into a flowing system is equal to the difference in concentration of the substance on each side of the system multiplied by the flow within the system. Cardiac output is thus usually calculated by dividing total-body VO_2 by the difference in oxygen content between arterial and mixed venous blood. Alternatively, CO_2 production can be used instead of VO_2 as the indicator. Arterial CO_2 can be derived noninvasively from end-tidal CO_2 whereas mixed venous CO_2 can be determined by rapid rebreathing into a bag until CO_2 levels have equilibrated.

Advantages
- 'Gold standard' for cardiac output estimation

Disadvantages
- For VO_2, this is invasive (requires measurement of mixed venous blood) and requires a leak-free open circuit or an unwieldy closed-circuit technique. VO_2 measurements via metabolic cart are unreliable if FiO_2 is high. Lung VO_2 is not measured by the pulmonary artery catheter technique (may be high in ARDS, pneumonia).
- For CO_2, it is noninvasive but requires normal lung function and is thus not generally applicable in ICU patients.

See also

CO_2 monitoring, p. 94; Blood gas analysis, p. 102; Pulmonary artery catheter—use, p. 120; Cardiac output—thermodilution, p. 124; Cardiac output—noninvasive (1), p. 128; Cardiac output—noninvasive (2), p. 130; Indirect calorimetry, p. 168; Fluid challenge, p. 272; Hypotension, p. 310; Heart failure—assessment, p. 322; Systemic inflammation/multiorgan failure, p. 486; Burns—fluid management, p. 512

Cardiac output—noninvasive (1)

Doppler ultrasound

An ultrasonic beam of known frequency is reflected by moving red blood corpuscles, with a shift in frequency proportional to the blood flow velocity. The actual velocity can be calculated from the Doppler equation, which requires the cosine of the vector between the direction of the ultrasonic beam and that of blood flow. This has been applied to blood flow in the ascending aorta and aortic arch (via a suprasternal approach), descending thoracic aorta (esophageal approach), and intracardiac flow (e.g., transmitral from an apical approach). Spectral analysis of the Doppler frequency shifts produces velocity–time waveforms, the area of which represents the 'stroke distance', i.e., the distance traveled by a column of blood with each left ventricular systole; (Fig. 8.3). The product of stroke distance and aortic (or mitral valve) cross-sectional area is stroke volume. Cross-sectional area can be measured echocardiographically; however, because both operator expertise and equipment are required, this additional measurement can be either ignored or assumed from nomograms to provide a reasonable *estimate* of stroke volume.

Advantages
- Quick, safe, minimally invasive,
- Reasonably accurate,
- Continuous (via esophageal approach),
- Other information on contractility, preload and afterload from waveform shape (Fig. 8.4)

Disadvantages
- Noncontinuous (unless via esophagus),
- Learning curve, operator dependent,
- May be unreliable in certain populations (e.g., poststernotomy)

Echocardiography

Echocardiography combines structural as well as dynamic assessment of the heart using ultrasound reflected off various interfaces. Transthoracic or transesophageal probes provide information on valve integrity, global (diastolic and systolic) and regional ventricular function, wall thickness, pericardial fluid or thickening, aortic dissection, ventricular volumes and ejection fraction, and pulmonary pressures. Often combined with integral Doppler ultrasound for cardiac output estimation derived from combined measurement of aortic diameter plus flow at various sites (e.g., left ventricular outflow tract, aorta, transmitral). Analytical software or formulas can also enable computation of cardiac output from estimations of ventricular volumes.

Advantages
- Noninvasive, safe, relatively quick
- Provision of other useful information on cardiac structure and function.

Disadvantages
- Expensive equipment, lengthy learning curve, interobserver variability
- Possible impairment of image quality from body habitus or pathology (e.g., emphysema)

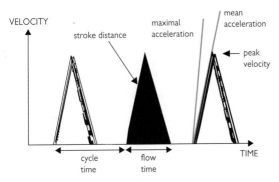

Fig. 8.3 Doppler blood flow velocity waveform variables

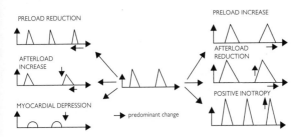

Fig. 8.4 Changes in Doppler flow velocity waveform shape

See also

Cardiac output—thermodilution, p. 124; Cardiac output—other invasive, p. 126; Cardiac output—noninvasive (2), p. 130; Fluid challenge, p. 272; Hypotension, p. 310; Heart failure—assessment, p. 322; Systemic inflammation/multiorgan failure, p. 486; Burns—fluid management, p. 512

Cardiac output—noninvasive (2)

Pulse contour analysis

The concept of this technique is that the contour of the arterial pressure waveform is proportional to stroke volume. However, it is also influenced by aortic impedance, so another cardiac output measuring technique (e.g., commercial devices utilizing COLD-Pulsion or LiDCO) must be used in tandem for initial calibration. Although it can then be used as a means of continuous cardiac output monitoring, frequent recalibration should be performed against the reference technique. This is particularly important when changes in impedance occur (e.g., with changes in cardiac output, vascular tone, body temperature).

Advantages
- Continuous flow monitoring used
- Data from arterial cannula already in situ for pressure monitoring

Disadvantages
- Changes in vascular compliance will affect accuracy, requiring frequent recalibration.
- Requires a good-quality, nonobstructed, and nondamped arterial waveform.
- There is debate about the relative quality of signal from the radial artery versus the femoral artery.

Thoracic bioimpedance

Impedance changes originate in the thoracic aorta when blood is ejected from the left ventricle. This effect is used to determine stroke volume from formulas utilizing the electrical field size of the thorax, baseline thoracic impedance and fluctuation related to systole, and ventricular ejection time. A correction factor for sex, height, and weight is also introduced. The technique simply uses four pairs of electrodes placed in proscribed positions on the neck and thorax. These are then connected to a dedicated monitor that measures thoracic impedance to a low-amplitude, high-frequency (70-kHz), 2.5-mA current applied across the electrodes.

Advantages
- Quick, safe, totally noninvasive
- Reasonably accurate in normal, spontaneously breathing subjects

Disadvantages
- Discrepancies in critically ill patients (especially those with arrhythmias, tachycardias, intrathoracic fluid shifts, anatomic deformities, aortic regurgitation)
- Metal within the thorax
- Inability to verify signal

See also

Cardiac output—thermodilution, p. 124; Cardiac output—other invasive, p. 126; Cardiac output—noninvasive (1), p. 128; Fluid challenge, p. 272; Hypotension, p. 310; Heart failure—assessment, p. 322; Systemic inflammation/multiorgan failure, p. 486; Burns—fluid management, p. 512

Chapter 9

Neurological monitoring

ICP monitoring

Indications

ICP monitoring is used to confirm the diagnosis of increased ICP and monitor treatment. ICP monitoring is indicated in patients with severe head injury (Glasgow Coma Scale [GCS], score, 3–8 points after resuscitation) and an admission CT scan revealing hematoma, contusion, edema, or compressed basal cisterns. ICP monitoring is also appropriate in the setting of severe head injury and a normal admission CT if two or more of the following features are present at admission: age >40 years, posturing, systolic blood pressure <90 mmHg. Also used in encephalopathy, postneurosurgery, and in select cases of intracranial hemorrhage and fulminant hepatic failure. Although increased ICP can be related to poor prognosis after head injury, the converse is not true. Sustained reduction of increased ICP (or maintenance of cerebral perfusion pressure [CPP]) in head injury may improve outcome, although large, controlled trials are lacking.

Methods of monitoring ICP

Ventricular monitoring

A catheter is inserted into the lateral ventricle via a burr hole. The catheter may be connected to a pressure transducer or may contain a fiberoptic pressure monitoring device. Fluid-filled pressure-transducing catheters are zeroed at the level of the external auditory canal. Fiberoptic catheters require calibration but do not need to be zeroed. Both systems may be tested for patency and damping by temporarily increasing the ICP (e.g., with a cough or by occluding a jugular vein). CSF may be drained through the ventricular catheter to reduce ICP.

Subdural monitoring

The dura is opened via a burr hole and a hollow bolt is inserted into the skull. The bolt may be connected to a pressure transducer or may admit a fiberoptic or highfidelity pressure monitoring device. A subdural bolt is easier to insert than a ventricular monitor. The main disadvantages of subdural monitoring are a tendency to underestimate ICP, damping effects, and the inability to withdraw CSF therapeutically for treatment of elevated ICP. Again, calibration and patency testing should be performed regularly.

Complications

- Infection, particularly after 5 days
- Hemorrhage, particularly with coagulopathy or difficult insertion

Using ICP monitoring

Normal ICP is <10 mmHg. An increased ICP is usually treated when >25 mmHg in head-injured patients. As ICP increases, there are often sustained increases in ICP to 50 to 100 mmHg, lasting for 5 to 20 min, increasing with frequency as the baseline ICP rises. This is associated with a 60% mortality. CPP is the difference between mean blood pressure and mean ICP. Treatment aimed at reducing ICP may also reduce mean blood pressure. It is important to maintain CPP at >50 to 60 mmHg.

See also
Intracranial hemorrhage, p. 378; Subarachnoid hemorrhage, p. 380; Increased ICP, p. 384; Head
injury (1), p. 506; Head injury (2), p. 508

Jugular venous bulb saturation

Retrograde passage of a fiberoptic catheter from the internal jugular vein into the jugular bulb enables continuous monitoring of jugular venous bulb saturation (SjO_2). This can be used in conjunction with other monitors of cerebral hemodynamics, such as middle CBF, cerebral AV lactate difference, and ICP to direct management. The jugular bulb saturation can also be used to calculate cerebral metabolism of oxygen ($CMRO_2$) and cerebral oxygen extraction ratio.

Principles of SjO_2 management

Normal values are approximately 65% to 70%. In the absence of anemia and with maintenance of normal SaO_2 values, values of SjO_2 >75% suggest hyperemia or global infarction with oxygen not being utilized. Values <54% correspond to cerebral hypoperfusion, whereas values <40% suggest global ischemia and are usually associated with increased cerebral lactate production. Knowledge of SjO_2 allows optimization of brain blood flow to avoid (1) either excessive or inadequate perfusion and (2) iatrogenically induced hypoperfusion through treating increased ICP aggressively with diuretics and hyperventilation. Studies in trauma patients have found (1) a higher mortality with episodes of jugular venous desaturation and (2) a significant relationship between CPP and SjO_2 when the CPP was <70 mmHg. Decreasing SjO_2 may be an indication to increase CPP, although no prospective, randomized trial has yet been performed to study the effect on outcome.

Approximately 85% of cerebral venous drainage passes down one of the internal jugular veins (usually the right). SjO_2 usually represents drainage from both hemispheres and is equal on both sides; however, after focal injury, this pattern of drainage may alter.

Insertion technique

- Insert catheter or introducer sheath (if used) rostrally in internal jugular vein.
- Calibrate fiberoptic catheter preinsertion.
- Insert catheter via introducer sheath; advance to jugular bulb.
- Withdraw introducer sheath (if used).
- Confirm (1) free aspiration of blood via catheter, (2) satisfactory light intensity reading, and (3) satisfactory positioning of catheter tip by lateral cervical radiograph (high in jugular bulb, above level of second cervical vertebra).
- Perform in vivo calibration; repeat calibration every 12 h.

Troubleshooting

If the catheter is situated too low in the jugular bulb, erroneous SjO_2 values may result from mixing of intracerebral and extracerebral venous blood. This could be particularly pertinent when CBF is low. Blood sampling must be done slowly to avoid mixing.

For fiberoptic catheters, ensure the light intensity reading is satisfactory; if too high, the catheter may be abutting against a wall; if low, the catheter may not be patent or may have a small clot over the tip. Before treating the patient, always confirm the veracity of low readings against a blood sample drawn from the catheter and measured in a co-oximeter.

Formulas

$$CMRO_2 = CBF \times 1.34 \times Hb(SaO_2 - SjO_2)$$

where SjO_2 is the jugular bulb oxygen saturation,
SaO_2 is arterial oxygen saturation (measured as a percentage),
$CMRO_2$ is the cerebral metabolism of oxygen,
CBF is cerebral blood flow, and
Hb is the hemoglobin concentration.

$$\text{Cerebral oxygen extraction ratio} = \frac{SaO_2 - SjO_2}{SaO_2}$$

$$CPP = \text{Mean systemic blood pressure} - ICP$$

See also

ICP monitoring, p. 134; Other neurological monitoring, p. 140; Intracranial hemorrhage, p. 378; Subarachnoid hemorrhage, p. 380; Increased ICP, p. 384; Head injury (1), p. 506; Head injury (2), p. 508

EEG monitoring

The electroencephalogram (EEG) reflects changes in cortical electrical function. This, in turn, is dependent on cerebral perfusion and oxygenation. EEG monitoring can be useful to assess epileptiform activity as well as cerebral well-being in patients who are sedated and paralyzed. EEG monitoring is essential in the treatment of status epilepticus. The conventional EEG can be used intermittently, but data reduction and artifact suppression are necessary to allow successful use of EEG recordings in the ICU.

Bispectral index (BIS) monitor

The BIS is a statistical index derived from the EEG and is expressed as a score between 0 and 100 points. Scores <50 points have been associated with anesthesia-induced unconsciousness. Assessment in the critically ill patient may be complicated by various confounding factors such as septic encephalopathy, head trauma, and hypoperfusion. A low score may be related to deep or excessive sedation, and may allow dose reduction (or cessation) of sedative agents, especially in paralyzed patients. The usefulness of BIS monitoring in the ICU remains unproved.

Other neurological monitoring

CBF

CBF can be measured by radio-isotopic techniques utilizing tracers such as X_n^{133} given IV or by inhalation. This remains a research tool in view of the radioactivity exposure and the usual need to move the patient to a gamma camera. However, portable monitors are now available. Middle cerebral artery (MCA) blood flow can be determined noninvasively by transcranial Doppler ultrasonography. The pulsatility index (PI) relates to cerebrovascular resistance, with an increase in PI indicating an increase in resistance and cerebral vasospasm.

Vasospasm can also be detected when the MCA blood flow velocity exceeds 120 cm/s, and severe vasospasm when velocities are >200 cm/s. Low values of common carotid end-diastolic blood flow and velocity have been shown to be highly discriminating predictors of brain death. Impaired reactivity of CBF to changes in PCO_2 (in healthy patients, 3% to 5% mmHg PCO_2 change) is another marker of poor outcome.

Near-infrared spectroscopy (NIRS)

- Near-infrared (700–1000 nm) light propagated across the head is absorbed by Hb (oxy- and deoxy-), myoglobin, and oxidized cytochrome aa_3 (the terminal part of the respiratory chain involved in oxidative phosphorylation).
- The sum of (oxy- + deoxy-) Hb is considered an index of cerebral blood volume (CBV) change, and the difference is an index of change in Hb saturation, assuming no variation occurs in CBV. CBV and flow can be quantified by changing FiO_2 and measuring the response.
- CBF is measured by a modification of the Fick principle. Oxyhemo-globin is the intravascular nondiffusible tracer, its accumulation being proportional to the arterial inflow of tracer. Good correlations have been found with the X_n^{133} technique.
- Cytochrome aa_3 cannot be quantified by NIRS, but its redox status may be followed to provide some indication of mitochondrial function.
- Movement artifact must be avoided and some devices require reduction of ambient lighting.

Lactate

The brain normally utilizes lactate as fuel; however, in states of severely impaired cerebral perfusion, the brain may become a net lactate producer, with venous lactate increasing above the arterial value. A lactate oxygen index can be derived by dividing the venous–arterial lactate difference by the arteriojugular venous oxygen difference. Values >0.08 are consistently seen with cerebral ischemia.

See also

Lactate, p. 170; Intracranial hemorrhage, p. 378; Subarachnoid hemorrhage, p. 380; Increased ICP, p. 384; Head injury (1), p. 506; Head injury (2), p. 508; Brain stem death, p. 550

Laboratory monitoring

Blood urea nitrogen (BUN) and creatinine

BUN and creatinine are measured in blood, urine, and, occasionally, in other fluids such as abdominal drainage fluid (e.g., ureteric disruption, fistulas).

BUN

A product of the urea cycle resulting from ammonia breakdown, BUN depends on adequate liver function for its synthesis, and adequate renal function for its excretion. Low levels are thus seen in cirrhosis, and high levels are seen in renal failure. Uremia is a clinical syndrome that includes lethargy, drowsiness, confusion, pruritus, and pericarditis resulting from high BUN (or, more correctly, nitrogenous waste products—azotemia).

The ratio of urine urea nitrogen to BUN may be useful in distinguishing oliguria of renal or prerenal origins. Higher ratios (>10:1) are seen in prerenal conditions (e.g., hypovolemia), whereas low levels (<4:1) occur with direct renal causes.

Twenty-four-hour measurement of urinary nitrogen excretion has been previously used as a guide to nutritional protein replacement but is currently not considered a useful routine tool.

Creatinine

A product of creatine breakdown, creatinine is predominantly derived from skeletal muscle and is also excreted renally. Low levels are found with malnutrition, and high levels with muscle breakdown (rhabdomyolysis) and impaired excretion (renal failure). In the latter case, a creatinine value >3 mg/dL suggests a creatinine clearance of <25 mL/min.

The usual ratio for BUN to creatinine is approximately 10:1. A much lower ratio in a critically ill patient is suggestive of rhabdomyolysis, whereas higher ratios are seen in cirrhosis, malnutrition, hypovolemia, and hepatic failure.

The ratio of urine to plasma creatinine may help distinguish between oliguria of renal or prerenal origins. Higher ratios (>40) are seen in prerenal conditions, and low levels (<20) are seen in direct renal causes.

Creatinine clearance is a measure of glomerular filtration. Once filtered, only small amounts of creatinine are reabsorbed. Normally it exceeds 80 mL/min.

Normal plasma ranges
BUN   5 to 20 mg/dL
Creatinine   0.7 to 1.5 mg/dL (depends on muscle mass, race, and diet)

See also

Continuous renal replacement therapy (1), p. 62; Continuous renal replacement therapy (2), p. 66; Peritoneal dialysis, p. 6; Nutrition—use and indications; Urinalysis, p. 166; Acute renal failure—diagnosis, p. 330; Acute renal failure—management, p. 332; Rhabdomyolysis, p. 530

Electrolytes (Na$^+$, K$^+$, Cl$^-$, HCO$_3^-$)

Electrolytes are measured accurately by direct-reading ion-specific electrodes from plasma or urine, although they are sensitive to interference by excess liquid heparin.

Sodium, potassium

Plasma concentrations poorly reflect intracellular concentrations (approximately 3–5 mmol/L for Na$^+$, 140–150 mmol/L for K$^+$) or total-body levels. Plasma potassium levels are affected by plasma pH; acidosis causes a shift of K$^+$ out of the cells wereas alkalosis will have the opposite effect.

Older measuring devices such as flame emission photometry or indirect potentiometry gave spuriously low plasma Na$^+$ levels with concurrent hyperproteinemia or hyperlipidemia. However, even ion-selective electrodes in machines using direct potentiometry can still report falsely low Na$^+$ levels in patients with hyperlipidemia.

Plasma Na$^+$ is also reduced by hyperglycemia as water is shifted out of cells because of the restriction of glucose to the extracellular space. This is not an artifact of the measurement, as with hyperproteinemia or hyperlipidemia, but rather a physiological effect on the plasma Na$^+$ concentration. To correct plasma Na$^+$ for hyperglycemia, add 2.4 mmol/L for each 100 mg/dL glucose over 100 mg/dL.

Urinary Na$^+$ excretion depends on intake, total-body balance, acid–base balance, hormones (including antidiuretic hormone, aldosterone, corticosteroids, atrial natriuretic peptide), drugs (particularly diuretics, nonsteroidal anti-inflammatory drugs (NSAIDs), and ACE inhibitors), and renal function.

In oliguria, a urinary Na$^+$ level <10 mmol/L suggests a prerenal cause whereas >20 mmol/L is seen with direct renal damage. This does not apply if diuretics have been given previously.

Chloride, bicarbonate

Bicarbonate levels vary with acid–base balance. For a constant PCO$_2$, an increase in Cl$^-$ will result in a decrease in HCO$_3^-$ and vice versa. Plasma Cl$^-$ thus tends to vary inversely with plasma HCO$_3^-$, keeping the total anion concentration normal. Increased [Cl$^-$], producing a hyperchloremic metabolic acidosis, may be seen with administration of large volumes of isotonic saline or isotonic saline containing colloid solutions.

Anion gap

The anion gap is the difference in charges between plasma anions (Na$^+$, K$^+$) and plasma cations (Cl$^-$, HCO$_3^-$). Normally this 'gap' is filled by protein (primarily albumin) and phosphate. However, in metabolic acidosis, unmeasured anions (e.g., lactate, ketones, sulfate, and certain toxins like salicylate, methanol, and ethylene glycol) will cause an increased anion gap, whereas a normal anion gap (associated with relative or absolute hyperchloremia) is found with Addison's disease, renal tubular acidosis, diarrhea, pancreatic/biliary fistula, acetazolamide, and ureterosigmoidostomy.

Normal plasma ranges

Na^+	135 to 145 mmol/L
K^+	3.5 to 5.3 mmol/L
Cl^-	95 to 105 mmol/L
HCO_3^-	23 to 28 mmol/L

$$\text{Anion gap} = \text{plasma } [Na^+] + [K^+] - [HCO_3^-] - [Cl^-]$$

Normal range (i.e., when albumin and phosphate are normal) is 12 to 16 mmol/L (if K^+ is omitted, normal range is 8–12 mmol/L).

If albumin and/or phosphate are abnormal, the 'normal range' for the anion gap (with K^+) is determined by the formula

$$2(\text{albumin}) + 0.5(\text{phosphate}) \pm 2$$

where albumin is measured in grams per deciliter and phosphate is measured in milligrams per deciliter.

Strong ion gap (SIG)

SIG quantifies missing ions after correcting for plasma proteins and lactate. Normally SIG is near zero.

$$SIG = [(Na^+ + K^+ + Ca^{2+} + Mg^{2+}) - (Cl^- + lactate^-)] - [(2.46 \times 10^{-8} \times PCO_2/10^{-pH} + (\text{albumin}) \times (0.123 \times pH - 0.631) + [PO_4] \times (0.309 \times pH - 0.469)]$$

where albumin is measured in grams per deciliter.

Osmolar gap

The osmolar gap is the difference between measured and calculated osmolality.

$$\text{Osmolar gap} = \text{Measured osmolality} - [(1.86 \times [Na^+]) + \text{glucose}/18 + \text{BUN}/2.8 + 9 + \text{ethanol}/4.6]$$

An osmolar gap >10 mOsm/L is abnormal and suggests a low-molecular weight substance, including mannitol and poisons such as methanol and ethylene glycol.

See also

Continuous renal replacement therapy (1), p. 62; Continuous renal replacement therapy (2), p. 66; Peritoneal dialysis, p. 68; Urinalysis, p. 166; Crystalloids, p. 176; Diuretics, p. 212; Tachyarrhythmias, p. 314; Bradyarrhythmias, p. 316; Acute renal failure—diagnosis, p. 330; Acute renal failure—management, p. 332; Vomiting/gastric stasis, p. 336; Diarrhea, p. 338; Acute liver failure, p. 360; Hypernatremia, p. 418; Hyponatremia, p. 420; Hyperkalemia, p. 422; Hypokalemia, p. 424; Metabolic acidosis, p. 436; Metabolic alkalosis, p. 438; Diabetic ketoacidosis, p. 444; Hyperosmolar diabetic emergencies, p. 446; Hypoadrenal crisis, p. 450; Poisoning—general principles, p. 454; Rhabdomyolysis, p. 530

Calcium, magnesium, and phosphate

Calcium

Plasma calcium levels have been traditionally corrected to plasma albumin levels. However, correction factors for Ca^{++} are unreliable, particularly at the low albumin levels seen in critically ill patients. Measurement of the ionized fraction is now considered more pertinent because it is the ionized fraction that is responsible for the extracellular actions of calcium being responsible for the symptomatology.

High calcium levels occur with hyperparathyroidism, certain malignancies, sarcoidosis, and tuberculosis, whereas low levels are seen in renal failure, severe pancreatitis, and hypoparathyroidism.

Magnesium

Plasma levels poorly reflect intracellular or whole-body stores, 65% of which is in bone and 35% in cells. The ionized fraction is approximately 50% of the total level.

High magnesium levels are seen with renal failure and excessive administration. This rarely requires treatment unless serious cardiac conduction problems or neurological complications (respiratory paralysis, coma) occur.

Low levels are common in the ICU and occur after severe diarrhea, diuretic therapy, and alcohol abuse, and accompany hypocalcemia.

Magnesium is used therapeutically for a number of conditions, including ventricular and supraventricular arrhythmias, eclampsia, seizures, asthma, and after myocardial infarction. Supranormal plasma levels of 3 to 5 mg/dL are often sought.

Phosphate

High levels are seen with renal failure and in the presence of an ischemic bowel. Low levels (sometimes <0.5 mg/dL) occur with critical illness, chronic alcoholism, and diuretic usage, and may possibly result in muscle weakness, failure to wean from mechanical ventilation, and myocardial dysfunction.

Normal plasma ranges

Calcium	8.5 to 10.5 mg/dL
Ionized calcium	1.05 to 1.2 mmol/L
Magnesium	1.7 to 2.4 mg/dL
Phosphate	2.3 to 4.3 mg/dL

See also

Cardiac function tests

The importance of biochemical markers of myocardial necrosis has been emphasized by a consensus document from the European Society of Cardiology and American College of Cardiology (see Fig. 10.1). The diagnosis of myocardial infarction (MI) was redefined as a typical increase and decrease in troponin, or a more rapid increase and decrease in creatine kinase (CK)-MB, with at least one of the following:

- Ischemic symptoms
- Development of pathological Q waves on ECG
- ECG ST elevation or depression
- Coronary intervention

Troponins

Troponins are bound to the actin filament within muscles and are involved in excitation–contraction coupling. Both cardiac troponin T and troponin I are coded by specific genes and are immunologically distinct from those in skeletal muscle. Neither is detectable in normal healthy individuals, but both are released into the bloodstream from cardiomyocytes damaged by necrosis, toxins, and inflammation. They become detectable by 4 to 6 h after myocardial injury, peak at 14 to 18 h, and persist for up to 12 days. Current assays are highly specific, because they use recombinant human cardiac troponin T as a standard.

Because of to their high sensitivity, plasma levels increase with other cardiac insults (e.g., tachycardia [SVT/VT], pericarditis, myocarditis, sepsis, heart failure, severe exertion, and pulmonary embolism). The degree of increase after MI or during critical illness correlates with a worse outcome.

A positive test is when the cardiac troponin T or I value exceeds the 99th percentile of values for a control group on one or more occasions during the first 24 h after the index clinical event. For cardiac troponin T, this is quoted as 0.05 to 0.1 ng/mL, although many labs now consider values >0.03 ng/mL as positive. Values for cardiac troponin I depend on the particular assay used (usually >0.5–1.5 ng/mL). The negative predictive value after AMI is probably strongest after 6 h. Sensitivity peaks at 12 h, but at the expense of a lower specificity. With renal dysfunction, higher levels are needed to diagnose myocardial damage resulting from impaired excretion.

Cardiac enzymes

CK is detectable in plasma within a few hours of myocardial injury. The cardiac-specific isoform (CK-MB) is used to distinguish cardiac muscle damage from skeletal muscle injury. CK and aspartate aminotransferase (AST) peak by 24 h and decrease over 2 to 3 days, whereas the increase and subsequent decrease in plasma lactate dehydrogenase (LDH) takes 1 to 2 days longer.

Brain (or B-type) natriuretic peptide (BNP)

Cardiomyocytes produce and secrete cardiac natriuretic peptides. Plasma levels increase in a variety of conditions, but high levels are predominantly associated with heart failure, and they increase in relation to severity. A sensitivity of 90% to 100% has been reported, whereas specificity is approximately 70% to 80%. Numerous commercial assays for BNP or pro-BNP are now available, each with their own diagnostic range. They are useful as a screening tool for patients presenting with dyspnea, for prognostication, and, potentially, for titration of therapy. Levels increase in the elderly, in renal failure, and in pulmonary diseases causing right ventricular overload (e.g., pulmonary embolus).

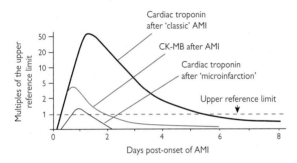

AMI = Acute myocardial infarction

Fig. 10.1 Timecourse of biomarkers for AMI.

Key papers

Antman E, et al. Myocardial infarction redefined—A consensus document of the Joint European Society of Cardiology/American College of Cardiology Committee for the Redefinition of Myocardial Infarction. *J Am Coll Cardiol* 2000; **36**:959–69.

McCullough PA, et al. B-type natriuretic peptide and clinical judgment in emergency diagnosis of heart failure: Analysis from Breathing Not Properly (BNP) Multinational Study. *Circulation* 2002; **106**:416–22.

See also

Acute coronary syndrome (1), p. 318; Acute coronary syndrome (2), p. 320; Heart failure—assessment, p. 322

Liver function tests

Hepatic metabolism proceeds via phase I enzymes (oxidation and phosphorylation) and then subsequently to phase II enzymes (glucuronidation, sulfation, acetylation). Phase I enzyme reactions involve cytochrome p. 450.

Markers of hepatic damage

- Alanine aminotransferase (ALT)
- AST
- LDH

Patterns and ratios of various enzymes are variable and unreliable diagnostic indicators. Measurement of ALT alone is usually sufficient. It is more liver specific but less sensitive than AST and has a longer half-life.

AST is not liver specific but is a sensitive indicator of hepatic damage. The plasma level is proportional to the degree of hepatocellular damage. Low levels occur in extrahepatic obstruction and inactive cirrhosis.

LDH is insensitive and nonspecific. Isoenzyme electrophoresis is needed to distinguish cardiac, erythrocyte, skeletal muscle, and liver injury.

Acute-phase reactants such as C-reactive protein (CRP) are also produced by the liver. Levels increase during critical illness and after hepatocellular injury.

Markers of cholestasis

- Bilirubin
- Alkaline phosphatase
- Gamma-glutamyl transpeptidase (γ-GTP)

Bilirubin is derived from Hb released from erythrocyte breakdown and conjugated with glucuronide by the hepatocytes. The conjugated fraction is watersoluble whereas the unconjugated fraction is lipidsoluble. Levels are increased with intra- and extrahepatic biliary obstruction (predominantly conjugated), hepatocellular damage, and hemolysis (usually mixed picture). Jaundice is detected at levels >3 mg/dL.

Alkaline phosphatase is released from bone, liver, intestine, and placenta. In the absence of bone disease (check Ca^{2+} and PO_4^{3-}) and pregnancy, increased levels usually indicate biliary tract dysfunction. Alkaline phosphatase can be fractionated to distinguish bone from liver origin.

Increased γ-GTP is a highly sensitive marker of hepatobiliary disease. Increased synthesis is induced by obstructive cholestasis, alcohol, various drugs and toxins, and acute and chronic hepatic inflammation.

Markers of reduced synthetic function

- Albumin
- Clotting factors
- Cholinesterase

Albumin levels decrease during critical illness as a result of protein catabolism, capillary leak, decreased synthesis, and dilution with artificial colloids.

Coagulation factors II, VII, IX, and X are liver synthesized. More than 33% of the functional hepatic mass must be lost before any abnormality is seen.

Indicators of function
- Lidocaine metabolites monoethylglycinerylidide (MegX)

Indicators of hepatic blood flow
- Indocyanine green clearance
- Bromosulfthalein clearance

Normal plasma ranges

Albumin	3.5 to 5.3 g/dL
Bilirubin	0.1 to 1.4 mg/dL
Conjugated bilirubin	0 to 0.3 mg/dL
ALT	7 to 35 U/L
Alkaline phosphatase	30 to 125 mU/mL
AST	7 to 45 U/L
γ-GTP	5 to 85 U/L
LDH	30 to 200 U/L

See also

Parenteral nutrition, p. 84; Jaundice, p. 358; Acute liver failure, p. 360; Chronic liver failure, p. 364; Acetaminophen poisoning, p. 458; HELLP syndrome, p. 542

Full blood count

Hb

Increased Hb occurs in polycythemia (primary and secondary to chronic hypoxemia) and in hemoconcentration. Anemia may be the result of reduced red cell mass (decreased red cell production or survival) or hemodilution. The latter is common in critically ill patients. In severe anemia there may be a hyperdynamic circulation that, if severe, may decompensate to cardiac failure. In this case, blood transfusion must be performed with extreme care to avoid fluid overload, or in association with plasmapheresis. Differential diagnosis of anemia includes
- Reduced mean corpuscular volume (MCV)
  - Iron deficiency (anisocytosis and poikilocytosis)
- Increased MCV
  - Vitamin B12 or folate deficiency
  - Alcohol excess
  - Liver disease
  - Hypothyroidism
- Normal MCV
  - Anemia of chronic disease
  - Bone marrow failure (e.g., acute folate deficiency)
  - Hypothyroidism
  - Hemolysis (increased reticulocytes and bilirubin)

White blood cells

An increased white cell count is extremely common in critical illness. Causes of changes in the differential count include those presented in (Table 10.1)

Table 10.1 Common causes of abnormal white blood cell count

Neutrophilia	Lymphocytosis	Eosinophilia
Bacterial infection	Brucellosis	Asthma
Trauma and surgery	Typhoid	Allergic conditions
Burns	Myasthenia gravis	Parasitemia
Hemorrhage	Hyperthyroidism	
Inflammation	Leukemia	
Steroid therapy		
Leukemia		
Neutropenia	**Lymphopenia**	
Viral infections	Steroid therapy	
Brucellosis	SLE	
Typhoid	Legionnaire's disease	
Tuberculosis	AIDS	
Sulfonamide treatment		
Severe sepsis		
Hypersplenism		
Bone marrow failure		

No specific guidelines exist regarding precautions for hospitalized patients with neutropenia (<1.0 × 10^9 /L). Common practice includes routine hand hygiene, no fresh fruit or flowers, and private rooms. Barriers (gown, mask, and glove), visiting limitations, and avoidance of unnecessary procedures (i.e., axillary rather than rectal temperature and removal of Foley catheters) may be used.

Platelets

Correct interpretation of platelet counts requires blood to be taken by a venepuncture. Arterial blood is commonly taken from an indwelling cannula but is not ideal. Thrombocytopenia is the result of decreased platelet production (bone marrow failure, vitamin B12, or folate deficiency), decreased platelet survival (idiopathic thrombocytopenic purpura [ITP], TTP, infection, hypersplenism, heparin therapy), increased platelet consumption (hemorrhage, disseminated intravascular coagulation [DIC]), or in vivo aggregation giving an apparent thrombocytopenia. This should be checked on a blood smear. Spontaneous bleeding is associated with platelet counts <20 × 10^9 platelets/L. Counts less than this should prompt an empiric platelet transfusion. Platelet transfusion is also required for invasive procedures or traumatic bleeds at counts <50 × 10^9 /L.

Normal ranges

Hb	13 to 17 g/dL (men),
	12 to 16 g/dL (women)
MCV	76 to 96 fL
White cell count	4 to 11 × 10^9/L
Neutrophils	2 to 7.5 × 10^9/L
Lymphocytes	1.3 to 3.5 × 10^9/L
Eosinophils	0.04 to 0.44 × 10^9/L
Basophils	0 to 0.1 × 10^9/L
Monocytes	0.2 to 0.8 × 10^9/L
Platelets	150 to 400 × 10^9/L

See also

Blood transfusion, p. 182; Blood products, p. 250; Hemothorax, p. 300; Hemoptysis, p. 302; Upper gastrointestinal hemorrhage, p. 342; Bleeding varices, p. 344; Lower intestinal bleeding and colitis, p. 346; Bleeding disorders, p. 398; Anemia, p. 402; Sickle cell disease, p. 404; Hemolysis, p. 406; Platelet disorders, p. 408; Neutropenia, p. 410; Leukemia, p. 412; Malaria, p. 494; Vasculitides, p. 498; Multiple trauma (1), p. 502; Multiple trauma (2), p. 504; Burns—fluid management, p. 512; Postpartum hemorrhage, p. 544

Coagulation monitoring

Basic coagulation screen

The basic screen consists of a platelet count, prothrombin time (PT), activated partial thromboplastin time (APTT), and thrombin time (TT). Close attention to blood sampling technique is very important for correct interpretation of coagulation tests. Drawing blood from indwelling catheters should, ideally, be avoided, because samples may be diluted or contaminated with heparin. The correct volume of blood must be placed in the sample tube to avoid dilution errors. Laboratory coagulation tests are usually performed on citrated plasma samples taken into glass tubes.

Specific coagulation tests

Activated clotting time (ACT)

Sample tube contains celite, which activates the contact system; thus, the ACT predominantly tests the intrinsic pathway. The ACT is prolonged by heparin therapy, thrombocytopenia, hypothermia, hemodilution, fibrinolysis, and high-dose aprotinin. Normal is 100 to 140 s.

TT

Sample tube contains lyophilized thrombin and calcium. Thrombin bypasses the intrinsic and extrinsic pathways such that the coagulation time tests the common pathway with conversion of fibrinogen to fibrin. The TT is prolonged by fibrinogen depletion (e.g., fibrinolysis or thrombolysis) and heparin via are antithrombin III-dependent interaction with thrombin. A high-dose TT is more sensitive to heparin anticoagulation than fibrinogen levels. Normal range is 12 to 16 s.

PT

Sample tube contains tissue factor (TF) and calcium. TF activates the extrinsic pathway. The PT is prolonged with coumarin anticoagulants, liver disease, and vitamin K deficiency. Normal range is 12 to 16 s. The international normalized ratio (INR) relates PT to control and is normally 1.

APTT

Sample tube contains kaolin and cephalin as a platelet substitute to activate the intrinsic pathway. The APTT is prolonged by heparin therapy, DIC, severe fibrinolysis, von Willebrand factor, factor VIII, factor X1, or factor XIII deficiencies. Normal range is 30 to 40 s.

D-dimers and fibrin degradation products (FDPs)

Fibrin fragments are released by plasmin lysis. FDPs can be assayed by an immunological method. They are often measured in the critically ill to confirm DIC. A level of 20 to 40 µg/mL is common postoperatively in sepsis, trauma, renal failure, and deep vein thrombosis (DVT). Increased levels do not distinguish fibrinogenolysis and fibrinolysis. Assay of the d-dimer fragment is more specific for fibrinolysis (e.g., in DIC), because it is only released after fibrin is formed.

Coagulation factor assays

Assays are available for all coagulation factors and may be used for diagnosis of specific defects. Because heparins inhibit factor Xa activity, the factor Xa assay is therefore the most specific method of controlling low-molecular weight heparin therapy. Because this assay is not dependent on contact system activation, it also avoids the effects of aprotinin when monitoring heparin therapy.

The coagulation cascade—a new concept

The traditional coagulation cascade consisting of extrinsic, intrinsic, and common pathways has been replaced in recent years by a cell-based model with the major initiating hemostasis event in vivo being the action of factor VIIa and TF at the site of injury (Fig. 10.2).

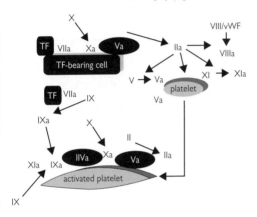

Fig. 10.2 Coagulation cascade.

See also

Bacteriology

Microbiology samples should, if possible, be taken prior to commencement of antimicrobial therapy. In severe infections, broad-spectrum antimicrobials should be started without awaiting results. Sampling sites include those suspected clinically of harboring infection or, if a specific site cannot be identified clinically, blood, urine, and sputum samples. In severe infection, indwelling intravascular catheters should be replaced and the catheter tips sent for culture. Samples should be sent to the laboratory promptly to allow early incubation and to prevent potentially misleading growth. Swabs must be sent in the appropriate transport media.

Blood cultures

To avoid skin contamination, the skin should be cleaned with alcohol and allowed to dry thoroughly before venepuncture. A 5 to 20-mL blood sample is withdrawn and divided into anaerobic and aerobic culture bottles. Larger volumes of blood per blood culture bottle are more sensitive in detecting bacteremia. In addition, cultures should be taken through indwelling intravascular catheters if catheter-related sepsis is suspected. All samples must be clearly labeled. Culture bottles are incubated and examined frequently for bacterial growth. Positive cultures must be interpreted in light of the clinical picture; an early pure growth from multiple bottles is likely to be significant, although cultures from critically ill patients may appear later or not at all as a result of antibiotic therapy. Any Gram-negative isolates or *S. aureus* are usually taken as significant.

Urine

Catheter specimens are usually obtained from the critically ill. The sampling site should be prepared aseptically prior to sampling. The specimen should be sent to the laboratory immediately and examined microscopically for organisms, casts, and crystals. Urine is plated onto culture medium with a calibrated loop and incubated for 18 to 24 h prior to examination. Bacteria >10⁸/L (or a pure growth of 10⁵/L) represent a significant growth. All catheter specimens show bacterial growth if the catheter has been in place for >2 days. Isolation of the same organism from blood confirms a significant culture.

Sputum

Sputum samples are easily contaminated during collection, particularly specimens from nonintubated patients. Suction specimens from intubated patients can be taken via a sterile suction catheter, protected catheter brush, or from specific lung segments via a bronchoscope. Gram-negative bacteria are frequently isolated from tracheal aspirates of intubated patients; only deep suction specimens are significant. Blood cultures should accompany sputum specimens in the diagnosis of pneumonia. Samples should be sent to the laboratory immediately.

Pus samples and wound swabs

Aspirated pus must be sent to the laboratory immediately or a swab sample may be taken and sent in transport medium. Pus is preferable for bacterial isolation.

Typical ICU-acquired nosocomial infections

- Pneumonia resulting from *P. aeruginosa, S. aureus, Klebsiella* spp., *Enterobacter* spp.
- Urinary infection with *Escherichia coli, P. aeruginosa, Klebsiella* spp., *Proteus* spp.
- Catheter related sepsis from *S. aureus*, coagulase-negative staphylococci.

See also

Pleural aspiration, p. 44; Fiberoptic bronchoscopy, p. 46; Chest physiotherapy, p. 48; Virology, serology, and assays, p. 160; Urinalysis, p. 166; Antimicrobials, p. 258; Atelectasis and pulmonary collapse, p. 282; Acute chest infection (1), p. 286; Acute chest infection (2), p. 288; Abdominal sepsis, p. 348; Pancreatitis, p. 354; Meningitis, p. 374; Tetanus, p. 392; Neutropenia, p. 410; Infection—diagnosis, p. 482; Infection—treatment, p. 484; Sepsis and septic shock—treatment, p. 488; HIV- related disease, p. 492; Malaria, p. 494; Burns—general management, p. 514; Pyrexia (1), p. 520; Pyrexia (2), p. 522

Virology, serology, and assays

Antibiotic assays

Antibiotic assays are usually performed for drugs with a narrow therapeutic range, such as aminoglycosides and vancomycin (see Table 10.2). Vancomycin trough levels are normally drawn 30 minutes prior to the fourth scheduled dose and as clinically required thereafter. Vancomycin peak levels are rarely useful. Aminoglycoside levels can be drawn between 8 to 24 hours after the first dose and are used to calculate the dosing interval with an aminoglycoside nomogram. Peak levels drawn 30 minutes after infusion may occasionally be useful in calculating peak-to-MIC (minimal inhibitory concentration) ratios.

Serology

A clotted blood specimen allows antibodies to viral and atypical antigens to be assayed. It is usual to send acute and convalescent (14 days) serum to determine increasing antibody titers. Single-sample titers may be used to determine previous exposure and carrier status.

Hepatitis B

Serology includes hepatitis B surface antigen as a screening test and hepatitis B core antigen to determine infectivity. There is a 10% carrier rate in south east Asians. Serology should be sent in all high-risk patients (e.g., jaundice, IV drug abuse, homosexuals, prostitutes, those with tattoos or unexplained hepatic enzyme abnormalities). In addition, hepatitis B status should be known in staff who experience accidental exposure to body fluids (e.g., through needlestick injury). Those who are not immune may be treated with immunoglobulin.

HIV

Because HIV-positive status carries consequences for lifestyle and insurance, it should rarely be assessed without prior counseling and consent. The CD4 count may be used to assess the likelihood of symptomatology being Acquired Immune Deficiency Syndrome (AIDS) related, although this will decrease further with acute critical illness. Again, consent should usually be sought pretesting. High-risk patients should be considered for testing (e.g., homosexual males, IV drug abusers, hemophiliacs, central African origin). In critically ill patients, such consent can rarely be obtained, and 'unconsented' testing may be used when management may change significantly with knowledge of the HIV status, or when organ donation is being considered. Most AIDS-related infections can be adequately treated without knowledge of the HIV status. Patients or staff who are recipients of a needlestick injury can be treated with antiretroviral therapies if risk is high.

Viral culture

Viral culture is most commonly used for cytomegalovirus (CMV). Samples of blood, urine, or bronchial aspirate may be sent for detection of early antigen fluorescent foci. Herpes virus infections may be detected by electron microscopy of samples (including pustule fluid) and adenovirus in immunosuppressed patients with a chest infection.

Fungi

Candida and *Aspergillus* can be assessed by culture ± antigen tests. *Cryptococcus* can be detected by Indian ink stain in biopsy samples.

Other tests

Other tests available to make microbiological diagnoses include antigen testing for certain bacteria (e.g., *Pneumococcus*), and polymerase chain reaction (PCR). which amplifies the microbial DNA. PCR is an extremely sensitive test for specific organisms; however, it is prone to environmental contamination (e.g., from airborne spores) and it cannot distinguish between colonization and infection.

Common serology for critically ill patients

- Hepatitis A
- Hepatitis B
- Hepatitis C
- HIV
- Cytomegalovirus
- *Mycoplasma pneumoniae*
- *Legionella pneumophila*

Table 10.2 Antibiotic therapeutic levels

	Trough (mg/L)	Peak (mg/L)
Amikacin	<8	30
Gentamicin	<2	4–10
Tobramycin	<2	4–10
Vancomycin	<20	30–50

See also

Bacteriology, p. 158; Urinalysis, p. 166; Antimicrobials, p. 258; Acute chest infection (1), p. 286; Acute chest infection (2), p. 288; Jaundice, p. 358; Acute liver failure, p. 360; Tetanus, p. 392; Botulism, p. 394; HIV-related disease, p. 492; Pyrexia (1), p. 520; Pyrexia (2), p. 522

Toxicology

Purpose

Samples are taken from blood, urine, emesis, or gastric lavage (depending on the drug or poison ingested) for
- Monitoring of therapeutic drug levels (usually plasma) and avoidance of toxicity (e.g., digoxin, aminoglycosides, lithium, phenytoin)
- Identification of unknown toxic substances (e.g., cyanide, amphetamines, opiates) causing symptomatology and/or pathology. Always take a urine sample for analysis.
- Confirmation of toxic plasma levels and monitoring of treatment effect (e.g., acetaminophen, aspirin)
- Medicolegal reasons (e.g., alcohol, recreational drugs after motor vehicle crash)

Samples

Confirm with chemistry laboratory ± local poison unit regarding which, how, and when body fluid samples should be taken for analysis (e.g., peak/trough levels for aminoglycosides, urine samples for out-of-hospital poisoning, repeat acetaminophen levels to monitor efficacy of treatment).

See also
Virology, serology, and assays, p. 160; Poisoning—general principles, p. 454

Miscellaneous monitoring

Urinalysis

Techniques

- Biochemical/metabolic
  - Colorimetric dipsticks are read manually from reference chart or by automated machine within 15 s to 2 min of dipping in urine (see manufacturer's instructions). Usually performed at the bedside.
  - Na and K levels can be measured in most analyzers used for plasma electrolyte measurement. Recalibration of the machine or special dilution techniques may be required.
  - Laboratory analysis is required for detection of urea, creatine nitrogen, osmolality drugs, protein crystals, casts and cell counts.
- Hematological—either by dipstick or laboratory testing
- Microbiological—M, C, S, antigen tests
- Renal disease—usually by microscopy and laboratory testing

Associated tests

Some of these investigations are performed in conjunction with a blood test (e.g., urine-to-plasma ratios of urea, creatinine, and osmolality to distinguish renal from prerenal causes of oliguria, 24-h urine collection plus plasma creatinine for creatinine clearance estimation).

Cautions

- White blood cells, proteinuria, and mixed bacterial growths are routine findings in catheterized patients and do not necessarily indicate infection.
- A 'positive' dipstick test for blood does not differentiate between hematuria, hemoglobinuria, or myoglobinuria.
- Only conjugated bilirubin is excreted into the urine.
- Urinary sodium and potassium levels are increased by diuretic usage.

Urinalysis tests
Biochemical/metabolic

pH	Dipstick
Glucose	Dipstick
Ketones	Dipstick
Protein	Dipstick, laboratory
Bilirubin	Dipstick
Sodium, potassium	Electrolyte analyzer, laboratory
Urea, creatinine, nitrogen	Laboratory
Osmolality	Laboratory
Specific gravity	Bedside gravimeter, laboratory
Myoglobin	Laboratory, positive dipstick to blood
Drugs, poisons	Laboratory

Hematological

Red blood cells	Microscopy, positive dipstick to blood
Hb	Laboratory, positive dipstick to blood
Neutrophils	Dipstick, laboratory

Microbiological

Bacteriuria	Microscopy, culture
TB	Microscopy, culture (early-morning specimens)
Legionnaire's disease	Laboratory

Nephrourological

Hematuria	Microscopy
Granular casts	Microscopy
Protein	Laboratory
Sodium, potassium	Electrolyte analyzer, laboratory
Malignant cells	Cytology

See also

Nutrition—use and indications, p. 80; Bacteriology, p. 158; Virology, serology, and assays, p. 160; Acute renal failure—diagnosis, p. 330; Hypernatremia, p. 418; Hyponatremia, p. 420; Hyperkalemia, p. 422; Hypokalemia, p. 424; Diabetic ketoacidosis, p. 444; Poisoning—general principles, p. 454; Infection—diagnosis, p. 482; Rhabdomyolysis, p. 530

Indirect calorimetry

Calorimetry refers to the measurement of energy production. Direct calorimetry is the measurement of heat production in a sealed chamber but is impractical for critically ill patients. Indirect calorimetry measures the rate of oxidation of metabolic fuels by detecting the volume of O_2 consumed and CO_2 produced. The ratio of VCO_2 to O_2 utilization (respiratory quotient or RQ) defines which fuels are being utilized (Table 11.1). Knowledge of the oxygen utilization by the various fuels allows the calculation of energy production. Carbohydrate and fat are oxidized to CO_2 and water, producing 15 to 17 kJ/g and 38 to 39 kJ/g respectively. Protein is oxidized to CO_2, water, and nitrogen (subsequently excreted as urea), producing 15 to 17 kJ/g.

Technique of indirect calorimetry

Inspiratory and mixed expiratory gases must be sampled. O_2 concentration may be measured by a fuel cell sensor or a fast response, paramagnetic sensor. CO_2 is usually measured by infrared absorption. Sensors may be calibrated with reference to known concentrations of standard gas or by burning a pure fuel with a predictable VO_2. Measurements are usually made at ambient temperature, pressure, and humidity prior to conversion to standard temperature, pressure, and humidity. To calculate metabolic rate (energy expenditure), inspired and expired minute volumes are required. It is common for one minute volume to be measured and the other derived from a Haldane transformation:

$$V_I = V_E \times \frac{N_E}{N_I}$$

The nitrogen concentrations are assumed to be the concentration of gas that is not O_2 or CO_2. Calculation of resting energy expenditure (REE) utilizes a modification of the Weir formula:

$$REE = (3.94 \ VO_2 + 1.11 \ VCO_2) \times 1440 \ min/day$$

Although it is possible to calculate the rate of protein metabolism by reference to the urinary urea concentration, and therefore to separate nonprotein from protein energy expenditure, the resulting modification is not usually clinically significant.

Errors associated with indirect calorimetry

• Underestimate VCO_2—H^+ ion loss, hemodialysis, hemofiltration
• Overestimate VCO_2—hyperventilation, HCO_3 infusion
• Underestimate VO_2—free radical production, unmeasured O_2 supply
• FiO_2 >0.6—small difference between inspired and expired O_2
• Loss of volume—circuit leaks, bronchopleural fistula

Use of indirect calorimetry

Indirect calorimetry is more accurate than formulas used to estimate REE. Measurement of REE and RQ may be helpful in formulating nutritional regimens to reduce VCO_2 in patients with chronic obstructive pulmonary disease (COPD) and patients on mechanical ventilation. It may also reduce the incidence of under- or overfeeding and decrease costs associated with TPN. However, there is no evidence that indirect caloprimetry improves outcomes, or decreases duration of mechanical ventilation or ICU/hospital length of stay.

Table 11.1 Respiratory quotients for various metabolic fuels

Fuel	RQ
Ketones	0.63
Fat	0.71
Protein	0.80
Carbohydrate	1.00

The whole-body RQ depends on the fuel or combination of fuels being utilized. Normally a combination of fat and carbohydrate are utilized with an RQ of 0.8. Lipogenesis associated with both sepsis and overfeeding may give an RQ of 1.1 to 1.3.

See also

Lactate

Measurement of blood lactate

Analyzers are available to allow rapid measurement of blood or plasma lactate on small samples using enzyme-based methods. A whole blood sample (venous or arterial, because there is no practical difference) is collected into a heparin fluoride tube to prevent coagulation and glycolysis (lactate production). Nitrite may be used in the sample tube to convert Hb to methemoglobin, thus avoiding uptake of oxygen during the enzyme reaction. The enzymatic method is specific for the L-isomer and will not, therefore, detect D-lactate (e.g., in short bowel syndrome). Normal arterial whole blood lactate concentrations vary among laboratories, but are generally <2 mmol/L. Lactate may also be measured from regional sites as an aid to the assessment of regional perfusion (e.g., arterial–jugular bulb difference).

Biochemistry of lactate production

Pyruvate is the end product of glycolysis. Most is then metabolized by pyruvate dehydrogenase to acetyl co-enzyme A (CoA), the major substrate for the Krebs cycle. However, in conditions of mitochondrial dysfunction (e.g., cellular hypoxia, sepsis), more pyruvate is converted to lactate by LDH. Although lactic acid results in acidosis, the addition of its sodium salt (sodium lactate) to the plasma is not acidifying. In continuous hemofiltration, older lactate-based replacement fluid contained lactate at 35 to 45 mmol/L. Use of these solutions, particularly in high volume, resulted in increased blood lactate levels without acidosis.

Causes of lactic acidosis

Lactic acidosis occurs when production of lactic acid is in excess of removal. The major sources are skeletal muscle, brain, lung, and white and red blood cells. Removal is mainly by metabolism in the liver, heart, and brain, although the kidney also excretes lactate. Hepatic removal is impaired by poor perfusion and acidosis. In the past, lactic acidosis has been classified as type A or type B. Type A refers to excess production when tissue oxygenation is inadequate. Type B occurs when there is no systemic tissue hypoxia. However, the value of this classification system has never been established and most cases of lactic acidosis have components of both types. Epinephrine may cause accelerated glycolysis and aerobic lactate production in excess of mitochondrial needs; this may produce increasing metabolic acidosis usually without signs of hypoperfusion. In sepsis, hyperlactatemia is probably multifactorial secondary to increased lactate production during anaerobic and aerobic metabolism and decreased lactate clearance. Treatment of metabolic acidosis with sodium bicarbonate solution may increase lactate production. A severe and persistent lactic acidosis is associated with a poor outcome.

Evidence of poor tissue perfusion may be obvious clinically. Calculation of arterial oxygen delivery may confirm inadequate tissue, but normal oxygen delivery does not guarantee adequacy of supply. For an increase in blood lactate to occur, lactate production and release must exceed hepatic, renal, and skeletal muscle uptake. Local hypoperfusion may occur despite normal blood lactate levels.

Key trial

Totaro RJ, Raper RF. Epinephrine-induced lactic acidosis following cardiopulmonary bypass. *Crit Care Med* 1997; **25**:1693–9.

See also

Continuous renal replacement therapy (1), p. 62; Continuous renal replacement therapy (2), p. 66; Blood gas analysis, p. 102; Arterial cannulation, p. 114; Other neurological monitoring, p. 140; Metabolic acidosis, p. 436; Systemic inflammation/multiorgan failure, p. 486

Colloid osmotic pressure

Colloid osmotic pressure (COP) is the pressure required to prevent net fluid movement between two solutions separated by a selectively permeable membrane when one contains a greater colloid concentration than the other. The selectively permeable membrane should impede the passage of colloid molecules but not small ions and water. COP is determined by the number of molecules rather than the type. However, most solutions exhibit nonideal behavior as a result of intermolecular interactions and electrostatic effects. Hence, COP cannot be inferred from plasma protein concentrations; it must be measured.

Measurement of COP

In a membrane oncometer, the plasma sample is separated from a reference 0.9% saline solution by a membrane with a molecular weight exclusion between 10,000 and 30,000 Da. The reference solution is in a closed chamber containing a pressure transducer. Saline will pass to the sample chamber by colloid osmosis, creating a negative pressure in the reference chamber. When the negative pressure prevents any further flow across the membrane, it is equal to the COP of the sample. Normal plasma COP is 25 to 30 mmHg.

Clinical use of COP measurement

Assessing significance of reduced plasma proteins

Plasma albumin levels are almost invariably reduced in critically ill patients. Causes include interstitial leakage, failed synthesis, and increased metabolism. However, the same group of patients often have increased levels of acute-phase proteins, which contribute to COP. Because there is no evidence that correction of plasma albumin levels is beneficial, many clinicians correct a plasma volume deficit with artificial colloid. This will contribute to COP while also reducing hepatic albumin synthesis. If COP is maintained at >20 mmHg, it is likely that reduced plasma albumin levels are of no significance.

Avoiding pulmonary edema

It has been suggested that a difference between COP and PAWP >6 mmHg minimizes the risk of pulmonary edema. However, in the face of severe capillary leak, it is unlikely that pulmonary edema can be avoided if plasma volumes are to be maintained compatible with circulatory adequacy. Conversely, a normal COP would not necessarily prevent pulmonary edema in severe capillary leak; the contribution of COP to fluid dynamics in this situation is much reduced.

Selection of appropriate fluid therapy

In patients with renal failure, the repeated use of colloid fluid may lead to a hyperoncotic state. This is associated with tissue dehydration and failure of glomerular filtration (thus prolonging renal failure). Measurement of a high COP in patients who have been treated with artificial colloids should direct the use of crystalloid fluids. It is important to note that excessive diuresis may also lead to a hyperoncotic state for which crystalloid replacement may be necessary.

See also

Continuous renal replacement therapy (1), p. 62; Continuous renal replacement therapy (2), p. 66; Liver function tests, p. 152; Fluid challenge, p. 272

Fluids

Crystalloids

Types
- Saline (e.g., 'normal', 0.9% saline; 'halfnormal', 0.45%)
- Lactate based (Ringer's lactate, Hartmann's solution)
- Dextrose (e.g., 5%, 10%, 20%, 50%)

Uses
- Crystalloid fluids—to provide the daily requirements of water and electrolytes. They should be given to critically ill patients as a continuous background infusion to supplement fluids given during feeding, or to carry drugs
- Higher concentration dextrose infusions—to prevent hypoglycemia
- Potassium chloride—to supplement crystalloid fluids
- Sodium bicarbonate—for correction of metabolic acidosis, urinary alkalinization, and so on

Routes
- IV

Notes

Many clinicians believe that a significant plasma volume deficit should be replaced at least partially with colloid solutions because crystalloids are rapidly lost from the plasma, particularly during periods of increased capillary leak (e.g., sepsis). Because most plasma substitutes are carried in saline solutions, any additional 0.9% saline crystalloid infusion is needed only to replace excess sodium losses.

The sodium content of 0.9% saline is equivalent to that of extracellular fluid (see Table 12.1). A daily requirement of 70 to 80 mmol sodium is normal, although there may be excess loss in sweat and from the gastrointestinal tract (see Table 12.2).

Ringer's lactate or Hartmann's solution have no practical advantage over 0.9% saline for fluid maintenance. They may, however, be useful if large volumes of crystalloid are used to avoid hyperchloremic acidosis.

Hyperchloremic acidosis may adversely affect coagulation and possibly renal function.

Five percent dextrose is used to supply IV water requirements. The 50 g/L glucose content ensures an isotonic solution, but only provides 200 KCal/L. The normal requirement is approximately 1.5 to 2 L/day. Water loss in excess of electrolytes is uncommon, but occurs in excess sweating, fever, hyperthyroidism, diabetes insipidus, and hypercalcemia.

Potassium chloride must be given slowly because rapid injection may cause fatal arrhythmias. No more than 40 mmol/h should be given, although 20 mmol/h is more usual. The frequency of infusion is dictated by plasma potassium measurements.

Table 12.1 Ion content of crystalloids (mmol/L)

	Na⁺	K⁺	HCO₃⁻	Cl⁻	Ca²⁺
0.9% saline (normal saline)	154			154	
Hartmann's	131	5	29	111	2
D5 half normal saline	77			77	

Table 12.2 Ion content of gastrointestinal fluids (mmol/L)

	Na⁺	K⁺	HCO₃⁻	Cl⁻
Gastric	20–80	5–20	150	100–150
Biliary	120–140	5–15	30–50	80–120
Pancreatic	120–140	5–15	70–110	40–80
Small bowel	120–140	5–15	20–40	90–130
Large bowel	100–120	5–15	20–40	90–130

See also

Nutrition—use and indications, p. 80; Urea and creatinine, p. 144; Electrolytes (Na⁺, K⁺, Cl⁻, HCO₃⁻), p. 146; Sodium bicarbonate, p. 178; Colloids, p. 180; Hypernatremia, p. 418; Hyponatremia, p. 420; Hyperkalemia, p. 422; Hypokalemia, p. 424; Metabolic acidosis, p. 436; Diabetic ketoacidosis, p. 444; Hyperosmolar diabetic emergencies, p. 446; Multiple trauma (1), p. 502; Multiple trauma (2), p. 504; Burns—fluid management, p. 512; Postoperative intensive care, p. 536

Sodium bicarbonate

Types
- Isotonic sodium bicarbonate, 1.26%
- Hypertonic sodium bicarbonate (1 mmol/mL), 8.4% (see Table 12.3)

Uses
- Correction of metabolic acidosis
- Alkalinization of urine
- Alkalinization of blood (e.g., for treatment of tricyclic antidepressant overdose)

Routes
- IV

Notes
Isotonic (1.26%) sodium bicarbonate may be used to correct acidosis associated with renal failure or to induce a forced alkaline diuresis. The hypertonic (8.4%) solution is rarely required in intensive care practice to increase blood pH in severe metabolic acidosis. Bicarbonate therapy is rarely effective when tissue hypoperfusion or necrosis is present.

Administration may be indicated as either specific therapy (e.g., alkaline diuresis for salicylate overdose) or if the patient is symptomatic (usually dyspneic) in the absence of tissue hypoperfusion (e.g., renal failure). $PaCO_2$ may increase if minute volume is not increased. Bicarbonate cannot cross the cell membrane without dissociation, so an increase in $PaCO_2$ may result in intracellular acidosis and depression of myocardial cell function.

The decrease in plasma ionized calcium may also cause a decrease in myocardial contractility. Significantly worse hemodynamic effects have been reported with bicarbonate compared with equimolar saline in patients with severe heart failure.

Convincing human evidence that bicarbonate improves myocardial contractility or increases responsiveness to circulating catecholamines in severe acidosis is lacking, although anecdotal success has been reported.

Acidosis relating to myocardial depression is related to intracellular changes that are not accurately reflected by arterial blood chemistry.

Excessive administration may cause hyperosmolality, hypernatremia, hypokalemia, sodium overload, and 'overshoot' alkalemia.

Sodium bicarbonate does have a place in the management of acid retention or alkali loss (e.g., chronic renal failure, renal tubular acidosis, fistulas, diarrhea). Fluid and/or potassium deficits should be corrected first.

Table 12.3 Ion content of sodium bicarbonate (mmol/L)

	Na^+	K^+	HCO_3^-	Cl^-	Ca^{2+}
1.26% sodium bicarbonate	150		150		
8.4% sodium bicarbonate	1000		1000		

See also

Blood gas analysis, p. 102; Electrolytes (Na^+, K^+, Cl^-, HCO_3^-), p. 146; Crystalloids, p. 176; Cardiac arrest, p. 270; Metabolic acidosis, p. 436; Salicylate poisoning, p. 456

Colloids

Types

- Albumin (e.g., 4.5%–5%, 20%–25% human albumin solution)
- Dextran (e.g., 6% Dextran 70; 10% Dextran 40)
- Hydroxyethyl starch (e.g., 6% hetastarch, in saline or balanced electrolyte solutions)

Uses

- Replacement of plasma volume deficit
- Prophylaxis of venous thrombosis (Dextran 40)

Routes

- IV

Side effects

- Dilution coagulopathy
- Anaphylaxis
- Interference with blood cross-matching (Dextran)

Notes

Smaller volumes of colloid are required for resuscitation with less contribution to edema. Maintenance of plasma COP is a useful effect not seen with crystalloids, but colloids contain no clotting factors or other plasma enzyme systems.

Albumin is the main provider of COP and has several other roles. There is no evidence that maintaining plasma albumin levels, as opposed to plasma COP with artificial plasma substitutes, is better. Albumin 20% to 25% is hyperoncotic and is used to provide colloid when salt restriction is necessary. This is rarely necessary in intensive care because plasma volume expansion is related to the weight of colloid infused rather than the concentration. Artificial colloids used with ultrafiltration or diuresis are just as effective in edema states.

In patients with capillary leak, albumin and smaller molecular weight colloids leak to the interstitium. In these cases it is perhaps better to use larger molecular weight colloids such as hydroxyethyl starch, although conclusive evidence is lacking.

Hetastarch is usually a 6% solution with a high degree of protection from metabolism because of its high degree of substitution (DS; proportion of glucose units substituted with hydroxyethyl groups) or a high ratio of C2 to C6 carbon atoms substituted (C2-to-C6 ratio). The molecular weight ranges vary, but molecular sizes are large enough to ensure a prolonged effect. These are the most useful colloids in capillary leak. Prolonged itching related to intradermal deposition and interference with coagulation are complications if excessive doses are used.

Hetastarch is available premixed in 0.9% saline or in a lactated electrolyte solution. In balanced lactated solution, hetastarch does not cause hyperchloremic acidosis or coagulopathy and may therefore be preferable to saline preparations.

Unique features of albumin
- Transport of various molecules
- Free radical scavenging
- Binding of toxins
- Inhibition of platelet aggregation

Relative persistence of colloid effect

Albumin	+++
Dextran 70	++
Dextran 40	+
Hetastarch (high molecular weight, high DS, low C2-to-C6 ratio)	++++

- Persistence is dependent on molecular size and protection from metabolism.
- High DS and high C2-to-C6 ratio protect hydroxyethyl starch from metabolism.
- All artificial colloids are polydisperse (i.e., there is a range of molecular sizes).

Key trials

The SAFE study investigators. A comparison of albumin and saline for fluid resuscitation in the intensive care unit. *N Engl J Med* 2004; J50:2247–56.

See also

Crystalloids, p. 176; Blood transfusion, p. 182; Blood products, p. 250; Basic resuscitation, p. 268; Fluid challenge, p. 272; Diabetic ketoacidosis, p. 444; Systemic inflammation/multiorgan failure, p. 486; Sepsis and septic shock treatment, p. 552; Anaphylactoid reactions, p. 498; Burns—fluid management, p. 512; Postoperative intensive care, p. 536

Blood transfusion

Blood storage

Blood cells are eventually destroyed as a result of oxidant damage during storage of whole blood. Because white cells and plasma enzyme systems are of importance in this cellular destruction, effects are correspondingly less severe for packed red cells. Blood used for transfusion in most of Europe is now routinely leukodepleted. Microaggregate formation is associated with platelets, white cells, and fibrin, and ranges in size from 20 to 170 μm. The risk of microaggregate damage is reduced with packed red cells. The use of filters can decrease the number of leukoaggregates in transfused blood. In addition to spherocytosis and hemolysis, prolonged storage depletes adenosine triphosphate (ATP) and di-phosphoglycerate (2,3-DPG) levels, thus decreasing oxygen delivery with transfused red cells. If whole blood is to be used in critically ill patients, it should be as fresh as possible.

Compatibility

In an emergency, with massive blood loss that threatens life, it is permissible to transfuse O-negative packed cells, but a sample must be taken for typing and cross-matching prior to transfusion. With modern laboratory procedures, it is possible to obtain ABO compatibility for group-specific transfusion within 5 to 10 min and a full cross-match in 30 min.

Hazards of blood transfusion

- Citrate toxicity—hypocalcemia is rarely a problem and the prophylactic use of calcium supplementation is not recommended
- Potassium load—potassium returns to cells rapidly, but hyperkalemia may be a problem if blood is stored at room temperature
- Sodium load—from citrate if the transfusion is massive
- Hypothermia—can be avoided by warming blood as it is transfused
- Jaundice—hemolysis of incompatible or old blood
- Pyrexia—immunological transfusion reactions to incompatible red or white cells or platelets
- DIC—partial activation of clotting factors and destruction of stored cells, either in old blood or when transfusion is incompatible
- Anaphylactoid reaction—urticaria is common and probably the result of a reaction to transfused plasma proteins. If severe, it may be treated by slowing the transfusion and giving chlorpheniramine 10 mg IV/intramuscularly (IM). In severe anaphylaxis, in addition to standard treatment, the transfusion should be stopped and saved for later analysis and a sample taken for further cross-matching
- Transmission of disease—including viruses, parasites (malaria), and prions
- Transfusion-related acute lung injury and other immune reactions; may be be severe and life threatening
- A multicenter trial suggested liberal transfusion in the critically ill produced less favorable outcomes, particularly in younger, less sick patients, than using a trigger Hb of 7 g/dL

Key trial

Hebert PC, Wells G, Blajchman MA, *et al.*, for the Transfusion Requirements in Critical Care Investigators. A multicenter, randomized, controlled clinical trial of transfusion requirements in critical care. *N Engl J Med* 1999; **340**:409–17.

See also

Calcium, magnesium, and phosphate, p. 148; Full blood count, p. 154; Coagulation monitoring, p. 156; Basic resuscitation, p. 268; Hemothorax, p. 300; Hemoptysis, p. 302; Upper gastrointestinal hemorrhage, p. 342; Bleeding varices, p. 344; Lower intestinal bleeding and colitis, p. 346; Bleeding disorders, p. 398; Anemia, p. 402; Hemolysis, p. 406; Malaria, p. 494; Anaphylactoid reactions, p. 498; Postoperative intensive care, p. 536; Postpartum hemorrhage, p. 544

Respiratory drugs

Bronchodilators

Types

- β_2-agonists (e.g., albuterol, epinephrine, terbutaline)
- Anticholinergics (e.g., ipratropium)
- Theophyllines (e.g., aminophylline)
- Steroids (e.g., hydrocortisone, prednisolone)
- Others (e.g., ketamine, isoflurane, halothane)

Uses

Relief of bronchospasm

Routes

- Inhaled (albuterol, epinephrine, terbutaline, ipratropium, isoflurane, halothane)
- Nebulized (albuterol, epinephrine, terbutaline, ipratropium)
- IV (epinephrine, terbutaline, ipratropium, aminophylline, hydrocortisone, ketamine)
- By mouth or per os (PO, aminophylline, prednisolone)

Side effects

- CNS stimulation (albuterol, epinephrine, terbutaline, aminophylline)
- Tachycardia (albuterol, epinephrine, terbutaline, aminophylline, ketamine)
- Hypotension (albuterol, terbutaline, aminophylline, isoflurane, halothane)
- Hyperglycemia (albuterol, epinephrine, terbutaline, hydrocortisone, prednisolone)
- Hypokalemia (albuterol, epinephrine, terbutaline, hydrocortisone, prednisolone)
- Lactic acidosis (albuterol, epinephrine)—rare

Notes

Selective β_2-agonists are usually given by inhalation via a pressurized aerosol or a nebulizer (see Table 13.1). Inhalation often gives rapid relief of bronchospasm, although the aerosol is of less benefit in severe asthma.

Nebulized drugs require a minimum volume of 4 mL and a driving gas flow of 6 to 8 L/min.

In extremis, epinephrine may be used IV, SC, or injected down the endotracheal tube. Because epinephrine is not selective, arrhythmias are more likely. However, the α-agonist effect may reduce mucosal swelling by vasoconstriction.

Ipratropium bromide has no systemic effects and does not depress mucociliary clearance. It is synergistic with β_2-agonists but has a slower onset of action.

Aminophylline is synergistic with β_2-agonists. Dosages must be adjusted according to plasma levels (range, 10–20 mg/L) because toxic effects may be severe. Dose requirements are reduced by heart failure, liver disease, chronic airflow limitation, fever, cimetidine, and erythromycin. Dose requirements are increased in children, and smokers, and in those with a moderate to high alcohol intake.

Table 13.1 Drug dosages

	Aerosol*	Nebulizer*	IV bolus	IV infusion
Albuterol	100–200 µg	2.5–5 mg		
Terbutaline	250–500 µg	5–10 mg	1.5–5 µg/min	
Epinephrine		0.5 mg		
Ipratropium		0.5 mg		
Aminophylline			5 mg/kg over 20 min	0.5 mg/kg/h
Hydrocortisone			200 mg qid	

*Aerosols and nebulizers are usually given four to six times daily, but may be given more frequently if necessary.
In extremis, epinephrine may be given as 0.1 to 0.5 mg SC, injected down the endotracheal tube, or by IV infusion.

See also

Steroids, p. 260; Chronic airflow limitation, p. 284; Asthma—general management, p. 294 Asthma—ventilatory management, p. 296

Respiratory stimulants

Types
- Drug antagonists (e.g., naloxone, flumazenil)
- CNS stimulants (e.g., doxapram)

Uses
- Acute respiratory failure resulting from failure of ventilatory drive
- Drug-induced ventilatory failure (e.g., as a result of excessive sedation or postoperatively)

Routes
- IV

Modes of action
- Naloxone—short-acting opiate antagonist
- Flumazenil—short-acting benzodiazepine antagonist
- Doxapram—generalized CNS stimulant with predominant respiratory stimulation at lower doses; stimulation of carotid chemoreceptors at very low doses with increased tidal volumes

Side effects
- Seizures (flumazenil, doxapram)
- Tachyarrhythmias (naloxone, flumazenil)
- Hallucinations (doxapram)

Notes
Respiratory stimulants are mainly used in patients with chronic airflow limitation who develop acute hypercapnic respiratory failure. Effects of doxapram are short lived, so infusion is necessary. After about 12 h of infusion, the effects on ventilatory drive are reduced. (See Table 13.2).

Naloxone may be used in respiratory depression resulting from opiates. Because it reverses all opiate effects, it may be better to reverse respiratory depression with nonspecific respiratory stimulants, leaving pain relief intact. It may need to be repeated when long-acting opiates are involved.

Because most benzodiazepines are long acting compared with flumazenil, repeated doses may be necessary.

Table 13.2 Drug dosages

IV infusion	IV bolus	IV
Naloxone	0.1–0.4 mg	
Flumazenil	0.2 mg over 15 min (0.1 mg/min to max 2 mg)	
Doxapram	1–1.5 mg/kg over 30 s	2–3 mg/min

Key papers

Greenstone M, Lasserson TJ. Doxapram for ventilatory failure due to exacerbations of chronic obstructive pulmonary disease. *Cochrane Database Syst Rev* 2003; CD000223. [Review].

See also

Opioid analgesics, p. 232; Sedatives, p. 236; Respiratory failure, p. 280; Sedative poisoning, p. 460; Postoperative intensive care, p. 536

Nitric oxide

Nitric oxide is now recognized as a fundamental mediator in many physiological processes. One of its most important effects is smooth muscle relaxation. Nitric oxide is the major local controller of vascular tone via effects on cyclic guanosine monophosphate (CGMP).

Inhaled nitric oxide

Nitric oxide is provided for inhalation via a proprietary delivery system. It is diluted with inspiratory gases at the inspiratory limb of the ventilator circuit to provide an inhaled concentration of 1 to 40 ppm, although most patients require less than 20 ppm. Inhalation produces vasodilatation at the site of gas exchange, may improve ventilation–perfusion matching, and may reduce pulmonary artery pressures. Randomized multicenter studies in patients with acute lung injury have revealed no long-term benefit or outcome improvement. Because nitric oxide works in ventilated lung units, its use may be most effective when lung inflation is optimized, such as after a recruitment maneuver or prone positioning.

Side effects

Nitric oxide is immediately bound to Hb, ensuring local effects only. There is no tolerance, but patients can become dependent on continued inhalation, with rebound pulmonary hypertension and hypoxemia on withdrawal. For this reason, withdrawal must be gradual. Excessive humidification of inspired gases may form nitric acid with nitric oxide. When nitric oxide is administered with high concentrations of inspired oxygen, nitrogen dioxide can be produced. This can be minimized by introducing nitric oxide at the inspiratory limb of the ventilator circuit.

Monitoring

Nitric oxide and nitrogen dioxide concentrations may be monitored conveniently with portable fuel cell analyzers or by chemiluminescence. It is important to monitor concentrations of both gases in the inspiratory limb of the ventilator circuit. Monitoring of nitrogen dioxide is important to ensure that toxic doses are not formed with the oxygen in the inspired gas and subsequently inhaled by the patient. Although it is extremely rare to see toxic nitrogen dioxide concentrations (>5 ppm), it is possible to remove nitrogen dioxide from the inspired gas by using a soda lime adsorber. Methemoglobin is formed when nitric oxide binds to Hb. Inhalation at doses of 40 ppm or less will rarely result in methemoglobinemia without a preexisting methemoglobin reductase deficiency.

Achieving the correct dose

Approximately 50% of patients with severe respiratory failure respond to nitric oxide. A positive response is usually defined as a 20% increase in oxygenation. However, the most effective dose varies. It is usual to start at 1 ppm for 10 min and monitor the change in the PaO_2-to-FiO_2 ratio. An increase should be followed by an increase in nitric oxide concentration to 5 ppm for a further 10 min. Thereafter, the dose is adjusted according to the response at 10 min intervals until the most effective dose is found.

Dose–response curves are extremely variable between patients and in single patients over time. It is imperative to assess the dose response as titrated against a therapeutic goal at daily intervals, aiming to keep the dose at the lowest effective level.

Scavenging

Because the concentrations used are so small, dilution of exhaled gases into the atmosphere is unlikely to produce important environmental concentrations. In the air-conditioned intensive care environment, air changes are so frequent that they make scavenging unnecessary.

Key trials

Dellinger RP, et al., for the Inhaled Nitric Oxide in ARDS Study Group. Effects of inhaled nitric oxide in patients with acute respiratory distress syndrome: Results of a randomized phase II trial. *Crit Care Med* 1998; **26**:15–23.

Lundin S, et al., for The European Study Group of Inhaled Nitric Oxide. Inhalation of nitric oxide in acute lung injury: Results of a European multicentre study. Intensive *Care Med* 1999; **25**:911–19.

See also

Vasodilators, p. 198; Acute respiratory distress syndrome (1), p. 290; Acute respiratory distress syndrome (2), p. 292

Surfactant

In ARDS there is decreased surfactant production, biochemical abnormality of the surfactant produced, and inhibition of surfactant function. The net result is alveolar and small-airway collapse. Surfactant also contributes to host defense against microorganisms. Surfactant replacement would be expected to exert therapeutic effects on lung mechanics, gas exchange, and host defense.

Instillation of surfactant (either as a liquid or nebulized) via the endotracheal tube into the lungs is associated with improved outcome in neonatal respiratory distress syndrome. Potential indications in adults include ARDS, pneumonia, chronic airflow limitation, and asthma. Multiple studies in ARDS have yet to demonstrate a mortality benefit, although this may be related to the type of surfactant, the volume used, or the delivery system.

Studies have demonstrated improved oxygenation with recombinant surfactant protein C and a trend to improved survival in patients with direct lung injury. Further studies are underway using recombinant surfactant protein C with phospholipids, and with surfactant proteins B and C. The surfactant is instilled into the lungs via an endotracheal catheter.

Complications of surfactant treatment have included increased cough, sputum production, bronchospasm, increased peak airway pressure, and adverse effects on pulmonary function. These can be minimized by adequate sedation and neuromuscular blockade before instilling surfactant.

Key trial

Spragg RG, Lewis JF, Walmrath HD, *et al.* Effect of recombinant surfactant protein C-based surfactant on the acute respiratory distress syndrome. *N Engl J Med* 2004; **351**:884–92.

See also

Acute respiratory distress syndrome (1), p. 290; Acute respiratory distress syndrome (2), p. 292

Cardiovascular drugs

Inotropes

Types
- Catecholamines (e.g., epinephrine, norepinephrine, dobutamine, dopamine)
- Phosphodiesterase (PDE) inhibitors (e.g., milrinone)
- Dopexamine
- Calcium sensitizers (e.g., levosimendan)
- Cardiac glycosides (e.g., digoxin [weak])

Modes of action
- Increase force of myocardial contraction, either by stimulating cardiac β_1 adrenoreceptors (catecholamines), decreasing cyclic adenosine monophosphate (cAMP) breakdown (PDE inhibitors), increasing calcium sensitivity (Ca sensitizers), directly increasing contractility (digoxin), or inhibiting neuronal reuptake of noradrenaline (dopexamine). All agents except digoxin have, to greater or lesser degrees, associated dilator or constrictor properties via β_1 and α_1 adrenoreceptors, dopaminergic receptors, or K_{ATP} channels.
- Digoxin may cause splanchnic vasoconstriction and, for an inotropic effect, requires plasma levels at the top of the therapeutic range.
- The increase in cardiac work is partially offset in those drugs possessing associated dilator effects.
- Other than epinephrine (when used for its vasoconstricting effect in cardiopulmonary resuscitation [CPR]) or digoxin (for long-term use in chronic heart failure), inotropes are usually given by continuous IV infusion, titrated for effect.

Uses
- Myocardial failure (e.g., post-MI, cardiomyopathy)
- Myocardial depression (e.g., sepsis)
- Augmentation of oxygen delivery in high-risk surgical patients

Side effects
- Arrhythmias (usually associated with concurrent hypovolemia)
- Tachycardia (usually associated with concurrent hypovolemia)
- Hypotension (related to dilator properties ± concurrent hypovolemia)
- Hypertension (related to constrictor properties)
- Anginal chest pain, or ST-segment and T-wave changes on ECG
- Hyperglycemia and lactic acidosis (epinephrine)

Notes
Epinephrine, norepinephrine, and dopamine should be given via a central vein because tissue necrosis may occur secondary to peripheral extravasation.

Table 14.1 Drug dosages

Epinephrine	Infusion starting from 0.05 µg/kg/min
Norepinephrine	Infusion starting from 0.05 µg/kg/min
Dobutamine	Infusion from 2–20 µg/kg/min
Dopamine	Infusion from 2–20 µg/kg/min
Dopexamine	Infusion from 0.5–6 µg/kg/min
Milrinone	Loading dose of 50 µg/kg over 10 min followed by infusion from 0.375–0.75 µg/kg/min
Digoxin	0.5 mg given PO or IV over 10–20 min. Repeat at 4 to 8 h intervals until loading achieved (assessed by clinical response). Maintenance dose thereafter is 0.0625–0.25 mg/day depending on plasma levels and clinical response.
Levosimendan	12–24 µg/kg over 10 min followed by 0.1 µg/kg/min for 24 h

See also

Intra-aortic balloon counterpulsation, p. 58; Cardiac output—thermodilution, p. 124; Cardiac output—other invasive, p. 126; Cardiac output—noninvasive (1), p. 128; Cardiac output—noninvasive (2), p. 130; Basic resuscitation, p. 268; Cardiac arrest, p. 270; Fluid challenge, p. 272 Hypotension, p. 310; Sepsis and septic shock—treatment, p. 488; Care of the potential organ donor, p. 554

Vasodilators

Types
- Nitrates (e.g., glyceryl trinitrate, isosorbide dinitrate)
- ACE inhibitors (e.g., captopril)
- Smooth muscle relaxants (e.g., sodium nitroprusside, hydralazine)
- α-Adrenergic antagonists (e.g., phentolamine)
- β_2-Adrenergic agonists (e.g., salbutamol)
- Calcium antagonists (e.g., nifedipine, diltiazem)
- Dopaminergic agonists (e.g., fenoldopam)
- PDE inhibitors (e.g., milrinone, sildenafil)
- Prostaglandins (e.g., epoprostenol [PGI_2] alprostadil [PGE_1])
- BNP analogues, (e.g., nesiritide)

Modes of action
- Increases cGMP concentration (by nitric oxide donation or by inhibiting cGMP breakdown), or act directly on dopaminergic receptors leading to vasodilatation
- Reduces (to varying degrees) ventricular preload and/or afterload
- Reduces cardiac work

Uses
- Myocardial failure (e.g., post-MI, cardiomyopathy)
- Angina/ischemic heart disease
- Systemic hypertension (specific causes, such as pheochromocytoma)
- Vasoconstriction
- Peripheral vascular disease/hypoperfusion
- Pulmonary hypertension (inhaled nitric oxide, prostaglandins, sildenafil)

Side effects
- Hypotension (often associated with concurrent hypovolemia)
- Tachycardia (often associated with concurrent hypovolemia)
- Symptoms including headache, flushing, postural hypotension
- Renal failure (ACE inhibitors)—especially with renal artery stenosis, hypovolemia, NSAIDs

Notes
Glyceryl trinitrate and isosorbide dinitrate reduce both preload and afterload. At higher doses the afterload effect becomes more prominent.

Tolerance to nitrates usually commences within 24 to 36 h unless intermittent oral dosing is used. Progressive increases in dose are required to achieve the same effect.

Prolonged (>24 to 36 h) dose-related administration of sodium nitroprusside can produce cyanide accumulation. This rarely occurs in patients with intact renal function and may manifest as unexplained lactic acidosis.

ACE inhibitor tablets can be crushed and given either sublingually (SL) or via a nasogastric tube.

Table 14.2 Drug dosages

Nitrates	Glyceryl trinitrate 2–40 mg/h Isosorbide dinitrate 2–40 mg/h
Sodium nitroprusside	20–400 µg/min
Hydralazine	5–10 mg by slow IV bolus, repeat after 20–30 min; alternatively, by infusion starting at 200–300 µg/min and reducing to 50–150 µg/min
ACE inhibitors	Captopril, 6.25-mg test dose increasing to 25 mg tid Enalapril, 2.5-mg test dose increasing to 40 mg qd Lisinopril: 2.5-mg test dose increasing to 40 mg qd
Nifedipine	5–20 mg PO
Phentolamine	2–5 mg IV slow bolus; repeat as necessary
Fenoldopam	Initially, 0.1–0.3 µg/kg/min; may be increased in increments of 0.05–0.1 µg/kg/min every 15 min; maximum reported dose, 1.6 µg/kg/min
Milrinone	Loading dose of 50 µg/kg over 10 min followed by infusion from 0.375–0.75 µg/kg/min
Epoprostenol, alprostadil	Infusion from 2–30 ng/kg/min
Nitric oxide	By inhalation, 2–40 ppm
Nesiritide	2-µg/kg bolus followed by infusion of 0.01–0.03 µg/kg/min
Sildenafil	50 mg PO; IV forms also available

See also

Blood pressure monitoring, p. 112; Cardiac output—thermodilution, p. 124; Cardiac output—other invasive, p. 126; Cardiac output—noninvasive (1), p. 128; Cardiac output—noninvasive (2), p. 130; Hypotensive agents, p. 202; Antianginal agents, p. 208; Nitric oxide, p. 190; Basic resuscitation, p. 268; Fluid challenge, p. 272; Hypertension, p. 312; Acute coronary syndrome (1), p. 318; Acute coronary syndrome (2), p. 320; Heart failure—assessment, p. 322; Heart failure—management, p. 324; Preeclampsia and eclampsia, p. 540

Vasopressors

Types

- α-adrenergic agents (e.g., norepinephrine, epinephrine, dopamine, ephedrine, phenylephrine, methoxamine)
- Drugs reducing production of cGMP (in septic shock; for example, methylthionine chloride [methylene blue])
- Vasopressin or synthetic analogues (e.g., terlipressin)

Modes of action

- Acting on peripheral α-adrenergic or vasopressin V1 receptors
- Blocking cGMP production (methylene blue)
- Increasing afterload, mainly by arteriolar vasoconstriction and restoration of vascular reactivity
- Venoconstriction

Uses

- To increase organ perfusion pressures, particularly in high-output, low-peripheral resistance states (e.g., sepsis, anaphylaxis)
- To raise coronary perfusion pressures in CPR (epinephrine, vasopressin)

Side effects/complications

- Increased cardiac work
- Decreased cardiac output, especially with agents in which pressor effects predominate
- Myocardial and splanchnic ischemia
- Increased myocardial irritability, especially with concurrent hypovolemia, leading to arrhythmias and tachycardia
- Decreased peripheral perfusion and distal ischemia/necrosis

Notes

Pressor agents should be avoided, if possible, in low cardiac output states because they may further compromise the circulation.

Methoxamine and phenylephrine are the 'purest' pressor agents; other α-adrenergic agents have inotropic properties to greater or lesser degrees. Ephedrine is similar to epinephrine, but its effects are more prolonged because it is not metabolized by monoamine oxidase.

Effects of pressor agents on splanchnic, renal, and cerebral circulations are variable and unpredictable. Pulmonary vascular resistance is also raised by these agents.

Methylthionine chloride (methylene blue) inhibits the nitric oxide—cGMP pathway. It is currently unlicensed as a pressor agent and its use has only been reported in a few small case series. A multicenter study of a nitric oxide synthase inhibitor (L-N-mono-methyl-arginine [L-NMMA]) was prematurely discontinued because of adverse outcomes.

Vasopressin (short half-life, infusion needed) and terlipressin (longer half-life, can be given by bolus) may be effective in treating catecholamine-resistant vasodilatory shock. Paradoxically, such patients respond to small doses that have no pressor effect in healthy people. Multicenter outcome studies are ongoing.

Excessive dosing of any pressor agent may lead to regional ischemia (e.g., cardiac, splanchnic). Digital ischemia may respond to prompt administration of IV prostanoids (e.g., PGE_1, PGI_2).

Table 14.3 Drug dosages

Norepinephrine	Infusion starting from 0.05 µg/kg/min
Epinephrine	Infusion starting from 0.05 µg/kg/min
Dopamine	Infusion from 5–20 µg/kg/min
Methoxamine	3–10 mg by slow IV bolus (rate of 1 mg/min)
Ephedrine	3–30 mg by slow IV bolus
Vasopressin	0.01–0.04 U/min
Terlipressin	0.25–0.5 mg bolus, repeated at 30-min intervals as necessary to a maximum of 2 mg

Key papers

Landry DW, et al. Vasopressin deficiency contributes to the vasodilation of septic shock. *Circulation* 1997; **95**:1122–5.

Lopez A, et al. Multiple-center, randomized, placebo-controlled, double-blind study of the nitric oxide synthase inhibitor 546C88: Effect on survival in patients with septic shock. *Crit Care Med* 2004; **32**:21–30.

Vasopressor agents

Types

- Vasodilators
- α-Adrenergic and β-adrenergic blockers

Modes of action

- Vasodilators reduce preload and afterload to variable degrees depending on type and dose.
- β-Blockers reduce the force of myocardial contractility.

Uses

- Hypertension—systemic and pulmonary
- Heart failure—to reduce afterload ± preload (caution with β-blockers)
- Control of blood pressure (e.g., dissecting aortic aneurysm)

Side effects/complications

- Excessive hypotension
- Heart failure (with β-blockers)
- Peripheral hypoperfusion (with β-blockers)
- Bronchospasm (with β-blockers)
- Decreased sympathetic response to hypoglycemia (with β-blockers)

Notes

In critically ill patients, it is often advisable to use short-acting β-blockers by infusion.

In routine ICU practice, β-blockers are used relatively infrequently because most have a long half-life and the negative inotropic effects are generally undesirable. Exceptions are esmolol, metoprolol, and labetalol, all of which have short half-lives and vasodilating properties.

Table 14.4 Drug dosages

Nitrates	Glyceryl trinitrate, 2–40 mg/h Isosorbide dinitrate, 2–40 mg/h
Sodium nitroprusside	20–400 µg/min
ACE inhibitors	Captopril, 6.25-mg test dose increasing to 25 mg tid Enalapril, 2.5-mg test dose increasing to 40 mg qd Lisinopril, 2.5-mg test dose increasing to 40 mg qd
Nifedipine	5–20 mg PO
Phentolamine	2–5-mg IV slow bolus; repeat as necessary
Esmolol	A titrated loading dose regimen commenced, followed by an infusion rate of 50–200 µg/kg/min
Propranolol	Initially given as slow IV 1-mg boluses repeated at 2-min intervals until effect is seen (to maximum 5 mg)
Labetalol	0.25–2 mg/min
Hydralazine	5–10 mg by slow IV bolus, repeat after 20–30 min; alternatively, by infusion starting at 200–300 µg/min and reducing to 50–150 µg/min

See also

Blood pressure monitoring, p. 112; Cardiac output—thermodilution, p. 124; Cardiac output—other invasive, p. 126; Cardiac output—noninvasive (1), p. 128; Cardiac output—noninvasive (2), p. 130; Vasodilators, p. 198; Basic resuscitation, p. 268; Fluid challenge, p. 272; Hypertension, p. 312; Preeclampsia and eclampsia, p. 540

Antiarrhythmics

Only antiarrhythmics likely to be used in the ICU setting are described. For supraventricular tachyarrhythmias use adenosine, verapamil, amiodarone, digoxin, β-blockers, and magnesium. For ventricular tachyarrhythmias use amiodarone, lidocaine, flecainide, bretylium, β-blockers, and magnesium.

Uses

- Correction of supraventricular and ventricular tachyarrhythmias, which either compromise the circulation or could potentially do so
- Differentiation between supraventricular and ventricular arrhythmias (adenosine)

Notes

All antiarrhythmic agents have side effects. With the exception of digoxin, most are negatively inotropic and may induce profound hypotension (e.g., verapamil, β-blockers) or bradycardia (e.g., β-blockers, amiodarone, digoxin, lidocaine). β-Blockers in particular should be used with caution because of these effects.

All AV blockers are contraindicated in reentry tachycardia (e.g., Wolff–Parkinson–White syndrome).

- Adenosine—very short acting; may revert paroxysmal SVT to sinus rhythm. Ineffective for atrial flutter and fibrillation, VT. Contraindicated in second-degree and third-degree heart block, sick sinus syndrome, asthma. May cause flushing, bronchospasm, and occasional severe bradycardia.
- Amiodarone—effective against all types of tachyarrhythmia. Usually given by IV infusion for rapid effect but requires initial loading dose. When converting from IV to oral dosing, initial high oral dosing (200 mg tid) is still required. Contraindicated in patients with thyroid dysfunction. Has low acute toxicity, although may cause severe bradycardia and, rarely, pulmonary fibrosis. Avoid with other class III agents (e.g., sotalol). Must be given via central vein as causes peripheral phlebitis.
- β-Blockers—For SVT, esmolol is preferred because of its short half-life, although may cause vasodilatation. Initially, increasing loading doses required; an infusion may be needed thereafter. Propranolol can be given by slow IV boluses of 1 mg repeated at 2 min intervals to a maximum of 5 mg). Do not give β-blockers with verapamil.
- Bretylium—May take 15 to 20 min to take effect; now used predominantly for resistant VF/VT. CPR should be continued for at least 20 min.
- Digoxin—slow acting, requires loading (1–1.5 g) to achieve therapeutic plasma levels, which can be monitored. Loading ideally given over 12 to 24 h, but can be done over 4 to 6 h. Contraindicated in second-degree and third-degree heart block. May cause severe bradycardia. Low K^+ and Mg^{2+} and markedly increased Ca^{2+} increase myocardial sensitivity to digoxin. Amiodarone increases digoxin levels.
- Lidocaine—10 mL 1%-solution contains 100 mg. No effect on SVT. Loading achieved by 1-mg/kg slow IV bolus followed by infusion. Contraindicated in second-degree and third-degree heart block. May cause bradycardia and CNS side effects (e.g., drowsiness, seizures).

- Verapamil—should not be given with β-blockers because profound hypotension and bradyarrhythmias may result. Pretreatment with 3 to 5 mL 10% calcium gluconate by slow IV bolus prevents the hypotensive effects of verapamil without affecting its antiarrhythmic properties.

Table 14.5 Modes of action (Vaughan–Williams classification)

Class	Action	Examples
I	Reduces rate of rise of action potential: Ia, increases action potential duration; Ib, shortens duration; Ic, little effect	Ia, disopyramide; Ib, lidocaine; Ic, flecainide
II	Reduces rate of pacemaker discharge	β-Blockers
III	Prolongs duration of action potential and hence length of refractory period	Amiodarone, sotalol
IV	Antagonizes transport of calcium across cell membrane	Verapamil, diltiazem

Table 14.6 Drug dosages

Adenosine	3-mg rapid IV bolus; if no response after 1 min, give 6 mg; if no response after 1 min give 12 mg
Amiodarone	5 mg/kg over 20 min (or 150–300 mg over 3 min in emergency) then IV infusion of 15 mg/kg/24 h in 5% glucose via central vein; reduce thereafter to 10 mg/kg/24h (approximately 600 mg/day) for 3–7 days, then maintain at 5 mg/kg/24 h (300–400 mg/day)
β-Blockers	Esmolol: a titrated loading dose regimen is commenced followed by an infusion rate of 50–200 µg/kg/min Propranolol: Initially given as slow IV boluses of 1 mg repeated at 2-min intervals until effect is seen, to a maximum of 5 mg Labetalol 0.25–2 mg/min
Bretylium	In emergency, 5 mg/kg by rapid IV bolus; if no response after 5 min, repeat or increase to 10 mg/kg
Digoxin	0.5 mg given IV over 10–20 min; repeat at 4–8 h intervals until loading achieved (assessed by clinical response); maintenance dose thereafter is 0.0625–0.25 mg/day depending on plasma levels and clinical response
Lidocaine	1-mg/kg slow IV bolus for loading then 2–4 mg/min infusion; should be weaned slowly over 24 h
$MgSO_4$	10–20 mmol over 1–2 h; can be given over 5 min in emergency
Verapamil	2.5 mg slow IV; if no response, repeat to a maximum of 20 mg; an IV infusion of 1–10 mg/h may be tried; 10% calcium gluconate solution should be readily available

See also

Defibrillation, p. 52; ECG monitoring, p. 110; Basic resuscitation, p. 268; Cardiac arrest, p. 270; Tachyarrhythmias, p. 314

Chronotropes

Types
- Anticholinergic agents (e.g., atropine, glycopyrrolate)
- β-Adrenergic agents (e.g., dobutamine, dopamine, isoproterenol)

Modes of action
- The anticholinergic drugs act by competitive antagonism of acetylcholine at peripheral muscarinic receptors and decrease atrioventricular conduction time.
- β-Adrenergic agents act by stimulating both β_1 and β_2 receptors

Uses
- Used in all types of bradycardia including third degree heart block
- High-dose atropine is used in CPR protocols for treatment of asystole.
- Isoproterenol is rarely used to treat polymorphic VI with a long baseline QT interval (e.g., torsades de pointes)

Side effects/complications
- Anticholinergic drugs produce dry mouth, reduction and thickening of bronchial secretions, and inhibition of sweating. Urinary retention may occur, but parenteral administration does not lead to glaucoma.
- β-Adrenergic agents can cause arrhythmias, tachycardia, and hypotension (related to dilator properties ± concurrent hypovolemia).

Notes
The anticholinergic agents are usually given by IV bolus, repeated as necessary.

They are frequently used as a bridge to temporary pacing but should not be considered a substitute. External or internal pacing should be readily accessible.

Atropine nebulizers have been used successfully in patients developing symptomatic bradycardia during endotracheal suction.

Neurological effects may be seen with atropine but not glycopyrrolate.

Anticholinergic agents are generally tried first, and β-adrenergic agents are used in refractory cases.

Anticholinergic agents require an innervated heart to work. Thus, in heart transplant patients, bradycardia must be treated with β-adrenergic agents.

Table 14.6 Drug dosages

Atropine	0.3–0.6-mg IV bolus; 3 mg is needed for complete vagal blockade
Glycopyrrolate	0.2–0.4-mg IV bolus
Dopamine	Infusion from 2–20 µg/kg/min
Dobutamine	Infusion from 2–20 µg/kg/min
Isoproterenol	Infusion from 0.2–2 µg/kg/min

See also

Temporary pacing (1), p. 54; Temporary pacing (2), p. 56; ECG monitoring, p. 110; Basic resuscitation, p. 268; Cardiac arrest, p. 270; Bradyarrhythmias, p. 316

Antianginal agents

Types
- Vasodilators (e.g., nitrates, calcium antagonists)
- β-Blockers
- Potassium channel openers (e.g., nicorandil)
- Aspirin, heparin, clopidogrel

Modes of action
- Calcium channel blockers cause competitive blockade of cell membrane and slow calcium channels leading to decreased influx of calcium ions into cells. This leads to inhibition of contraction and relaxation of cardiac and smooth muscle fibers, resulting in coronary and systemic vasodilatation.
- Nitrates may cause efflux of calcium ions from smooth muscle and cardiac cells, and also increase cGMP synthesis, resulting in coronary and systemic vasodilatation.
- β-Blockers inhibit β-adrenoreceptor stimulation, reducing myocardial work and oxygen consumption. This effect is somewhat offset by compensatory peripheral vasoconstriction.
- Potassium channel openers are not yet available in the United States. They cause vasodilatation by relaxation of vascular smooth muscle. The potassium channel opening action works on the arterial circulation whereas a nitrate action provides additional vasodilatation.
- Although aspirin, heparin, and clopidogrel have no direct antianginal effect, patients with unstable angina benefit from the reduction in platelet aggregation and thrombus formation.

Uses
- Angina pectoris

Side effects
- See 'vasodilators' and 'vasopressor agents'.
- Nicorandil is contraindicated in hypotension and cardiogenic shock. It should be avoided in hypovolemia. Headache and flushing are the major reported side effects. Rapid and severe hyperkalemia has been reported after cardiac surgery.

Notes
Combination therapy involving IV nitrates, calcium antagonists, β-blockade, and heparinization has been shown to be beneficial in unstable angina. Thrombolytic therapy confers no added advantage.

Angina may occasionally be worsened by a 'coronary steal' phenomenon during which blood flow is diverted away from stenosed coronary vessels.

Table 14.7 Drug dosages

Glyceryl trinitrate	0.3 mg SL, 0.4–0.8 mg by buccal spray, 2–40 mg/h by IV infusion
Isosorbide dinitrate	10–20 mg tid orally, 2–40 mg/h by IV infusion
Nifedipine	5–20 mg PO; capsule fluid can be aspirated then injected down nasogastric tube or given SL.
Propranolol	Given either orally at doses of 10–100 mg tid or IV as slow bolus of 1 mg repeated at 2-min intervals to a maximum of 5 mg until effect is seen; can be repeated every 2–4 h as necessary
Clopidogrel	75 mg PO qd; for acute coronary syndrome, initial dose is 300 mg PO, followed by 75 mg PO qd
Aspirin	75–150 mg PO qd

See also

Acute coronary syndrome (1), p. 318; Acute coronary syndrome (2), p. 320

Renal drugs

Diuretics

Types
- Loop diuretics (e.g., furosemide, bumetanide, torsemide)
- Osmotic diuretics (e.g., mannitol)
- Thiazides (e.g., metolazone)
- Potassium-sparing diuretics (e.g., amiloride, spironolactone)

Uses
- To increase urine volume
- To control chronic edema (thiazides, loop diuretics)
- To control hypertension (thiazides)
- To promote renal excretion (e.g., forced diuresis, hypercalcemia)

Routes
- IV (mannitol, furosemide, bumetanide, torsemide)
- PO (metolazone, furosemide, bumetanide, amiloride, spironolactone)

Modes of action
- Osmotic diuretics—reduce distal tubular water reabsorption
- Thiazides—inhibit the Na/Cl transporters in the distal tubule. This increases excretion of sodium and hence water. Potassium loss is an important side effect
- Loop diuretics—inhibit Na^+ and Cl^- reabsorption in the ascending loop of Henle
- Potassium-sparing diuretics—inhibit distal tubular Na^+ and K^+ exchange

Side effects
- Ototoxicity (bumetanide and furosemide)
- Hypovolemia
- Hyponatremia or hypernatremia
- Hypokalemia
- Edema formation (mannitol)
- Reduced catecholamine effect (thiazides)
- Hyperglycemia (thiazides)
- Metabolic alkalosis (loop diuretics)
- Hypomagnesemia (loop diuretics)
- Pancreatitis (rare, furosemide)

Notes
Diuretics do not prevent renal failure and should not be thought of as a treatment for oliguria. Instead, they are helpful in managing volume overload. Use of diuretics has not been shown to improve outcome in critically ill patients.

If there is inadequate glomerular filtration, mannitol is retained and passes to the extracellular fluid, thereby promoting edema formation.

Bumetanide may be used in porphyria for which thiazides and other loop diuretics are contraindicated.

Potassium-sparing diuretics should be avoided with ACE inhibitors because there is an increased risk of hyperkalemia.

Table 15.1 Drug dosages

	Oral	IV	Infusion
Mannitol		100 g over 20 min q 6 h	
Metolazone	5–10 mg qd		
Furosemide	20–40 mg q 6–24 h	5–80 mg q 6–24 h	1–10 mg/h
Torsemide	5–20 mg q 6–24 h	5–20 mg q 6–24 h	1–5 mg/h
Bumetanide	0.5–1 mg q 6–24 h	0.5–2 mg q 6–24 h	1–5 mg/h
Amiloride	5–10 mg q 12–24 h		
Spironolactone	100–400 mg qd		

Key study

Uchino S, Doig GS, Bellomo R, et al. Diuretics and mortality in acute renal failure. *Crit Care Med* 2004; **32**:1669–77.

Agents used for renal protection

Types
- N-acetylcysteine
- Dopamine (DA) agonists (e.g., dopamine, fenoldopam)

Notes

Several studies have shown that N-acetylcysteine plus hydration reduces contrast nephropathy compared with hydration alone in high-risk patients undergoing contrast studies. Two doses of 1200 mg orally twice daily of N-acetylcysteine may be more effective in preventing contrast nephropathy than single-dose N-acetylcysteine, especially in people who receive high volumes of nonionic, low-osmolality contrast. However, a study of 50 healthy volunteers with normal renal function found that N-acetylcysteine could independently decrease serum creatinine without any effect on glomerular filtration rate. Thus, the role of N-acetylcysteine to prevent acute renal failure remains unclear.

The effects of dopamine are dependent on the dose infused. Dopamine was used widely at low doses in an attempt to secure preferential DA_1 stimulation and increase renal perfusion; however, three meta-analyses and a large multicenter, randomized, controlled study comparing 'renal-dose' dopamine showed no difference in the incidence of renal failure. The widespread use of low-dose dopamine (<3 µg/kg/min) has thus diminished considerably in recent years. Higher doses increase cardiac contractility via β_1 stimulation and produce vasoconstriction via α stimulation. Dopamine agonists may also increase urine output because of natriuresis and diuresis by enhanced Na^+ transport in the ascending loop of Henle.

Key trials and studies

Bellomo R, for the Australian and New Zealand Intensive Care Society (ANZICS) Clinical Trials Group. Low-dose dopamine in patients with early renal dysfunction: A placebo-controlled randomised trial. *Lancet* 2000; **356**:2139–43.
Hoffmann U, Fischereder M, Kruger B, *et al.* The value of N-acetylcysteine in the prevention of radiocontrast agent-induced nephropathy seems questionable. J Am Soc *Nephrol* 2004; **15**:407–10.

See also

Diuretics, p. 212; Oliguria, p. 328; Acute renal failure—management, p. 332

Gastrointestinal drugs

H₂ blockers and proton pump inhibitors

Types
- H₂ antagonists (e.g., famotidine, ranitidine, cimetidine)
- Proton pump inhibitors (e.g., omeprazole)

Modes of action
These agents inhibit secretion of gastric acid, reducing both volume and acid content, either by antagonism of the histamine H₂ receptor or by inhibiting H^+K^+-adenosin triphosphatase (ATPase), which fuels the parietal cell proton pump on which acid secretion depends.

Uses
- Peptic ulceration, gastritis, duodenitis
- Reflux esophagitis
- Prophylaxis against stress ulceration
- Upper gastrointestinal hemorrhage of peptic/stress ulcer origin
- With nonsteroidal anti-inflammatory agents in patients with dyspepsia

Side effects/complications
- The major concern voiced against these agents is the increased risk of nosocomial pneumonia by removal of the acid barrier. However, a multicenter randomized controlled trial (RCT) comparing ranitidine with sucralfate showed no difference in pneumonia rate and a lower incidence of gastrointestinal bleeding
- H₂ antagonists are rare, but include arrhythmias, altered liver function tests, and confusion (in the elderly)
- Proton pump inhibitors alter liver function tests

Notes
Although licensed and frequently used for stress ulcer prophylaxis, overwhelming supportive evidence is scanty. Enteral nutrition has been shown to be as effective. No adequately powered study of proton pump inhibitors has yet to be performed in ICU patients.

Some studies have shown efficacy in upper gastrointestinal hemorrhage secondary to stress ulceration or peptic ulceration.

Dosages should be modified in renal failure.

Cimetidine can affect metabolism of other drugs—in particular, warfarin, phenytoin, theophylline, and lidocaine (related to hepatic cytochrome P450-linked enzyme systems). This does not occur with ranitidine.

Omeprazole can delay elimination of diazepam, phenytoin, and warfarin.

Table 16.1 Drug dosages

Famotidine	20 mg bid by slow IV bolus
Cimetidine	200–400 mg qid by slow IV bolus, 400 mg bid PO
Omeprazole	40 mg IV qd (over 20–30 min), 20–40 mg PO

Key trial

Cook D, Guyatt G, Marshall J, et al. A comparison of sucralfate and ranitidine for the prevention of upper gastrointestinal bleeding in patients requiring mechanical ventilation. Canadian Critical Care Trials Group. N Engl J Med 1998; **338**:791–7.

See also

Upper gastrointestinal endoscopy, p. 76; Sucralfate, p. 220; Antacids, p. 220; Upper gastrointestinal hemorrhage, p. 342; Bleeding varices, p. 344; Bowel perforation and obstruction, p. 346

Sucralfate

Modes of action

- Sucralfate is a basic aluminium salt of sucrose octasulfate and is probably not absorbed from the gastrointestinal tract.
- It exerts a cytoprotective effect by preventing mucosal injury. A protective barrier is formed over both normal mucosa and any ulcerous lesion, providing protection against penetration of gastric acid, bile, and pepsin, as well as irritants such as aspirin and alcohol.
- It directly inhibits pepsin activity and absorbs bile salts.
- It has weak antacid activity.

Uses

- Peptic ulceration, gastritis, duodenitis
- Reflux esophagitis
- Prophylaxis against stress ulceration

Side effects/complications

- Constipation
- Reduced bioavailability of many drugs given orally (e.g., digoxin, phenytoin, oral antibiotics)
- Caution against use in renal failure because of risk of increased aluminium absorption

Notes

Although licensed for stress ulcer prophylaxis, overwhelming supportive evidence is scanty. Enteral nutrition and gastric acid blockers have been shown to be as effective.

Evidence for a reduced incidence of nosocomial pneumonia compared with H_2 blocker therapy is also conflicting. Significant reduction in nosocomial pneumonia has been shown compared with a combination of H_2 blocker plus antacid, but not against H_2 blocker alone. Indeed, a large multicenter randomized, controlled trial comparing ranitidine with sucralfate showed no difference in pneumonia rate and a lower incidence of gastrointestinal bleeding with ranitidine.

Antacids should not be given for 30 min before or after sucralfate.

Table 16.2 Drug dosages

Sucralfate	1 g qid PO or via nasogastric tube

Key trial

Cook D, Guyatt G, Marshall J, et al. A comparison of sucralfate and ranitidine for the prevention of upper gastrointestinal bleeding in patients requiring mechanical ventilation. Canadian Critical Care Trials Group. *N Engl J Med* 1998; **338**:791–7.

See also

Upper gastrointestinal endoscopy, p. 76; H$_2$ blockers and proton pump inhibitors, p. 218; Antacids, p. 220; Upper gastrointestinal hemorrhage, p. 342; Bleeding varices, p. 344; Bowel perforation and obstruction, p. 346

Antiemetics

Types
- Phenothiazines (e.g., prochlorperazine, chlorpromazine)
- Benzamides (e.g., metoclopramide)
- (5HT$_3$) receptor antagonists (e.g., ondansetron, granisetron)

Modes of action
- Phenothiazines increase the threshold for vomiting at the chemoreceptor trigger zone via central DA$_2$-dopaminergic blockade. At higher doses there may also be some effect on the vomiting center.
- Metoclopramide acts centrally and by increasing gastric motility.
- Ondansetron is a highly selective 5HT$_3$ (serotonin) receptor antagonist. Its precise mode of action is unknown, but it may act both centrally and peripherally.

Uses
- Nausea
- Vomiting

Side effects/complications
- Dystonic or dyskinetic reactions, oculogyric crises (prochlorperazine, metoclopramide)
- Arrhythmias (metoclopramide, prochlorperazine)
- Headaches, flushing (ondansetron)
- Postural hypotension (prochlorperazine)
- Rarely, neuroleptic malignant syndrome (prochlorperazine, metoclopramide)

Notes
The initial choice should fall between prochlorperazine or metoclopramide. Prochlorperazine is preferable when vomiting is related to drugs and metabolic disturbances acting at the chemoreceptor trigger zone whereas metoclopramide should be tried first if a gastrointestinal cause is implicated.

Metoclopramide and prochlorperazine dosage should be reduced in renal and hepatic failure.

Ondansetron dosage should be reduced in hepatic failure.

Table 16.3 Drug dosages

Prochlorperazine	5–10 mg tid PO, 12.5 mg qid IM or by slow IV bolus (note: not licensed for IV use)
Metoclopramide	10 mg tid by slow IV bolus, IM or PO
Ondansetron	4–8 mg tid by slow IV bolus, IM or PO
Granisetron	1–3 mg by slow IV bolus up to maximum 9 mg/24 h

See also

Enteral nutrition, p. 82; Vomiting/gastric stasis, p. 336

Gut motility agents

Types

- Metoclopramide
- Erythromycin

Modes of action

- Metoclopramide probably acts by blocking peripheral DA_2-dopaminergic receptors.
- Erythromycin is a motilin agonist that acts on antral enteric neurons.

Uses

- Ileus, large nasogastric aspirates
- Vomiting

Side effects/complications

- Dystonic or dyskinetic reactions, oculogyric crises (metoclopramide)
- Arrhythmias (metoclopramide and erythromycin)
- Cholestatic jaundice (erythromycin)

Notes

Metoclopramide dosing should be reduced in renal failure and hepatic failure, whereas erythromycin dosing should be reduced in hepatic failure.

Table 16.4 Drug dosages

| Metoclopramide | 10 mg tid by slow IV bolus, IM or PO |
| Erythromycin | 250 mg qid PO or IV |

See also

Enteral nutrition, p. 82; Vomiting/gastric stasis, p. 336; Bowel perforation and obstruction, p. 346

Antidiarrheals

Types
- Loperamide
- Codeine phosphate

Modes of action
- Loperamide and codeine phosphate bind to gut wall opiate receptors, reducing propulsive peristalsis and increasing anal sphincter tone.

Side effects/complications
- Abdominal cramps, bloating
- Constipation (if excessive amounts given)

Notes
Should not be used when abdominal distension develops, particularly with ulcerative colitis or pseudomembranous colitis, or as sole therapy in infective diarrhea.

Caution with loperamide in liver failure, and codeine in renal failure.

Table 16.5 Drug dosages

| Loperamide | 2 capsules (20 mL) initially, then 1 capsule (10 mL) after every loose stool for up to 5 days |
| Codeine phosphate | 30–60 mg q 4–6 h PO, IM, or by slow IV bolus |

See also

Enteral nutrition, p. 82; Diarrhea, p. 338

Anticonstipation agents

Types
- Laxatives (e.g., lactulose, propantheline, castor oil)
- Bulking agents (e.g., dietary fiber [bran], hemicelluloses [methylcellulose, ispaghula husk])
- Suppositories (e.g., glycerine)
- Enemata (e.g., warmed normal saline, olive oil, or arachis oil retention enemata)

Modes of action
- Laxatives include
  - Antispasmodic agents such as anticholinergics (e.g., propantheline)
  - Nonabsorbable disaccharides (e.g., lactulose), which soften the stool by an osmotic effect and by lactic acid production from a bacterial fermenting effect
  - Irritants, such as castor oil, which is hydrolyzed in the small intestine releasing ricinoleic acid
- Bulking agents, which are hydrophilic and thus increase the water content of the stool

Side effects/complications
- Bloating and abdominal distension
- Diarrhea if excessive amounts given

Notes
Surgical causes presenting as constipation, such as bowel obstruction, must be excluded. Other measures should be taken if possible to improve bowel function (e.g., reducing concurrent opiate dosage, correcting electrolyte levels, starting enteral nutrition).

The agent of choice is lactulose.

Larger doses of lactulose are used in hepatic failure because the pH of the colonic contents is reduced. This lowers formation and absorption of ammonium ions and other nitrogenous products into the portal circulation. A proven benefit in patients has not been shown.

Anthraquinone glycosides (e.g., senna) and liquid paraffin are no longer recommended for routine use.

Table 16.6 Drug dosages

Lactulose	15–50 mL tid PO

See also

Enteral nutrition, p. 82; Failure to open bowels, p. 340

Neurological drugs

Opioid analgesics

Types
- Natural opiates (e.g., morphine, codeine)
- Semisynthetic (e.g., oxycodone, hydromorphone)
- Synthetic (e.g., fentanyl, alfentanil, remifentanil)

Uses
- Analgesia—Strong analgesics are extracts from opium or synthetic substances with similar properties. They are useful for continuous pain rather than sharp, intermittent pain.
- Sedation
- Mild vasodilatation in heart failure (morphine)
- Antidiarrheal (codeine)

Routes
- IV (morphine, hydromorphone, fentanyl, alfentanil, remifentanil)
- IM/SC (morphine, codeine, hydromorphone, meperidine)
- PO (morphine, codeine, oxycodone, hydromorphone)
- Epidural (morphine, hydromorphone, fentanyl, alfentanil)

Side effects
- Respiratory depression
- CNS depression
- Addiction (rare in the critically ill)
- Withdrawal syndrome (withdraw slowly)
- Stimulation of the vomiting center
- Appetite loss
- Dry mouth
- Decreased gastric emptying and gut motility
- Histamine release and itching
- Increased muscular tone

Notes

Morphine is poorly absorbed from the gastrointestinal tract and is therefore usually administered parenterally. It is metabolized to morphine-6-glucuronide in the liver, and is six times more potent than morphine and accumulates in renal failure.

Hydromorphone has fewer renally excreted active metabolites than morphine and may be safe in mild to moderate renal impairment; however, in severe renal failure, fentanyl (which has no renally excreted metabolites) is the opioid of choice.

Codeine is a weak analgesic but is favored by some in head injury because it is less sedative than morphine.

Fentanyl and alfentanil are good, short-acting analgesics with poor sedative quality. They cause severe respiratory depression and muscular rigidity. Remifentanil is ultrashort acting and the patient may experience rebound pain if the infusion is stopped temporarily.

Table 17.1 Drug dosages

	Bolus	Infusion
IV		
Morphine	0.1–0.2 mg/kg	0.05–0.07 mg/kg/h
Hydromorphone	10–40 µg/kg	5–20 µg/kg
Fentanyl	5–7.5 µg/kg	5–20 µg/kg/h
Alfentanil	15–30 µg/kg	20–120 µg/kg/h
Remifentanil	1 µg/kg	0.05–2 µg/kg/min
Other routes		
Morphine	10 mg IM/SC every q 4 h	5–20 mg PO every q 4 h
Codeine	30–60 mg IM every q 4 h	30–60 mg PO every q 4 h
Hydromorphone	1–4 mg IM/SC every q 4 h	2–8 mg PO every q 4 h
Oxycodone	No parenteral route	5–30 mg PO every q 4 h

Note that these dosages are a guide only and may need to be altered widely according to individual circumstances. The correct dose of an opiate analgesic is generally enough to ablate pain.

See also

IPPV—failure to tolerate ventilation, p. 12; Nonopioid analgesics, p. 234; Sedatives, p. 236; Pain, p. 534; Postoperative intensive care, p. 536

Nonopioid analgesics

Types
- NSAIDs (e.g., aspirin, ibuprofen, ketorolac)
- Acetaminophen
- Ketamine
- Nitrous oxide
- Local anesthetics (e.g., lidocaine, bupivacaine)

Uses
- Pain associated with inflammatory conditions (aspirin, ibuprofen, ketorolac)
- Postoperative pain and musculoskeletal pain (aspirin, ibuprofen, ketorolac, acetaminophen, ketamine, nitrous oxide, lidocaine, bupivacaine)
- Opiate sparing effect (aspirin, ibuprofen, ketorolac used with strong analgesics)
- Antipyretic (aspirin, ibuprofen, acetaminophen)

Routes
- IV (ketamine, ketorolac)
- IM (ketorolac)
- PO (aspirin, ibuprofen, ketorolac, acetaminophen)
- PR (aspirin, acetaminophen)
- Local/regional (lidocaine, bupivacaine)
- Inhaled (nitrous oxide)

Side effects
- Gastrointestinal bleeding (aspirin, ibuprofen, ketorolac)
- Renal dysfunction (ibuprofen, ketorolac if any hypovolemia)
- Reduced platelet aggregation (aspirin, ibuprofen, diclofenac)
- Reduced prothrombin formation (aspirin, ibuprofen, ketorolac)
- Myocardial depression (lidocaine, bupivacaine)
- Hypertension and tachycardia (ketamine)
- Seizures (lidocaine, bupivacaine)
- Hallucinations and psychotic tendencies (ketamine—prevented by concurrent use of benzodiazepines or droperidol)

Notes

Acetaminophen overdose can cause severe hepatic failure resulting from the effects of alkylating metabolites. Although normally removed by conjugation with glutathione, stores are rapidly depleted in overdose.

Nonsteroidal anti-inflammatory agents should generally be avoided in patients with renal dysfunction, gastrointestinal bleeding or coagulopathy.

Ketamine is a derivative of phencyclidine, and is used as an IV anesthetic agent. In subanesthetic doses, it is a powerful analgesic. It has several advantages over opiates in that it is associated with good airway maintenance, allows spontaneous respiration, and provides cardiovascular stimulation. It is also a bronchodilator.

Nitrous oxide is a powerful, short-acting analgesic used to cover short, painful procedures. It may be useful when delivered via an intermittent positive-pressure breathing system as an adjunct to chest physiotherapy. Nitrous oxide should not be used in cases of undrained pneumothorax because it may diffuse into the pneumothorax, resulting in tension.

Table 17.2 Drug dosages

Aspirin	600 mg PO/PR q 4 h
Ibuprofen	300–800 mg PO q 8 h
Ketorolac	10 mg PO q 4–6 h
	15 –30 mg IV, IM q 6 h
Sulindac	200 mg PO q 12 h
Acetaminophen	0.5–1 g PO/PR q 4–6 h
Ketamine	5–25 µg/kg/min IV
Lidocaine	Maximum, 200 mg
Bupivacaine	Maximum, 150 mg*

* Local anesthetic doses vary according to the area to be anesthetized. Maximum doses may be increased if epinephrine is used locally.

See also

Opioid analgesics, p. 232; Salicylate poisoning, p. 456; Rheumatic disorders, p. 496; Pyrexia (1), p. 520; Pyrexia (2), p. 522; Pain, p. 534; Postoperative intensive care, p. 536

Sedatives

Types
- Benzodiazepines (e.g., diazepam, midazolam, lorazepam)
- Major tranquilizers (e.g., chlorpromazine, haloperidol)
- Anesthetic agents (e.g., propofol, isoflurane)
- α_2 agonists (e.g., clonidine, dexmedetomidine)

Uses
- Sedation and anxiolysis

Routes
- IV (diazepam, midazolam, lorazepam, chlorpromazine, haloperidol, propofol, dexmedetomidine)
- IM (diazepam, chlorpromazine, haloperidol)
- PO (diazepam, lorazepam, chlorpromazine, haloperidol, clonidine)
- Inhaled (isoflurane)

Side effects
- Hypotension (diazepam, midazolam, chlorpromazine, haloperidol, propofol, clonidine, dexmedetomidine)
- Respiratory depression (diazepam, midazolam, chlorpromazine, haloepridol, propofol)
- Arrhythmias (chlorpromazine, haloperidol)
- Dry mouth (clonidine, dexmedetomidine)
- Extrapyramidal disorder (chlorpromazine, haloperidol)
- Fluoride toxicity (isoflurane)

Notes

Sedation is necessary for most ICU patients. Although the appropriate use of sedative drugs can provide comfort, most have cardiovascular and respiratory side effects. Objective assessment of the depth of sedation is necessary to ensure that comfort does not give way to excessively and dangerously deep levels of sedation. All sedatives are potentially cumulative, so doses must be kept to a minimum.

Benzodiazepines have the advantage of being amnesic. Diazepam is mainly administered as an emulsion in intralipids because organic solvents are extremely irritating to veins. Midazolam is shorter acting than diazepam, although 10% of patients are slow metabolizers. All benzodiazepines accumulate in renal failure. Therefore, care must be taken to avoid excessive dosage by regular reassessment of need. Some patients sustain unpredictable, severe respiratory depression with hypotension.

Propofol used in subanesthetic doses is short acting, although effects are cumulative when infusions are prolonged or with coexisting hepatic or renal failure. It is given as an emulsion in 10% intralipid, so large volumes contribute significantly to calorie intake.

Because chlorpromazine and haloperidol antagonize catecholamines, they may cause vasodilatation and hypotension. Dystonic reactions and arrhythmias are also occasionally seen.

α_2 Antagonists also provide analgesia and are synergistic with opiates. Dexmedetomidine causes minimal respiratory depression, and the patient can be easily roused. Bradycardia and hypotension may occur, especially with the loading dose.

Isoflurane is largely exhaled unchanged and is therefore short acting. Cumulative effects have been recorded with prolonged use, carrying the theoretical risk of fluoride toxicity. Exhaled isoflurane should be scavenged.

Table 17.3 Drug dosages

	Bolus	**Infusion**
Diazepam	0.05–0.15 mg/kg	Excessive half-life
Midazolam	50 µg/kg	10–50 µg/kg/h
Lorazepam	1 mg PRN	
Propofol	0.5–2 mg/kg	1–3 mg/kg/h
Chlorpromazine	12.5–100 mg	Excessive half-life
Clonidine		100–150 µg/min
Dexmedetomidine		Loading infusion of 6.0 µg/kg/h over 10 min, followed by maintenance infusion of 0.2–0.7 µg/kg/h

Note that these dosages are a guide only and may need to be altered widely according to individual circumstances. PRN, pro re nata (as needed).

Monitoring sedation

Frequent, objective reassessment of sedation depth with corresponding adjustment of infusion doses is necessary to avoid severe cardiovascular and respiratory depression. Daily interruption of sedative infusions decreases the duration of mechanical ventilation and the length of stay in the ICU. Simple sedation scores are available to aid assessment. A number of sedation scales have become widely accepted, such as the Ramsay Scale, the Sedation Agitation Scale (SAS), and the Richmond Agitation Sedation Scale (RASS; see p. 580).

Key trials

Ely EW, et al. Monitoring sedation status over time in ICU patients: The reliability and validity of the Richmond Agitation Sedation Scale (RASS). *JAMA* 2003; **289**:2983–91.
Kress JP, et al. Daily interruption of sedative infusions in critically ill patients undergoing mechanical ventilation. *N Engl J Med* 2000; **342**:1471–7.

See also

IPPV—failure to tolerate ventilation, p. 12, opioid analgesics, p. 232; Agitation/confusion, p. 370; Sedative poisoning, p. 460; Postoperative intensive care, p. 536; Sedation scale—RAAS, p. 582

Muscle relaxants

Types
- Depolarizing (e.g., succinylcholine)
- Nondepolarizing (e.g., pancuronium, atracurium, vecuronium)

Mode of action
- Succinylcholine is structurally related to acetylcholine and causes initial stimulation of muscular contraction, seen clinically as fasciculation. During this process, the continued stimulation leads to desensitization of the postsynaptic membrane of the neuromuscular junction with efflux of potassium ions. Subsequent flaccid paralysis is short acting (2–3 min) and cannot be reversed by anticholinesterase drugs. Prolonged effects are seen when there is congenital or acquired pseudocholinesterase deficiency.
- Nondepolarizing muscle relaxants prevent acetylcholine from depolarizing the postsynaptic membrane of the neuromuscular junction by competitive blockade. Reversal of paralysis is achieved by anticholinesterase drugs such as neostigmine. They have a slower onset and longer duration of action than the depolarizing agents.

Uses
- To facilitate endotracheal intubation
- To facilitate mechanical ventilation when optimal sedation does not prevent patient interference with the function of the ventilator

Routes
- IV

Side effects
- Hypertension (succinylcholine, pancuronium)
- Bradycardia (succinylcholine)
- Tachycardia (pancuronium)
- Hyperkalemia (succinylcholine)

Notes
Modern intensive care practice and developments in ventilator technology have rendered the use of muscle relaxants less common. Furthermore, it is rarely necessary to paralyze muscles fully to facilitate mechanical ventilation.

The requirement for muscle relaxants should be reassessed frequently. Ideally, relaxants should be stopped intermittently to allow depth of sedation to be assessed. If mechanical ventilation proceeds smoothly when relaxants have been stopped, they probably should not be restarted.

Succinylcholine is contraindicated in spinal neurological disease, hepatic disease, and for 5 to 50 days after burns.

Cisatracurium is noncumulative and popular for infusion. Nonenzymatic (Hoffman) degradation allows clearance independent of renal or hepatic function, although effects are prolonged in hypothermia.

Table 17.4 Drug dosages

	Bolus	Infusion
Succinylcholine	0.6–1.5 mg/kg	0.5–10 mg/min
Pancuronium	0.04–0.1 mg/kg	0.1 mg/kg q30–60 min
Cisatracurium	0.15–0.2 mg/kg	3 µg/kg/min
Vecuronium	0.08–0.1 mg/kg	Excessive half-life

See also

IPPV—failure to tolerate ventilation, p. 12; Endotracheal intubation, p. 36; Sedatives, p. 236; Postoperative intensive care, p. 536

Anticonvulsants

Types
- Benzodiazepines (e.g., lorazepam, diazepam, clonazepam)
- Phenytoin
- Carbamazepine
- Sodium valproate
- Magnesium sulfate
- Thiopental

Uses
- Control of status epilepticus
- Intermittent seizure control
- Myoclonic seizures (clonazepam, sodium valproate)

Routes
- IV (lorazepam, diazepam, clonazepam, phenytoin, sodium valproate, magnesium sulfate, thiopental)
- PO (diazepam, clonazepam, phenytoin, carbamazepine, sodium valproate)
- PR (diazepam)

Side effects
- Sedation (benzodiazepines, thiopentone)
- Respiratory depression (benzodiazepines, thiopentone)
- Nausea and vomiting (phenytoin, sodium valproate)
- Ataxia (phenytoin, carbamazepine)
- Visual disturbance (phenytoin, carbamazepine)
- Hypotension (diazepam, thiopentone)
- Arrhythmias (phenytoin, carbamazepine)
- Pancreatitis (thiopentone)
- Hepatic failure (sodium valproate)

Notes
Common insults causing seizures include cerebral ischemic damage, space-occupying lesions, drugs or drug/alcohol withdrawal, metabolic encephalopathy (including hypoglycemia), and neurosurgery. Anticonvulsants provide control of seizures but do not replace removal of the cause when this is possible.

Onset of seizure control may be delayed by up to 24 h with phenytoin, but a loading dose is usually given during the acute phase of seizures.

Magnesium sulfate is especially useful in eclamptic seizures (and in their prevention).

Phenytoin has a narrow therapeutic range and a nonlinear relationship between dose and plasma levels. It is therefore essential to monitor plasma levels frequently. Enteral feeding should be stopped 1 h before and 2 h after oral phenytoin is administered. IV use should only occur if the ECG is monitored continuously.

Carbamazepine has a wider therapeutic range than phenytoin and there is a linear relationship between dose and plasma levels. It is not, therefore, critical to monitor plasma levels frequently.

Plasma concentrations of sodium valproate are not related to effects, so monitoring of plasma levels is not useful.

Table 17.5 IV drug dosages

	Bolus	Infusion
Lorazepam	4 mg	
Diazepam	2.5 mg repeated to 20 mg	
Phenytoin	18 mg/kg at <50 mg/min	100 mg of q 8 h
Magnesium sulfate	20 mmol over 10–20 min	5–10 mmol/h
Sodium valproate	400–800 mg	
Clonazepam	1 mg	1–2 mg/h
Thiopental	1–3 mg/kg	Lowest possible dose

Key trial

Magpie Trial Collaboration Group. Do women with pre-eclampsia, and their babies, benefit from magnesium sulphate? The Magpie Trial: A randomised placebo-controlled trial. *Lancet* 2002; **359**:1877–90.

Treiman VA, for the Veterans Affairs Status Epilepticus Cooperative Study Group. A comparison of four treatments for generalized convulsive status epilepticus. *N Engl J Med* 1998; **339**:792–8.

Which anticonvulsant for women with eclampsia? Evidence from the Collaborative Eclampsia Trial. *Lancet* 1995; **345**:1455–63.

Neuroprotective agents

Types

- Diuretics (e.g., mannitol, furosemide)
- Steroids (e.g., dexamethasone)
- Calcium antagonists (e.g., nimodipine)
- Barbiturates (e.g., thiopental)

Uses

- Reduction of cerebral edema (mannitol, furosemide, dexamethasone)
- Prevention of cerebral vasospasm (nimodipine)
- Reduction of cerebral metabolic rate (thiopental)

Routes

- IV

Notes

Cerebral protection requires generalized sedation and abolition of seizures to reduce cerebral metabolic rate, cerebral edema, and neuronal damage during ischemia and reperfusion.

Mannitol reduces cerebral interstitial water by the osmotic load. The effect is transient and at its best when the blood–brain barrier is intact. Interstitial water is mainly reduced in normal areas of brain and this may accentuate cerebral shift. Repeated doses accumulate in the interstitium and may eventually increase edema formation. Mannitol should only be given four to five times in 48 h. In addition to its osmotic effect, there is some evidence of cerebral vasoconstriction resulting from a reduction in blood viscosity and free radical scavenging.

The loop diuretic effect of furosemide encourages salt and water loss. There may also be a reduction of CSF chloride transport, reducing the formation of CSF.

Dexamethasone reduces edema around space-occupying lesions such as tumors. Steroids are not useful in head injury or after a cerebrovascular accident (CVA), but benefit has been shown if given early after spinal injury. Steroids encourage salt and water retention and must be withdrawn slowly to avoid rebound edema.

Nimodipine is used to prevent cerebral vasospasm during recovery from cerebrovascular insults. As a calcium channel blocker it also prevents calcium ingress during neuronal injury. This calcium ingress is associated with cell death. It is commonly used in the management of subarachnoid hemorrhage for 5 to 14 days.

Thiopental reduces cerebral metabolism, thus prolonging the time that the brain may sustain an ischemic insult. However, it also reduces CBF, although blood flow is redistributed preferentially to ischemic areas. Thiopental acutely reduces ICP, and this is probably the main cerebroprotective effect. Seizure control is a further benefit. Despite these effects, barbiturate coma has not been shown to improve outcome in cerebral insults of various causes.

Table 17.6 Drug dosages

	Bolus	Infusion
Mannitol	0.5–2 g q 6 h	
Furosemide		1–5 mg/h
Dexamethasone	4 mg q 6 h	
Nimodipine	60 mg PO q 4 h	
Thiopental	1.5–3.5 mg/kg	Lowest possible dose

Key trials

Allen GS, et al. Cerebral arterial spasm: A controlled trial of nimodipine in patients with subarachnoid hemorrhage. N Engl J Med 1983; **308**:619–24.

Bracken MB, et al. Administration of methylprednisolone for 24 or 48 hours or tirilazad mesylate for 48 hours in the treatment of acute spinal cord injury. Results of the Third National Acute Spinal Cord Injury Randomized Controlled Trial. National Acute Spinal Cord Injury Study. JAMA 1997; **277**:1597–604.

Effect of intravenous corticosteroids on death within 14 days in 10 008 adults with clinically significant head injury (MRC CRASH Trial): Randomised placebo-controlled trial. Lancet 2004; **364**:1321–8.

See also

ICP monitoring, p. 134; Jugular venous bulb saturation, p. 136; EEG monitoring, p. 138; Other neurological monitoring, p. 140; Basic resuscitation, p. 268; Generalized seizures, p. 372; Intracranial hemorrhage, p. 378; Subarachnoid hemorrhage, p. 380; Increased ICP, p. 384; Head injury (1), p. 506; Head injury (2), p. 508

Hematological drugs

Anticoagulants

Types
- Heparin
- Low-molecular weight heparin (e.g., dalteparin)
- Direct thrombin inhibitors (e.g., argatroban, lepirudin, bivalirudin)
- Anticoagulant prostanoids (e.g., epoprostenol, alprostadil)
- Sodium citrate
- Warfarin
- Drotrecogin alfa (activated)

Modes of action
- Heparin potentiates naturally occurring antithrombin, reduces the adhesion of platelets, to injured arterial walls, binds to platelets, and promotes in vitro aggregation.
- Low-molecular weight heparin appears specifically to influence factor Xa activity; its simpler pharmacokinetics allow for a smaller (two thirds) dose to be administered to the same effect.
- Direct thrombin inhibitors are AT (antithrombin)-independent and will inhibit clot-bound thrombin (whereas heparin will not). These agents are not susceptible to circulating inhibitors (e.g., PF4 (platelet factor 4), heparinase) and effective in states of acquired or inherited antithrombin deficiency. More important, direct thrombin inhibitors do not cause and can be used to treat heparin-induced thrombocytopenia syndrome (HIT lepirudin and argatroban have been approved for this purpose).
- The effects of the prostanoids depend on the balance between TXA_2 (thromboxane A_2) and PGI_2.
- Sodium citrate chelates ionized calcium.
- Warfarin produces a controlled deficiency of vitamin K-dependent coagulation factors (II, VII, IX, and X).
- Drotrecogin alfa (activated) is a recombinant form of activated protein C, an endogenous anticoagulant.

Uses
- Maintenance of an extracorporeal circulation
- Prevention or treatment of thromboembolism
- Acute coronary syndrome
- Severe sepsis (Drotrecogin alfa)

Routes
- IV (heparins, anticoagulant prostanoids, sodium citrate, activated Drotrecogin alfa)
- SC (heparins)
- PO (warfarin)

Side effects
- Bleeding
- Hypotension (anticoagulant prostanoids)
- Heparin-induced thrombocytopenia
- Hypocalcemia, hypernatremia, and metabolic alkalosis (sodium citrate)

Notes
Alprostadil has similar effects to epoprostenol but is less potent. Because it is metabolized in the lungs, systemic vasodilatation effects are usually minimal. This may be an important advantage in patients with hypotension.

Major uses in intensive care are for anticoagulation of filter circuits, digital vasculitis/ischemia, and pulmonary hypertension.

For extracorporeal use, citrate has advantages over heparin in that it has no known antiplatelet activity, is readily filtered by a hemofilter (reducing systemic anticoagulation), and is easily reversed by calcium administration (e.g., after filtering).

Warfarin is given orally and needs 48 to 72 h to develop its effect. It can be reversed by FFP or low doses (1 mg) of vitamin K.

Drotrecogin alfa (activated) has antiinflammatory and profibrinolytic properties in addition to its anticoagulant actions.

Drug dosages

Heparin

Dose requirement is variable to produce an APTT of 1.5 to 3 times control. This usually requires 500 to 2000 IU/h with an initial loading dose of 3000 to 5000 IU.

Low-molecular weight heparin

For DVT prophylaxis give 2500 IU SC q12h. For anticoagulation of an extracorporeal circuit, a bolus of 35 IU/kg is given IV followed by an infusion of 13 IU/kg. The dose is adjusted to maintain antifactor Xa activity at 0.5 to 1 IU/mL (or 0.2–0.4 IU/mL if there is a high risk of hemorrhage). For pulmonary embolism give 200 IU/kg SC daily (or 100 IU/kg q12h if at risk of bleeding).

Direct thrombin inhibitors

For HIT, argatroban 2 µg/kg/min to start (considerably lower doses may be effective in critically ill patients). Maintenance dose, measure APTT after 2 h, adjust dose until the steady-state APTT is 1.5 to 3.0 times the initial baseline value, not exceeding 100 s. Dosage should not exceed 10 µg/kg/min. Dosing precautions are recommended in patients with hepatic dysfunction. Dose adjustment is apparently not required in the presence of renal impairment, but experience is limited.

Lepirudin 0.1 to 0.4 mg/kg bolus followed by 0.1 to 0.15 mg/kg/h infusion. Caution should be used in patients with renal insufficiency because the drug is cleared by the kidney and its anticoagulant effect is not easily reversed.

Anticoagulant prostaglandins

Usual range of 2.5 to 10 ng/kg/min. If used for an extracorporeal circulation, the infusion should be started 30 min prior to commencement.

Warfarin

Start at 10 mg/day orally for 2 days then 1 to 6 mg/day according to INR. For DVT prophylaxis, pulmonary embolus, mitral stenosis, atrial fibrillation, and tissue valve replacements, the INR should be maintained between 2 and 3. For recurrent DVT or pulmonary embolus and mechanical valve replacements, the INR is generally kept between 2 and 3.5 (possibly even higher), depending on the type of valve.

Drotrecogin alpha (activated)

For sepsis, an infusion of 24 µg/kg/h is given for 96 h.

See also

Extracorporeal respiratory support, p. 34; Continuous renal replacement therapy (2), p. 66; Plasma exchange, p. 70; Coagulation monitoring, p. 156; Thrombolytics, p. 248; Pulmonary embolus, p. 306; Acute coronary syndrome (1), p. 318; Acute coronary syndrome (2), p. 320; Clotting disorders, p. 400; Hyperosmolar diabetic emergencies, p. 446; Sepsis and septic shock—treatment, p. 246; Postoperative intensive care, p. 536

Thrombolytics

Types
- rt-PA; (alteplase, reteplase, tenecteplase)
- Streptokinase
- Urokinase

Modes of action
- Activate plasminogen to form plasmin, which degrades fibrin

Uses
- Life-threatening venous thrombosis
- Life-threatening pulmonary embolus
- AMI
- Acute ischemic stroke (alteplase)
- To unblock indwelling vascular access catheters

Routes
- IV

Side effects
- Bleeding, particularly from invasive procedures
- Hypotension and arrhythmias
- Embolization from preexisting clot as it is broken down
- Anaphylactoid reactions (anistreplase, streptokinase, urokinase)

Contraindications/Cautions (absolute)
- Previous intracranial hemorrhage
- Known structural cerebral vascular lesion
- Known malignant intracranial neoplasm
- Ischemic stroke within 3 months (not acute stroke within 3 h)
- Suspected aortic dissection
- Active bleeding or bleeding diathesis
- Significant closed-head or facial trauma within 3 months

Contraindications/Cautions (relative)
- Poorly controlled or chronic, sustained hypertension (systolic blood pressure >180 mmHg)
- Ischemic stroke more than 3 months previously
- Dementia or other intracranial pathology
- Traumatic or prolonged CPR (>10 mins) or major surgery (within <3 weeks)
- Recent (within 2–4 weeks) internal bleeding
- Noncompressible vascular puncture
- For streptokinase and anistreplase, prior exposure (>5 days previously) or prior allergic reactions to these agents
- Pregnancy
- Active peptic ulcer
- Current use of anticoagulants—the higher the INR, the higher the risk of bleeding
- Proliferative diabetic retinopathy

Notes

In AMI they are of most value when used within 12h of onset. They may require adjuvant therapy (e.g., aspirin with streptokinase or heparin with rt-PA) to maximize the effect in AMI.

In acute ischemic stroke and in the absence of contraindications, alteplase may be beneficial, provided treatment is initiated within 3 h of clearly defined symptom onset. Patients should have a neurological deficit that they themselves find sufficiently significant to warrant being exposed to the risks of thrombolytic therapy. Neurological deficits should not be rapidly resolving or occurring after seizure. CT scan should be negative for hemorrhage or major early infarct signs (e.g., diffuse swelling).

Anaphylactoid reactions to streptokinase are not uncommon, particularly in those who have had streptococcal infections, and patients should not be exposed twice between 5 days and 1 year of receiving the last dose.

Table 18.1 Drug dosages

Alteplase (rt-PA)	For AMI, 10 mg in 1–2 min, 50 mg in 1 h, and 40 mg over 2 h IV
Anistreplase	Single IV injection of 30 U over 4–5 min
Streptokinase	In AMI, 1.5 mu over 60 min; severe venous thrombosis, 250,000 U over 30 min followed by 100,000 U/h for 24–72 h
Urokinase	For unblocking indwelling vascular catheters, 5000–37,500 IU are instilled; for thromboembolic disease, 4400 IU/kg is given over 10 min followed by 4400 IU/kg/h for 12–24 h

See also

Coagulation monitoring, p. 156; Coagulants and antifibrinolytics, p. 252; Pulmonary embolus, p. 306; Acute coronary syndrome (1), p. 318

Blood products

Types
- Plasma (e.g., FFP)
- Platelets
- Concentrates of coagulation factors (e.g., cryoprecipitate, factor VIII concentrate, factor IX complex)

Uses
- Vitamin K deficiency (FFP, factor IX complex)
- Hemophilia (cryoprecipitate)
- von Willebrand's disease (cryoprecipitate)
- Fibrinogen deficiency (cryoprecipitate)
- Christmas disease (factor IX complex)

Routes
- IV

Notes

A unit (150 mL) of FFP is usually collected from one donor and contains all coagulation factors including 200 U factor VIII, 200 U factor IX, and 400 mg fibrinogen. FFP is stored at −30°C and should be infused within 2 h once defrosted.

Platelet concentrates are viable for 3 days when stored at room temperature. If they are refrigerated, viability decreases. They must be infused quickly via a short line set with no filter. Indications for platelet concentrates include platelet count $<10 \times 10^9$, or $<50 \times 10^9$ with spontaneous bleeding, or to cover invasive procedures and spontaneous bleeding with platelet dysfunction. They are less useful in conditions associated with immune platelet destruction (e.g., ITP).

A 15-mL vial of cryoprecipitate contains 100 U factor VIII, and 250 mg fibrinogen, factor XIII, and von Willebrand factor, and is stored at −30°C. In hemophilia, cryoprecipitate is given to achieve a factor VIII level >30% of normal.

Factor VIII concentrate contains 300 U factor VIII per vial. In severe hemorrhage resulting from hemophilia, 10 to 15 U/kg are given every 12 h.

Factor IX complex is rich in factors II, IX, and X. It is formed from pooled plasma, so FFP is preferred.

See also

Coagulation monitoring, p. 156; Blood transfusion, p. 182; Anticoagulants, p. 246; Bleeding disorders, p. 398; Clotting disorders, p. 400; Postoperative intensive care, p. 536; Postpartum hemorrhage, p. 544

Coagulants and antifibrinolytics

Types
- Vitamin K
- Protamine
- Tranexamic acid
- Activated factor VII

Uses
- To reverse a prolonged PT (e.g., malabsorption, oral anticoagulant therapy, antibiotics, or critical illness [vitamin K])
- To reverse the effects of heparin (protamine)
- Bleeding from raw surfaces (e.g., prostatectomy, dental extraction [tranexamic acid])
- Bleeding from thrombolytics (tranexamic acid)
- Bleeding from major trauma or hemophilia (factor VIIa)

Routes
- IV (vitamin K, protamine, tranexamic acid, factor VIIa)
- PO (vitamin K, tranexamic acid)

Notes
The effects of vitamin K are prolonged, so it should be avoided when patients are dependent on oral anticoagulant therapy. A dose of 10 mg is given orally or by slow IV injection daily. In life-threatening hemorrhage 5 to 10 mg is given by slow IV injection with other coagulation factor concentrates. If INR is >7 or in less severe hemorrhage, 0.5 to 2 mg may be given by slow IV injection with minimal lasting effect on oral anticoagulant therapy.

Protamine has an anticoagulant effect of its own in high doses. Protamine 1 mg neutralizes 100 IU unfractionated heparin if given within 15 min. Less is required if given later because heparin is excreted rapidly. Protamine should be given by slow IV injection according to the APTT. Total dose should not exceed 50 mg. Protamine injection may cause severe hypotension.

Tranexamic acid has an antifibrinolytic effect by antagonizing plasminogen. The usual dose is 1 to 1.5 g every 6 to 12 h orally or by slow IV injection.

Recombinant factor VIIa is licensed for use in hemophilia, but a number of case series in major trauma, orthopedic, and cardiac surgery report benefit in severe, intractable bleeding that had not responded to standard measures. The dose is 4500 IU/kg over 2 to 5 min, followed by 3000 to 6000 IU/kg, depending on the severity of bleeding.

See also

Coagulation monitoring, p. 156; Anticoagulants, p. 246; Thrombolytics, p. 248; Aprotinin, p. 254; Bleeding disorders, p. 398; Clotting disorders, p. 400; Postoperative intensive care, p. 536; Postpartum hemorrhage, p. 544

Aprotinin

The role of serine protease inhibitors in coagulation and anticoagulation is complicated because of their effects at various points in the coagulation pathway. Aprotinin is a naturally occurring, nonspecific serine protease inhibitor with an elimination half-life of about 2 h. Prevention of systemic bleeding with aprotinin does not promote coagulation within the extracorporeal circulation and may even contribute to the maintenance of extracorporeal anticoagulation.

Modes of action

The effects of aprotinin on the coagulation cascade are dependent on the circulating plasma concentrations (expressed as kallikrein inactivation units per milliliter—kIU/mL) because the affinity of aprotinin for plasmin is significantly greater than that for plasma kallikrein. At a plasma level of 125 kIU/mL, aprotinin inhibits fibrinolysis and complements activation. Inhibition of plasma kallikrein requires higher doses to provide plasma levels of 250 to 500 kIU/mL.

- Plasma kallikrein inhibition—reduces blood coagulation mediated via contact with anionic surfaces and, in the critically ill patient, improves circulatory stability via reduced kinin activation
- Prevention of inappropriate platelet activation—neutrophil activation (complement or kallikrein mediated) causes a secondary activation of platelets. Important in this platelet–neutrophil interaction is the release of cathepsin G by neutrophil degranulation. It has been demonstrated recently that aprotinin can significantly inhibit the platelet activation, resulting from purified cathepsin G, with this mechanism forming a direct inhibition of inappropriate neutrophil-mediated platelet activation.

Uses

The main role of aprotinin in the management of the extracorporeal circulation has been to prevent bleeding associated with heparinization. High-dose aprotinin given during cardiopulmonary bypass procedures has been shown to reduce postoperative blood loss dramatically. However, it has also been shown to increase significantly the risk of postoperative acute renal failure.

Table 18.2 Drug dosages

Aprotinin loading dose of 2×10^6 kIU followed by 500,000 kIU/h

See also

Extracorporeal respiratory support, p. 34; Continuous renal replacement therapy (2), p. 66; Anticoagulants, p. 246; Postoperative intensive care, p. 536

Miscellaneous drugs

Antimicrobials

Types

- Penicillins (e.g., nafcillin, piperacillin, ampicillin)
- Cephalosporins (e.g., ceftriaxone, cefepime, cefuroxime)
- Carbapenems (e.g., imipenem, meropenem)
- Aminoglycosides (e.g., gentamicin, amikacin, tobramycin)
- Quinolones (e.g., ciprofloxacin)
- Glycopeptides (e.g., vancomycin)
- Macrolides (e.g., erythromycin, clarithromycin)
- Other antibacterials (e.g., clindamycin, metronidazole, linezolid, trimethoprim–sulfamethoxazole [TMP-SMX], rifampin)
- Antifungals (e.g., amphotericin, flucytosine, fluconazole, caspofungin, Voriconazole, itraconazole)
- Antivirals (e.g., acyclovir, ganciclovir)

Uses

- Treatment of infection
- Prophylaxis against infection (e.g., perioperatively)
- Local choice of antimicrobial varies. However, as a guide, the following choices are common:
- Pneumonia (hospital-acquired Gram negative)—cefepime, meropenem or piperacillin/tazobactam (± vancomycin if methicillin-resistant *S. aureus* [MRSA] likely)
- Pneumonia (community acquired)—ceftriaxone and clarithromycin
- Systemic sepsis—cefepime ± tobramycin (and metronidazole if anaerobes likely, and vancomycin if MRSA likely)

Route

- Generally IV in critically ill patients

Side effects

- Hypersensitivity reactions (all)
- Seizures (high-dose penicillins; high-dose metronidazole, ciprofloxacin)
- Gastrointestinal disturbance (cephalosporins, erythromycin, clindamycin, vancomycin, TMP-SMX, rifampin, metronidazole, ciprofloxacin, amphotericin, flucytosine)
- Vestibular damage (aminoglycosides)
- Renal failure (aminoglycosides, teicoplanin, vancomycin, ciprofloxacin, rifampin, amphotericin, acyclovir)
- Erythema multiforme (TMP-SMX)
- Leucopenia (cotrimoxazole, metronidazole, ciprofloxacin, flucytosine, acyclovir)
- Thrombocytopenia (linezolid)
- Peripheral neuropathy (metronidazole)

Notes

Appropriate, broad-spectrum, empirical therapy for serious infections should be instituted in a timely fashion. Inadequate initial antimicrobial therapy increases mortality.

Specific drug choices should be determined by likely organisms, taking into account known community and hospital infection and resistance patterns. Empiric antimicrobial therapy should be tailored according to microbial sensitivities, usually based on advice from the microbiology laboratory.

Up to 10% of penicillin-allergic patients are also cephalosporinallergic.

Table 19.1 Drug dosages (intravenous)

Nafcillin	500 mg–2 g q 4–6 h
Ampicillin	500 mg–1 g q 6 h
Piptazobactam	4.5 g q 6–8 h
Cefotaxime	1–4 g q 8 h
Ceftazidime	2 g q q 8 h
Ceftriaxone	1–4 g q daily
Cefepime	1 g q 6–12 h
Gentamicin*	4–7 mg/kg daily (dosing intervals determined by levels)
Amikacin*	15–20 mg/kg daily (dosing intervals determined by levels)
Tobramycin*	4–7 mg/kg daily (dosing intervals determined by levels)
Erythromycin	500 mg–1g q 6–12 h
Metronidazole	500 mg q 8 h
Clindamycin	300–600 mg q 6 h
Ciprofloxacin	200–400 mg q 12 h
TMP-SMX	20 TMP/kg/day divided q 6 h in *Pneumocystis carinii* pneumonia
Imipenem	1–2 g q 6–8 h
Meropenem	500 mg–1g q 8 h
Rifampin	600 mg daily
Vancomycin	1 g 12 h (monitor levels)
Linezolid	600 mg q 12 h
Amphotericin	250 µg–1.5 mg/kg daily
Flucytosine	25–50 mg/kg q 6 h
Fluconazole	200–400 mg daily
Caspofungin	70 mg stat then 50–70 mg daily
Voriconazole	6 mg/kg q 12 h on first day then 3–4 mg/kg q 12 h
Itraconazole	200 mg q 12 h for 2 days then 200 mg daily
Acyclovir	5–10 mg/kg q 8 h
Ganciclovir	5 mg/kg q 12 h

Most antimicrobials need dose adjustment for renal or hepatic failure.
* Individualization is critical with aminoglycoside dosing because of the low therapeutic index.

Table 19.2 Common choices for specific organisms

S. aureus	Nafcillin
MRSA	Teicoplanin, vancomycin, linezolid
Streptococcus pneumoniae	Cefuroxime, benzylpenicillin
N. meningitidis	Ceftriaxone, cefotaxime, benzylpenicillin
Haemophilus influenzae	Cefuroxime, cefotaxime
E. coli	Ampicillin, ceftazidime, gentamicin, ciprofloxacin, meropenem
Klebsiella spp.	Ceftazidime, cefepime, ciprofloxacin, gentamicin, meropenem
P. aeruginosa	Ceftazidime, cefepime, ciprofloxacin, gentamicin, meropenem, piptazobactam

Key papers

Ibrahim E, Sherman G, Ward S, Fraser V, Kollef M. The influence of inadequate antimicrobial treatment of bloodstream infections on patient outcomes in the ICU setting. *Chest* 2000; **118**: 146–55.

Steroids

Uses

- Anti-inflammatory—often given in high dose for their anti-inflammatory effect (e.g., asthma), allergic and anaphylactoid reactions, vasculitic disorders, rheumatoid arthritis, inflammatory bowel disease, neoplasm-related cerebral edema, the fibroproliferative phase of ARDS, pneumococcal meningitis, *Pneumocystis* pneumonia, laryngeal edema (e.g., after repeated intubation), and after spinal cord injury. They do not improve outcome in cerebral edema after head injury or cardiorespiratory arrest, and they may be harmful in cerebral malaria and sepsis (at high dose).
- A multicenter trial has shown improved outcomes with 'low-dose' hydrocortisone (50 mg qid for 1 week) in septic shock patients with depressed adrenal function (subnormal plasma cortisol response to ACTH (adrenal corticotropic hormone), often despite 'normal' or increased plasma levels). Some patients with hypotension not responding to catecholamines will improve with corticosteroid therapy.
- Replacement therapy is needed for patients with Addison's disease and after adrenalectomy or pituitary surgery. In the longer term, fludrocortisone is usually also required for its mineralocorticoid sodium retaining effect. Higher replacement doses are needed in chronic steroid takers (i.e., >2 weeks within the last year) undergoing a stress (e.g., surgery) infection.
- Immunosuppressive—after organ transplantation

Side effects/complications

- Sodium and water retention (especially with mineralocorticoids)
- Hypoadrenal crisis if stopped abruptly after prolonged treatment
- Immunosuppressive—possibly increased infection risk (q.v.)
- Neutrophilia
- Impaired glucose tolerance/diabetes mellitus
- Hypokalemic alkalosis
- Osteoporosis, proximal myopathy (long-term use)
- Increased susceptibility to peptic ulcer disease and gastrointestinal bleeding

Notes

The perceived heightened risk of systemic infection appears exaggerated. Chronic steroid users generally appear no more affected than the general population. Studies in ARDS and sepsis revealed no greater incidence of infection after steroid administration. Oral fungal infection is relatively common with inhaled steroids, but systemic and pulmonary fungal infection is predominantly seen in the severely immunocompromised (e.g., AIDS, postchemotherapy) and not in those taking high-dose steroids alone.

The choice of corticosteroid for short-term anti-inflammatory effect is probably irrelevant, provided the dose is sufficient. Chronic hydrocortisone should be avoided for anti-inflammatory use because of its mineralocorticoid effect, but it is appropriate for adrenal replacement.

Prednisone and cortisone are inactive until metabolized by the liver to prednisolone and hydrocortisone respectively. Glucocorticoids antagonize the effects of anticholinesterase drugs.

The role of steroids in critical illness myopathy remains a contentious issue.

Table 19.3 Relative potency and activity

Drug	Glucocorticoid activity	Mineralo-corticoid activity	Equivalent anti-inflammatory dose (mg)
Cortisone	++	++	25
Dexamethasone	++++	—	0.75
Hydrocortisone	++	++	20
Methylprednisolone	+++	+	4
Prednisolone	+++	+	5
Prednisone	+++	+	5
Fludrocortisone	+	++++	—

Table 19.4 Drug dosages

Drug	Replacement dose	Anti-inflammatory dose
Dexamethasone	—	4–20 mg tid IV
Hydrocortisone	20–30 mg daily; for shock, 50–100 mg q 6–8 h	100–200 mg qid IV
Methylprednisolone	—	500 mg–1 g IV daily
Prednisolone	2.5–15 mg daily	40–60 mg qd PO
Fludrocortisone	0.05–0.3 mg daily	—

Weaning

Acute use (<3–4 days)	Can stop immediately
Short-term use (≥3–4 days)	Wean over 2–5 days
Medium-term use (weeks)	Wean over 1–2 weeks
Long-term use (months/years)	Wean slowly (months to years)

Key papers

Annane D, Sebille V, Charpentier C, et al. Effect of treatment with low doses of hydrocortisone and fludrocortisone on mortality in patients with septic shock. *JAMA* 2002; **288**:862–71.

Bracken MB, et al. Administration of methylprednisolone for 24 or 48 hours or tirilazad mesylate for 48 hours in the treatment of acute spinal cord injury. Results of the Third National Acute Spinal Cord Injury Randomized Controlled Trial. National Acute Spinal Cord Injury Study. *JAMA* 1997; **277**:1597–604.

de Gans J, van de Beek D, European Dexamethasone in adulthood bacterial meningitis Study Investigators. Dexamethasone in adults with bacterial meningitis. *N Engl J Med* 2002; **347**:1549–56.

Effect of intravenous corticosteroids on death within 14 days in 10 008 adults with clinically significant head injury (MRC CRASH Trial): Randomised placebo-controlled trial. *Lancet* 2004; **364**:1321–8.

Prasad K, Garner P. Steroids for treating cerebral malaria. *Cochrane Database Syst Rev* 2000; (2):CD000972. [Review].

Prostaglandins

Types
- Epoprostenol (prostacyclin, PGI$_2$)
- Alprostadil (PGE$_1$)

Modes of action
- Stimulate adenyl cyclase, thus increasing platelet cAMP concentration, which inhibits phospholipase and cyclooxygenase and thus reduces platelet aggregation (epoprostenol is the most potent inhibitor known)
- Reduce platelet procoagulant activity and release of heparin neutralizing factor
- May have a fibrinolytic effect
- Pulmonary and systemic vasodilator by relaxation of vascular smooth muscle

Uses
- Anticoagulation, particularly for extracorporeal circuits, either as a substitute or in addition to heparin
- Pulmonary hypertension
- Microvascular hypoperfusion (including digital vasculitis)
- Hemolytic uremic syndrome
- Acute respiratory failure (by inhalation)

Side effects/complications
- Hypotension
- Bleeding (particularly at cannula sites)
- Flushing, headache

Notes

Epoprostenol is active on both pulmonary and systemic circulations.

Although alprostadil is claimed to be metabolized in the lung and have only pulmonary vasodilating effects, decreases in systemic blood pressure are not uncommonly seen, especially if metabolism is incomplete.

Avoid extravasation into peripheral tissues because solution has high pH.

Effects last up to 30 min after discontinuation of the drug.

Prostaglandins may potentiate the effect of heparin.

Recent studies have shown improvement in gas exchange by selective pulmonary vasodilatation after inhalation of epoprostenol at doses of 10 to 15 ng/kg/min. The efficacy appears similar to that of nitric oxide inhalation but is not as rapid.

Table 19.5 Drug dosages

Epoprostenol	2–20 ng/kg/min
Alprostadil	2–20 ng/kg/min

See also

Continuous renal replacement therapy (2), p. 66; Plasma exchange, p. 70; Vasodilators, p. 198; Nitric oxide, p. 190; Anticoagulants, p. 246; Acute respiratory distress syndrome (1), p. 290; Acute respiratory distress syndrome (2), p. 292; Clotting disorders, p. 400; Vasculitides, p. 496

Novel therapies in sepsis

Greater understanding of the pathophysiology of sepsis has stimulated the development and investigation of agents that modulate different components of the inflammatory response. These drugs have been targeted at triggers (e.g., endotoxin), cytokines (e.g., tumour necrosis factor, interleukin [IL]-1), and effector cells and their products (e.g., neutrophils, free oxygen radicals, nitric oxide), or aim to boost a general anti-inflammatory response (e.g., steroids). An increasing area of research is in replacement or augmentation of endogenous anti-inflammatory systems (e.g., activated protein C, antithrombin-III, IL-10) because there is an increasing realization of the degree of disruption and imbalance between pro- and anti-inflammatory substances.

Unfortunately, because of deficiencies in trial design and size, choice of appropriate patient, timing of drug administration, dosage, and lack of standardization of concurrent therapies, only two agents ('low-dose' hydrocortisone and activated protein C) have been shown to produce outcome benefit in reasonably sized multicenter trials. For many other products, promising results from posthoc subgroup analysis and from tightly controlled small patient studies have not been reproduced. Concern over cost has highlighted the potential budgetary implications of any successful therapy, although, in terms of life years, the cost–benefit will be comparable with other commonly used therapies.

Uses
- Sepsis
- Multiple-organ dysfunction

Drotrecogin alfa (activated)
Drotrecogin alfa (activated) is a recombinant form of protein C and has anti-inflammatory, anticoagulant, and fibrinolytic properties. Its beneficial effects in adult sepsis are most likely to be related to its anti-inflammatory properties. A large, prospective, randomized, controlled trial demonstrated outcome benefit for patients with severe sepsis treated within 48 h of presentation with a 96-h infusion of 24 µg/kg/h drotrecogin. Most benefit was seen in those with a higher risk of death. Subsequent studies have failed to show benefit in lower risk adults (Acute Physiology and Chronic, Health Evaluation [APACHE] score <25 points) or in children. The major side effect is bleeding, so caution should be exercised in those at high risk of potentially catastrophic bleeding (e.g., concurrent coagulopathy) or a recent history of surgery, major trauma, head injury, and/or peptic ulcer disease.

Corticosteroids
Large, randomized multicenter studies of high-dose methylprednisolone showed either no benefit or a trend to harm. However, subsequent studies with lower doses of corticosteroids (e.g., 50 mg qid hydrocortisone) revealed earlier resolution of shock and improved survival in those patients with an impaired (<250 nmol/L [9 µg/dL]) increase in plasma cortisol to a synthetic ACTH challenge.

Examples of drugs investigated in multicenter studies

- Corticosteroids (methylprednisolone, hydrocortisone)
- Polyclonal immunoglobulin
- Antiendotoxin antibody (HA-1A, E5)
- Antitumor necrosis factor antibody
- Tumor necrosis factor-soluble receptor antibody
- IL-1 receptor antagonist
- Platelet activating factor (PAF) antagonists, PAF-ase
- Bradykinin antagonists
- Naloxone
- Ibuprofen
- N-acetylcysteine, procysteine
- L-NMMA
- Antithrombin III
- TF pathway inhibitor
- Drotrecogin alpha

Key trials

Annane D, et al. Effect of treatment with low doses of hydrocortisone and fludrocortisone on mortality in patients with septic shock. *JAMA* 2002; **288**:862–71.

Bernard GR, for the PROWESS Study Group. Efficacy and safety of recombinant human activated protein C for severe sepsis. *N Engl J Med*, **344**:699–709.

See also

Sepsis and septic shock—treatment, p. 488

Resuscitation

Basic resuscitation

In any severe cardiorespiratory disturbance, the order of priority should be (1) to secure the *airway*; (2) to maintain *breathing* (manual ventilation if necessary), and (3) to restore the *circulation* (with external cardiac massage if necessary). Initial assessment of the patient should include patency of the airway, palpation of the pulses, measurement of blood pressure, presumptive diagnosis, and consideration of treatment of the cause.

Airway protection

The airway should be opened by lifting the jaw forward and tilting the head back slightly. The head tilt should be avoided if a cervical spine injury is a concern. The mouth and pharynx should be cleared by suction, and loose-fitting dentures removed. If necessary an oropharyngeal (Guedel) airway may be inserted.

Manual ventilation

After the airway is opened, the patient who is not breathing requires manual ventilation with a self-inflating bag and mask (Ambu bag). One hundred percent oxygen should be delivered. If the patient breathes inadequately (poor arterial saturation; hypercapnia; rapid, shallow breathing), ventilatory support should continue.

Circulation

If pulses are not palpable or are weak, or if the patient has severe bradycardia, external cardiac massage is required and treatment should continue as for a cardiac arrest. Hypotension should be treated initially with a fluid challenge, although life-threatening hypotension may require treatment with epinephrine in doses of 0.05 to 0.2 mg at 1- to 2-min intervals IV until a satisfactory blood pressure is restored. Such treatment should not be prolonged without circulatory monitoring to ensure adequacy of cardiac output as well as correction of hypotension.

Venous access

Venous access must be secured early during basic resuscitation. Large-bore cannulas are necessary (e.g., 14 G). In cases of hemorrhage, two cannulas are required. Small peripheral veins should be avoided; antecubital veins are appropriate if nowhere else is available. In very difficult patients, a Seldinger approach to the femoral vein or a central vein may be appropriate. The latter has the advantage of providing for central venous monitoring.

See also

Oxygen therapy, p. 2; Ventilatory support—indications, p. 4; Endotracheal intubation, p. 36; Central venous catheter—insertion, p. 118; Colloids, p. 180; Inotropes, p. 196; Vasopressors, p. 200; Fluid challenge, p. 272; Hypotension, p. 310

Cardiac arrest

As with basic resuscitation, the order of priority is ABC—*airway*, *breathing*, and *circulation*—followed by drug treatment. If the cardiac arrest is witnessed, a precordial thump may revert VT or VF. Initial management of the airway and respiration is as for basic resuscitation. When intubation is attempted, it should be effected after adequate preoxygenation and quickly to avoid hypoxemia.

Cardiac massage

External cardiac massage provides minimal circulatory support during cardiac arrest. A compression rate of 100/min with a compression depth of approximately 2 inches is recommended. Once an advanced airway is established (endotracheal tube (ETT), laryngeal mask airway (LMA)), manual breaths should be provided at a rate of 8 to 10 breaths/min, and compressions should occur without pausing for ventilation.

Defibrillation

Defibrillation should be performed urgently if VT or VF cannot be excluded. It is important to restart cardiac massage immediately after defibrillation without waiting for the ECG to recover. Cerebral damage continues while there is no blood flow.

Drugs

Few drugs are necessary for first-line cardiac arrest management. Drugs should be given via a large vein because vasoconstriction and poor flow create a delay in injections given via small peripheral veins reaching the central circulation. Access should be secured early during the resuscitation; if venous access cannot be secured, double doses of some drugs may be given via the endotracheal tube.

Epinephrine

The α constrictor effects predominate during cardiac arrest, helping to maintain diastolic blood pressure and thus coronary and cerebral perfusion. Epinephrine should be given irrespective of rhythm at 1 mg (10 mL 1:10,000 solution) every 3 to 5 min while CPR continues.

Vasopressin

A recent randomized, controlled trial comparing vasopressin and epinephrine showed improved outcomes with vasopressin for patients in asystolic out-of-hospital cardiac arrest. The dose of vasopressin is 40 IU and may be repeated in 3 min if the first dose is ineffective.

Atropine

A single 3-mg dose is given early in asystole or to treat bradycardia.

Calcium chloride

Calcium chloride is used in pulseless electrical activity if there is hyperkalemia, hypocalcemia, or calcium antagonist use. A dose of 10 mL of a 10% solution is usual. The main disadvantage of calcium is the reduction of reperfusion of ischemic brain and promotion of cytosolic calcium accumulation during cell death.

Bicarbonate

Bicarbonate is used only if resuscitation is prolonged to correct temporarily a potentially lethal pH. A dose of 50 mL 8.4% solution is given. The main disadvantage is that intracellular and respiratory acidosis are exacerbated unless ventilation is increased and the cause of the metabolic acidosis is not corrected.

Key trial

Wenzel V, for the European Resuscitation Council Vasopressor During CPR Study. A comparison of vasopressin and epinephrine for out-of-hospital cardiopulmonary resuscitation. *N Engl J Med* 2004; **350**:105–13.

Fluid challenge

Hypovolemia must be treated urgently to avoid the serious complication of organ failure. An adequate circulating volume must be provided before considering other methods of circulatory support. Clinical signs of hypovolemia (reduced skin turgor, low central venous pressure (CVP), oliguria, tachycardia, and hypotension) are late indicators. Lifting the legs of a supine patient and watching for an improvement in the circulation is a useful indicator of hypovolemia. A high index of suspicion must be maintained; normal heart rate, blood pressure, and central venous pressure do not exclude hypovolemia, and the central venous pressure is particularly unreliable in pulmonary vascular disease, right ventricular disease, isolated left ventricular failure, and valvular heart disease. The absolute central venous pressure or PAWP are also difficult to interpret because peripheral venoconstriction may maintain these filling pressures despite hypovolemia; indeed, they may decrease in response to fluid. The response to a fluid challenge is the safest method of assessment.

Choice of fluid

The aim of a fluid challenge is to produce a significant (200 mL) and rapid increase in plasma volume. Colloid fluids (e.g., hydroxyethyl starch) will increase plasma volume more rapidly than crystalloids. Crystalloid fluids are also rapidly lost from the circulation. Packed red cells have a high hematocrit and do not adequately expand the plasma volume.

Assessing the response to a fluid challenge

Ideally, the response of central venous pressure, or stroke volume and PAWP, should be monitored during a fluid challenge. Fluid challenges should be repeated while the response suggests continuing hypovolemia. However, if such monitoring is not available, it is reasonable to assess the clinical response to up to two fluid challenges (200 mL each).

Central venous pressure response

The change in central venous pressure after a 200-ml fluid challenge depends on the starting blood volume (Fig. 20.1). A 3-mmHg increase in central venous pressure is significant and is probably indicative of an adequate circulating volume. However, a positive response may sometimes occur in the vasoconstricted patient with a lower blood volume. It is important to assess the clinical response as well. If inadequate, it is appropriate to monitor stroke volume and PAWP before further fluid challenges or before considering further circulatory support.

Stroke volume and PAWP response

In the inadequately filled left ventricle, a fluid challenge will increase the stroke volume. Failure to increase the stroke volume with a fluid challenge may represent an inadequate challenge, particularly if the PAWP fails to increase significantly (3 mmHg). This indicates that cardiac filling was inadequate and the fluid challenge should be repeated. Such a response may also be seen in right heart failure, pericardial tamponade, and mitral stenosis. It is important to monitor stroke volume rather than cardiac output during a fluid challenge. If the heart rate decreases appropriately in response to a fluid challenge, the cardiac output may not increase despite an increase in stroke volume.

Increases in intrathoracic pressure from intermittent positive-pressure breaths decreases preload. These responses to changes in preload can be evaluated using the cyclic systolic or pulse pressure variation with positive-pressure breaths. Significant fluctuation in systolic or pulse pressure predicts increases in stroke volume with subsequent fluid loading.

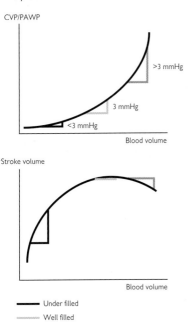

Fig. 20.1 Central venous pressure and stroke volume response to fluid challenge.

See also

Central venous catheter—use, p. 116; Pulmonary artery catheter—use, p. 120; Cardiac output—thermodilution, p. 124; Cardiac output—other invasive, p. 126; Cardiac output—noninvasive (1), p. 128; Cardiac output—noninvasive (2), p. 130; Lactate, p. 170; Colloids, p. 180; Hypotension, p. 310; Oliguria, p. 328; Metabolic acidosis, p. 436; Diabetic ketoacidosis, p. 444; Systemic inflammation/multiorgan failure, p. 486; Sepsis and septic shock—treatment, p. 488; Burns—fluid management, p. 512; Postoperative intensive care, p. 536

Respiratory disorders

Dyspnea

Dyspnea is defined as difficulty in breathing. The respiratory rate may be increased or decreased, although the respiratory effort is usually increased with the use of accessory muscles. The patient may show signs of progressive fatigue and impaired gas exchange.

Table 21.1 Common ICU causes

Respiratory	Respiratory failure
Circulatory	Heart failure, hypoperfusion, pulmonary embolus, severe anemia
Metabolic	Acidosis
Central	Stimulants (e.g., aspirin)
Anaphylactic	Upper airway obstruction, bronchospasm
Psychiatric	Anxiety

Principles of management
1. Provide O_2 therapy to maintain SaO_2 (ideally >90%–95%).
2. Correct abnormality when possible.
3. Support therapy until recovery.
    • Mechanical (e.g., positive-pressure ventilation, CPAP)
    • Pharmacological treatment (e.g., bronchodilators, vasodilators)
4. Relieve anxiety.

A psychiatric cause of dyspnea is only made after exclusion of other treatable causes.

Dual coexisting pathologies should be considered (e.g., lower respiratory ctract infection and hypovolemia).

See also

Airway obstruction

Causes

- In the lumen (e.g., foreign body, blood clot, vomitus, sputum plug)
- In the wall (e.g., epiglottitis, laryngeal edema, anaphylaxis, neoplasm)
- Outside the wall (e.g., trauma [facial, neck], thyroid mass, hematoma)

Presentation

- In spontaneously breathing patient—stridor, dyspnea, fatigue, cyanosis
- In ventilated patient (resulting from intraluminal obstruction)—increased peak airway pressures, decreased V_T, hypoxemia, hypercapnia

Diagnosis

- Chest and lateral neck radiograph
- Fiberoptic laryngoscopy/bronchoscopy
- CT scan

Management

Presentation outside ICU/operating room

1. High FiO_2
2. If collapsed or in extremis, immediate orotracheal intubation. If impossible, emergency cricothyroidotomy or tracheostomy.
3. If symptomatic but not in extremis, consider cause and treat as appropriate (e.g., fiberoptic or rigid bronchoscopy for removal of foreign body, surgery for thyroid mass). Elective orotracheal intubation or tracheostomy may be required.
4. With acute epiglottitis, the use of a tongue depressor or nasoendoscopy may precipitate complete obstruction so should be undertaken in an operating room ready to perform emergency tracheostomy. The responsible organism is usually *H. influenzae*, and early treatment with ampicillin–sulbactam should be instituted. Acute epiglottitis is recognized in adults, even in those of advanced age.
5. Consider Heliox (80%He/20%O_2 or 70%He/30%O_2) to reduce viscosity and improve airflow.

Presentation within ICU/operating room

1. If intubated:
   - High FiO_2
   - Pass suction catheter down the endotracheal tube, assess ease of passage and the contents suctioned. If the tube is patent, attempt repeated suction interspersed with 5-mL boluses of 0.9% saline. Urgent fiberoptic bronchoscopy may be necessary for diagnosis and, if possible, removal of a foreign body. If this cannot be removed by fiberoptic bronchoscopy, urgent rigid bronchoscopy should be performed by an experienced operator. If the endotracheal tube is obstructed, remove the tube, oxygenate by face mask then reintubate.

2. If not intubated:
   - As for out-of-ICU presentation
   - If recently extubated, consider laryngeal edema. Postextubation laryngeal edema is unpredictable, although occurs more commonly after prolonged or repeated intubation. The incidence may be reduced by proper tethering of the endotracheal tube and prevention of excessive coughing. If diagnosed (by nasendoscopy), dexamethasone 4 mg × 3 doses over 24 h may reduce the swelling, although reintubation is often necessary in the interim.

See also

Respiratory failure

Respiratory failure is defined as impaired pulmonary gas exchange leading to hypoxemia and/or hypercapnia.

Table 21.2 Common ICU causes

Central	CVA, drugs (e.g., opiates, sedatives), increased ICP, trauma
Brain stem/spinal cord	Trauma (at or above phrenic level), tetanus, Pickwickian syndrome, motor neuron disease
Neuropathy	Guillain–Barré, critical illness polyneuropathy
Neuromuscular	Muscle relaxants, organophosphorus poisoning, myasthenia gravis
Chest wall/muscular	Flail chest, heart failure, myopathy (including critical illness and disuse myopathy)
Airways	Upper airway obstruction, airway disruption, asthma, anaphylaxis
Parenchymal	Pneumonia, ARDS, fibrosis, pulmonary edema
Extrapulmonary	Pneumothorax, pleural effusion, hemothorax
Circulatory	Pulmonary embolus, heart failure, Eisenmenger intracardiac shunt

Types of respiratory failure
- Type I: Hypoxemic—often parenchymal in origin
- Type II: Hypoxemic, hypercapnic—often mechanical in origin

Principles of management
1. Ensure SaO_2 compatible with survival (i.e., usually >80%, preferably >90%–95%)
2. Correct abnormality when possible (e.g., drain pneumothorax, relieve/bypass obstruction).
3. Support therapy until recovery.
   - Positive-pressure ventilation
   - Noninvasive respiratory support
   - Pharmacological treatment (e.g., bronchodilators, antibiotics, opiate antagonists, respiratory stimulant)
   - General measures (e.g., hydration, airway humidification, removal of secretions, physiotherapy, bronchoscopy)
4. Unless the patient is symptomatic (e.g., drowsy, dyspneic) while being mechanically ventilated, the $PaCO_2$ may be left elevated to minimize ventilator trauma (permissive hypercapnia). Higher $PaCO_2$ values may also be tolerated if the patient is chronically hypercapnic (type II respiratory failure). Minute ventilation should ultimately be titrated to pH levels (not $PaCO_2$) in patients with chronic hypercapnia.

See also

Atelectasis and pulmonary collapse

A collapsed lobe or segment is usually visible on a CXR. Macroatelectasis is also evident as volume loss. In microatelectasis, the CXR may be normal but the alveolar–arterial oxygen difference will be high. Atelectasis reduces lung compliance and PaO_2, and increases work of breathing. This may result in poor gas exchange, increased airway pressures, reduced V_T, and, if severe, circulatory collapse.

Causes
- Collapsed lobe/segment—bronchial obstruction (e.g., sputum retention, foreign body, blood clot, vomitus, misplaced endotracheal tube)
- Macroatelectasis—air space compression by heavy, edematous lung tissue, external compression (e.g., pleural effusion, hemothorax), sputum retention
- Microatelectasis—inadequate depth of respiration, nitrogen washout by 100% oxygen with subsequent absorption of oxygen occurring at a rate greater than replenishment

Sputum retention
Excess mucous (sputum) normally stimulates coughing. If ciliary clearance is reduced (e.g., smoking, sedatives) or mucous volume is excessive (e.g., asthma, bronchiectasis, cystic fibrosis, chronic bronchitis), sputum retention may occur. Sputum retention may also be the result of inadequate coughing (e.g., chronic obstructive lung disease, pain, neuromuscular disease) or increased mucous viscosity (e.g., hypovolemia, inadequate humidification of inspired gas).

Preventive measures
- Sputum hydration—maintenance of systemic hydration and humidification of inspired gases (e.g., nebulized saline/bronchodilators, heated water bath, heat–moisture exchanging filter)
- Cough—requirement of inspiration to near-total lung capacity, glottic closure, contraction of abdominal muscles, and rapid opening of the glottis. Dynamic compression of the airways and high-velocity expiration expels secretions. The process is limited if total lung capacity is reduced, abdominal muscles are weak, pain limits contraction, or small airways collapse on expiration. It is usual to flex the abdomen on coughing, and this should be simulated in supine patients by drawing the knees up. This also limits pain in patients with an upper abdominal wound.
- Physiotherapy—postural drainage, percussion and vibration, hyperinflation, intermittent positive-pressure breathing, incentive spirometry, or manual hyperinflation
- Maintenance of lung volumes—increased V_T, CPAP, PEEP, positioning to reduce compression of lung tissue by edema

Management
Specific management depends on the cause and should be corrective. All measures taken for prevention should continue. If there is lobar or segmental collapse with obstruction of proximal airways, bronchoscopy may be useful to allow directed suction, foreign body removal, and saline instillation. Patients with high FiO_2 may deteriorate from the effects of excessive lavage or suction reducing minute ventilation.

See also

Chronic obstructive pulmonary disease

Many patients requiring ICU admission for a community-acquired pneumonia have chronic respiratory failure. An acute exacerbation (which may or may not be infection related) results in decompensation and symptomatic deterioration. Infections resulting in acute exacerbations include viruses, *H. influenzae*, *Klebsiella*, and *S. aureus* in addition to *S. pneumoniae*, *Mycoplasma pneumoniae*, and *L. pneumophila*. Otherwise, patients with coincidental COPD are admitted for other reasons or as a prophylactic measure in view of their limited respiratory function (e.g., for elective postoperative ventilation).

Management of COPD exacerbations

- Bronchodilators—short acting β_2 agonists (e.g., albuterol) and/or ipratropium
- Corticosteroids—Exact regimens will vary depending on severity and clinical response. Prednisone 30 to 40 mg PO daily for mild exacerbations; methylprednisolone 2 mg/kg, then 0.5 to 1 mg/kg q6h for severe cases.
- Antibiotics as appropriate
- Supplemental oxygen therapy/ventilatory support

Problems in managing COPD patients in the ICU

- Disability as a result of chronic ill health
- Fatigue, muscle weakness, and decreased physiological reserve leading to earlier need for ventilatory support; increased difficulty in weaning; and greater physical dependency on support therapies
- Psychological dependency on support therapies
- More prone to pneumothoraces
- Usually have greater levels of sputum production
- Right ventricular dysfunction (cor pulmonale)

Notes

Trials of noninvasive ventilatory support have shown considerable success in avoiding intubation and mechanical ventilation. Accept lower than usual target levels of PaO_2 (e.g., 88%–90%). Accept higher than normal target levels of $PaCO_2$ if patient is known or suspected to have chronic CO_2 retention on the basis of elevated plasma bicarbonate levels on admission to hospital. Watch for the development of auto-PEEP in ventilated patients.

Weaning ventilator support for the patient with COPD

- An early trial of extubation may be worthwhile before the patient becomes ventilator dependent.
- Weaning may be a lengthy procedure. Daily trials of spontaneous breathing may reveal faster than anticipated progress.
- Provide plentiful encouragement and psychological support. Setting daily targets and early mobilization may be advantageous.
- Do not tire by prolonged spontaneous breathing. Consider gradually increasing periods of spontaneous breathing interspersed by periods of rest. Ensure a good night's sleep.

- Use patient appearance and lack of symptoms (e.g., tachypnea, fatigue) rather than specific blood gas values to judge the duration of spontaneous breathing.
- Early tracheostomy may benefit when difficulty in weaning is expected.
- The patient may cope better with a tracheostomy mask than CPAP.
- Addition of extrinsic PEEP or CPAP may prevent early airway closure and thus reduce the work of breathing. However, this should be done with caution because of the risk of increased air trapping.
- Consider heart failure as a cause of difficulty in weaning.

Key trials

Antonelli M, *et al.* A comparison of noninvasive positive-pressure ventilation and conventional mechanical ventilation in patients with acute respiratory failure. N Engl J Med 1998; 339:429–35.

Brochard L, *et al.* Noninvasive ventilation for acute exacerbations of chronic obstructive pulmonary disease. N Engl J Med 1995; 333:817–22.

Epstein SK, Ciubotaru RL. Independent effects of etiology of failure and time to reintubation on outcome for patients failing extubation. Am J Respir Crit Care Med 1998; 158:489–93.

See also

Oxygen therapy, p. 2; Ventilatory support—indications, p. 4; IPPV—complications of ventilation, p. 14; Positive end expiratory pressure (1), p. 22; Positive end expiratory pressure (2), p. 24; Continuous positive airway pressure, p. 26; Noninvasive respiratory support, p. 32; Lung recruitment, p. 28; Endotracheal intubation, p. 36; Minitracheotomy, p. 40; Fiberoptic bronchoscopy, p. 46; Chest physiotherapy, p. 48; Blood gas analysis, p. 102; Bronchodilators, p. 186; Chronic airflow limitation, p. 284; Acute lower respiratory tract infection (1), p. 286; Acute lower respiratory tract infection (2), p. 288; Postoperative intensive care, p. 536

Acute lower respiratory tract infection (1)

Patients may present to intensive care as a result of an acute lower respiratory tract infection or may develop infection as a complication of intensive care management. Typical features include fever, cough, purulent sputum production, breathlessness, pleuritic pain, and bronchial breath sounds. Urgent investigation includes arterial gases, CXR, blood count, and cultures of blood and sputum. In community-acquired pneumonia, acute-phase antibody titers should be taken.

Diagnosis and initial antimicrobial treatment

Basic resuscitation is required if there is cardiorespiratory compromise. Appropriate treatment of the infection depends on CXR and culture findings; however, empiric 'best guess' antibiotic treatment should be started before culture results are available. Choice of antibiotics depends on the setting and risk factors for resistant organisms. General guidelines are provided here. Antibiotic treatment guidelines for pneumonia are available at www.thoracic.org. Treatment also includes physiotherapy and methods to aid sputum clearance.

Clear CXR

Acute bronchitis is associated with cough, mucoid sputum, and wheeze. In previously healthy patients, a viral etiology is most likely and there is often an upper respiratory prodrome. Symptomatic relief is usually all that is required. Viral pneumonia may be confused by the presence of bacteria in the sputum, but secondary bacterial infection is common.

Pulmonary cavitation on CXR

Cavitation should alert to the possibility of anaerobic infection (sputum is often foul smelling). S. aureus, K. pneumoniae, or TB are also associated with cavitation. Appropriate antibiotics include metronidazole or clindamycin for anaerobic infection, nafcillin for S. aureus, and cefepime and tobramycin for K. pneumoniae. Broader coverage is needed for hospital-acquired infection (e.g., vancomycin for MRSA). Local antibiotic resistance patterns should be considered. A foreign body or pulmonary infarct should also be considered when there is a single abscess.

Consolidation on CXR

The recent history is important for deciding the cause of a pneumonia:
- Hospital-acquired pneumonia—enteric (Gram-negative) organisms treated with cefepime ± tobramycin. If resistant S. aureus is a concern, add vancomycin or linezolid.
- Recent aspiration—The utility of adding anaerobic coverage (i.e., metronidazole) in settings of aspiration is controversial.
- Community-acquired pneumonia in a previously healthy individual— S. pneumoniae (often lobar, acute onset) or atypical pneumonia (insidious onset, known community outbreaks, renal failure, and electrolyte disturbance in Legionnaire's disease). Appropriate antibiotic therapy is cefuroxime and clarithromycin.
- Pneumonia complicating influenza—S. aureus treated with nafcillin (or vancomycin when methicillin resistance is likely). Both S. aureus and H. influenzae are common in those debilitated by chronic disease (e.g., alcoholism, diabetes, chronic airflow limitation, or the elderly).

- Immunosuppressed—opportunistic infections (e.g., TB, *Pneumocystis carinii*, herpes viruses, CMV, or fungi)

Table 21.3 Antimicrobial treatment

Drug	Dose	Organism
Acyclovir	5–10 mg/kg q 8h IV	*Herpes viruses*
Amphotericin B	250 μg–1.5 mg/kg daily	Fungi
Ampicillin–sulbactam	1–2 g ampicillin (1.5–3 g ampicillin–sulbactam) q 6h	*H. influenzae*, Gram-negative spp.
Cefepime	1 g q 6–12h IV	*K. pneumoniae P. aeruginosa* Gram-negative spp.
Cefuroxime	750 mg–1.5 g q 8h IV	*S. pneumoniae*, *H. influenzae*, Gram-negative spp.
Clarithromycin	500 mg q 12h PO	Atypical pneumonia, *S. Pneumoniae*
Erythromycin	1 g q 6–12h (500 mg q 6h PO if less severe)	Atypical pneumonia, *S. Pneumoniae*
Clindamycin	300–600 mg q 6h IV	Anaerobes, Gram-negative spp.
TMP-SMX	20 TMP/kg/day divided q 6h	*P. carinii*
Nafcillin	500 mg–2g q 4–6h	*S. aureus*
Ganciclovir	5 mg/kg q 12h IV (over 1 h)	CMV
Tobramycin	4–7 mg/kg daily (dosing intervals determined by levels)	*K. pneumoniae*, *P. aeruginosa* Gram-negative spp.
Metronidazole	500 mg q 8h IV	Anaerobes
Vancomycin	1–2 g q 12h (monitor levels)	MRSA
Linezolid	600 mg q 12h IV or PO	MRSA

Key trial

Iregui M, *et al.* Clinical importance of delays in the initiation of appropriate antibiotic treatment for ventilator-associated pneumonia. *Chest* 2002; **122**:262–8.

See also

Oxygen therapy, p. 2; Ventilatory support—indications, p. 4; IPPV—complications of ventilation, p. 14; Positive end expiratory pressure (1), p. 22; Positive end expiratory pressure (2), p. 24; Continuous positive airway pressure, p. 26; Noninvasive respiratory support, p. 32; Lung recruitment, p. 28; Endotracheal intubation, p. 36; Minitracheotomy, p. 40; Fiberoptic bronchoscopy, p. 46; Chest physiotherapy, p. 48; Blood gas analysis, p. 102; Bronchodilators, p. 186; Chronic airflow limitation, p. 284; Acute lower respiratory tract infection (1), p. 286; Acute lower respiratory tract infection (2), p. 288; Postoperative intensive care, p. 536

Acute lower respiratory tract infection (2)

Laboratory diagnosis

The following samples are required for laboratory diagnosis:

- Sputum (e.g., cough specimen, endotracheal tube aspirate, protected brush specimen, bronchoalveolar lavage specimen)
- Blood cultures
- Serology (in community-acquired pneumonia)
- Urine for antigen tests (if *Legionella*, *Candida*, or pneumococcus suspected)

Bronchoalveolar lavage is recommended to diagnose ventilator associated pneumonia because sputum/endotracheal tube aspirates may be misleading.

In severe pneumonia, empiric antibiotic therapy should not be withheld while awaiting results. Specimens should, however, be taken before starting antibiotics.

Microbiological yield is usually very low, especially if antibiotic therapy has started before sampling.

When cultures are positive, there is often multiple growth. Separating pathogenic organisms from colonizing organisms may be difficult.

In hospital-acquired pneumonia, known nosocomial pathogens are the likely source (e.g., local Gram-negative flora, MRSA).

Continuing treatment

Antibiotics should be adjusted according to sensitivities when available. Failure to respond to treatment in 72 h should prompt consideration of infections more common in the immunocompromised patient or other diagnoses.

Long durations of antimicrobial therapy are usually not required to obtain clinical and microbiologic cure. A recent multicenter study showed no difference in outcome between 8 and 15 days of treatment. Optimum duration of therapy for nonfermenting Gram-negative bacilli is still controversial.

In atypical or pneumococcal pneumonia, 10 to 14 days of antibiotic treatment is usual (although no evidence base exists to indicate the optimal duration of therapy).

Key trial

Chastre J, for the PneumA Trial Group. Comparison of 8 vs 15 days of antibiotic therapy for ventilator-associated pneumonia in adults: A randomized trial. JAMA 2003; 290:2588–98.

See also

Acute respiratory distress syndrome (1)

ARDS is the respiratory component of multiple-organ dysfunction. It may be predominant in the clinical picture or be of lesser clinical importance in relation to dysfunction of other organ systems.

Etiology

ARDS may occur as part of the exaggerated inflammatory response after a major exogenous insult that may be either direct (e.g., chest trauma, inhalation injury) or distant (e.g., peritonitis, major hemorrhage, burns). Histology reveals aggregation and activation of neutrophils and platelets, patchy endothelial and alveolar disruption, interstitial edema, and fibrosis. Classically, the acute phase is characterized by increased capillary permeability, and the fibroproliferative phase (after 7 days) by a predominant fibrotic reaction. However, more recent data would suggest such distinctions are not so clear-cut; there may be evidence of markers of fibrosis as early as day 1.

Definitions

Acute lung injury

- A clinical scenario consistent with acute lung injury
- PaO_2/FiO_2 <300 mmHg, regardless of PEEP
- With bilateral infiltrates on CXR
- With PAWP <18 mmHg

ARDS

As in previous list, but PaO_2/FiO_2 ≤200 mmHg

Prognosis

Prognosis depends in part on the underlying insult, the presence of other organ dysfunctions, and the age and chronic health of the patient. Predominant single-organ ARDS carries a mortality of 30% to 50%; there does appear to have been some improvement during the last decade.

Some deterioration on lung function testing is usually detectable in survivors of ARDS, even in those who are relatively asymptomatic. Recent studies indicate that a significant proportion of survivors of ARDS have physical and/or psychological sequelae at 1 year.

Key trials

Bernard GR, for the American–European Consensus Conference on ARDS. Definitions, mechanisms, relevant outcomes, and clinical trial coordination. Am J Respir Crit Care Med. 1994; 149:818–24.

Herridge MS, Cheung AM, for the Canadian Critical Care Trials Group. One-year outcomes in survivors of the acute respiratory distress syndrome. N Engl J Med 2003; 348:683–93.

Marshall RP, *et al*. Fibroproliferation occurs early in the acute respiratory distress syndrome and impacts on outcome. Am J Respir Crit Care Med 2000; 162:1783–8.

See also

Acute respiratory distress syndrome (2)

General management

1. Remove the cause whenever possible (e.g., drain pus, start antibiotic therapy, fix long-bone fracture).
2. Sedate with an opiate–benzodiazepine combination because mechanical ventilation is likely to be prolonged. Doses should be kept to the lowest possible, but consistent with adequate sedation.
3. Muscle relaxation may be indicated in severe ARDS to improve chest wall compliance, gas exchange, and tolerance to high airway pressures.
4. With regards to hemodynamic monitoring and support, no definitive hemodynamic strategy has been defined.

Respiratory management

- Maintain adequate gas exchange with increased FiO_2 and, depending on severity, either noninvasive respiratory support (e.g., CPAP, BiPAP) or invasive positive-pressure ventilation. General agreement exists for minimizing V_T (6–7 mL/kg ideal body weight) and plateau inspiratory pressures (≤30 cmH_2O) if possible. Specific modes may be utilized, such as pressure-controlled inverse ratio ventilation. Early work with high-frequency ventilation in the adult population is promising, but definitive evidence for a survival benefit does not yet exist. There is no consensus regarding the upper desired level of FiO_2 and PEEP. The ideal PEEP in patients with ARDS is unknown, and likely varies with individual patients. A recent study of PEEP levels conducted by the ARDSnet investigators showed no outcome benefit with higher PEEP levels.
- Nonventilatory respiratory support techniques such as ECMO or $ECCO_2R$ can be used in severe ARDS, but have yet to show convincing benefit over conventional ventilatory techniques.
- Blood gas values should be aimed at maintaining survival without striving to achieve normality. Permissive hypercapnia, during which pH values are allowed to decrease, sometimes to <7.2, has been associated with outcome benefit in small studies. Acceptable levels of SaO_2 are controversial. In general, values ≥90% to 95% are targeted, but in severe ARDS this may be relaxed to 80% to 85% or even lower, provided organ function remains adequate.
- Patient positioning may provide improvements in gas exchange but has not been shown to increase survival. This includes kinetic therapy using special rotational beds, and prone positioning with the patient being turned frequently through 180°. Care has to be taken during prone positioning to prevent tube displacement and shoulder injuries.
- Inhaled nitric oxide or epoprostenol improves gas exchange in some 50% of patients, although no outcome benefit has been shown.
- High-dose steroids commenced at 7 to 10 days may be beneficial in 50% to 60% of patients, at least in terms of improving gas exchange.
- Surfactant therapy is currently not indicated for ARDS.
- Ventilator trauma is ubiquitous. Multiple pneumothoraces are common and may require multiple chest drains. They may be difficult to diagnose by radiography and, despite the attendant risks, CT scanning may reveal undiagnosed pneumothoraces and aid correct placement of chest drains.

Key trials

Acute Respiratory Distress Syndrome Network. Ventilation with lower tidal volumes compared with traditional tidal volumes for acute lung injury and the acute respiratory distress syndrome. *N Engl J Med* 2000; **342**:1301–8.

ALVEOLI Trial. Higher versus lower positive end-expiratory pressures in patients with the acute respiratory distress syndrome. *N Engl J Med* 2004; **351**:327–36.

Derdak, S, Mehta S, Stewart T, *et al.* High frequency oscillatory ventilation for acute respiratory distress syndrome in adults. *Am J Respir Crit Care Med* 2002; **166**:801–8.

Gattinoni L, *et al.*, for the Prone–Supine Study Group. Effect of prone positioning on the survival of patients with acute respiratory failure. *N Engl J Med* 2001; **345**:568–73.

Hickling KG, *et al.* Low mortality rate in adult respiratory distress syndrome using low-volume, pressure-limited ventilation with permissive hypercapnia: A prospective study. *Crit Care Med* 1994; **22**:1568–78.

Meduri GU, *et al.*, Effect of prolonged methylprednisolone therapy in unresolving acute respiratory distress syndrome: a randomized controlled trial. *JAMA* 1998; **280**:159–65.

See also

Oxygen therapy, p. 2; Ventilatory support—indications, p. 4; IPPV—complications of ventilation, p. 14; Positive end expiratory pressure (1) Positive end expiratory pressure (2), p. 24; Continuous positive airway pressure, p. 26; Lung recruitment, p. 28; Prone positioning, p. 30; Extracorporeal respiratory support, p. 34; Endotracheal intubation, p. 36; Blood gas analysis, p. 102; Bacteriology, p. 158; Virology, serology, and assays, p. 160; Colloid osmotic pressure, p. 172; Colloids, p. 180; Bronchodilators, p. 186; Nitric oxide, p. 190; Surfactant, p. 192; Antimicrobials, p. 258; Steroids, p. 260; Basic resuscitation, p. 268; Acute lower respiratory tract infection (1), p. 286; Acute lower respiratory tract infection (2), p. 288; Acute respiratory distress syndrome (2), p. 292; Inhalation injury, p. 304; Infection—diagnosis, p. 482; Infection—treatment, p. 484; Systemic inflammation/multiorgan failure, p. 486; Sepsis and septic shock—treatment, p. 488; Multiple trauma (1), p. 502; Multiple trauma (2), p. 504; Pyrexia (1), p. 520; Pyrexia (2), p. 522

Asthma—general management

Pathophysiology

The pathophysiology of asthma is acute bronchospasm and mucus plugging, often secondary to an insult such as infection. The patient may progress to fatigue, respiratory failure, and collapse. The onset may develop slowly over days, or occur rapidly within minutes to hours.

Clinical features

- Dyspnea, wheeze (expiratory ± inspiratory), difficulty in talking, use of accessory respiratory muscles, fatigue, agitation, cyanosis, coma, collapse are the usual clinical features.
- Pulsus paradoxus is a poor indication of severity; a fatiguing patient cannot generate significant respiratory swings in intrathoracic pressure.
- A 'silent' chest is also a late sign suggesting severely limited airflow.
- Pneumothorax and lung/lobar collapse.

Management of asthma

Asthmatics must be managed in a well-monitored area. If clinical features are severe, they should be admitted to an ICU where rapid institution of mechanical ventilation is available. Monitoring should comprise, as a minimum, pulse oximetry, continuous ECG, regular blood pressure measurement, and blood gas analysis. If severe, an intra-arterial cannula ± central venous access should be inserted.

1. High $FiO_2 \geq 0.60$ should be used to maintain $SpO_2 \geq 95\%$
2. Nebulized β_2-agonist (e.g., albuterol) may be repeated every 2 to 4 h or, in severe attacks, administered continuously
3. IV steroids for 24 h then switch to oral. Nebulized ipratropium bromide may give additional benefit.
4. IV bronchodilators (e.g., terbutaline, magnesium sulfate).
5. Exclude pneumothorax and lung/lobar collapse.
6. Ensure adequate hydration and fluid replacement.
7. Commence antibiotics (e.g., cefuroxime ± clarithromycin) if strong evidence of bacterial infection. Green sputum does not necessarily indicate a bacterial infection.
8. If no response to previous measures or if patient is in extremis, consider
   - Epinephrine IV, SC, or by nebulizer
   - Mechanical ventilation
   - Heliox (80%He/20%O_2 or 70%He/30%O_2) to reduce viscosity and improve airflow
   - Anecdotal success has been reported with subanesthetic doses of a volatile anesthetic agent such as isoflurane, which both, calms/sedates and bronchodilates.

Indications for mechanical ventilation

- Increasing fatigue and obtundation
- Respiratory failure—increasing $PaCO_2$, decreasing PaO_2
- Cardiovascular collapse

Facilitating endotracheal intubation

Summon senior assistance. Preoxygenate with 100% oxygen. Perform rapid sequence induction with succinylcholine and etomidate or ketamine. 'Breathing down' with an inhalational anesthetic (e.g., isoflurane) preintubation should only be attempted by an experienced clinician. To minimize barotrauma, extreme care should be taken to avoid excess air trapping, high airway pressures, and high tidal volumes, especially when bagging the patient after intubation.

Table 21.4 Drug dosage

Epinephrine	0.5 mL 1:1000 solution SC
	2 mL 1:10,000 solution by nebulizer
	0.02–1 µg/kg/min IV
Hydrocortisone	100–200 mg qid
Methylprednisolone	2 mg/kg, then 0.5–1 mg/kg q6h for up to 5 days
Ipratropium bromide	250–500 µg qid by nebulizer
Prednisolone	40–60 mg qd initially
Albuterol	2.5–5 mg by nebulizer
Magnesium sulfate	1.2–2.0 g IV over 20 min

See also

Oxygen therapy, p. 2; Ventilatory support—indications, p. 4; Endotracheal intubation, p. 36; Pulse oximetry, p. 92; Blood gas analysis, p. 102; Bacteriology, p. 158; Bronchodilators, p. 186; Sedatives, p. 236; Steroids, p. 260; Dyspnea, p. 276; Asthma—ventilatory management, p. 296; Anaphylactoid reactions, p. 498

Asthma—ventilatory management

Early period

1. Initially, give low V_T (5 mL/kg) breaths at low rate (5–10 breaths/min) to assess degree of bronchospasm and air trapping. Slowly increase V_T (to 7–8 mL/kg) and/or increase rate, taking care to avoid significant air trapping and high inspiratory pressures. Low rates with prolonged I:E ratio may be advantageous. Avoid very short expiratory times. Do not strive to achieve normocapnia.
2. Administer muscle relaxants for a minimum 2 to 4 h, until severe bronchospasm has abated and gas exchange improved. Although atracurium may cause histamine release, it does not appear clinically to worsen bronchospasm.
3. Sedate with either standard medication or with agents such as ketamine or isoflurane that have bronchodilating properties. Ketamine given alone may cause hallucinations whereas isoflurane carries a theoretical risk of fluoride toxicity.
4. If significant air trapping remains, consider ventilator disconnection and forced manual chest compressions every 10 to 15 min.
5. If severe bronchospasm persists, consider injecting 1 to 2 mL 1:10,000 epinephrine down endotracheal tube or instituting a low-dose epinephrine drip.

Maintenance

1. Ensure adequate rehydration.
2. Generous humidification should be given to loosen mucus plugs. Use a heat–moisture exchanger plus either hourly 0.9% saline nebulizers or instillation of 5 mL 0.9% saline down the endotracheal tube.
3. Physiotherapy assists mobilization of secretions and removal of mucus plugs. Hyperventilation should be avoided.
4. With improvement, gradually normalize ventilator settings (V_T, rate, I:E ratio) to achieve normocapnia before allowing patient to waken and breathe spontaneously.
5. Consider pneumothorax or lung/lobar collapse if acute deterioration occurs.
6. If mucus plugging constitutes a major problem, instillation of a mucolytic (N-acetyl cysteine) may be considered, although this may induce further bronchospasm. Bronchoscopic removal of plugs should only be performed by an experienced operator.

Assessment of air trapping (PEEPi)

- Measure PEEPi using the end-expiratory hold feature on the ventilator.
- No pause between expiratory and inspiratory sounds
- An increasing $PaCO_2$ may respond to reductions in minute volume that will lower the level of PEEPi.

Weaning

- Bronchospasm may increase on decreasing sedation, resulting from awareness of endotracheal tube and increased coughing.
- May need trial of extubation while still on high FiO_2.
- Consider extubation under inhalational or short-acting IV sedation.
- Space out intervals between β-agonist nebulizers. Convert other antiasthmatic drugs to oral medication. Theophylline doses should be adjusted to ensure therapeutic levels.

See also

Oxygen therapy, p. 2; Ventilatory support—indications, p. 4; Endotracheal intubation, p. 36; Pulse oximetry, p. 92; Blood gas analysis, p. 102; Bacteriology, p. 158; Bronchodilators, p. 186; Sedatives, p. 236; Steroids, p. 260; Dyspnea, p. 276; Asthma—general management, p. 294; Anaphylactoid reactions, p. 498

Pneumothorax

Pneumothorax is a significant collection of air in the pleural space that may occur spontaneously, after trauma (including iatrogenic), with asthma, and in COPD, and is a common sequel of ventilator trauma.

Clinical features

- May be asymptomatic
- Dyspnea, pain
- Decreased breath sounds, hyperresonant, asymmetrical chest expansion—may be difficult to assess in a ventilated patient
- Respiratory failure and deterioration in gas exchange
- Increasing airway pressures and difficulty in ventilating.
- Cardiovascular deterioration with mediastinal shift (tension)

Diagnosis

- CXR—most easily seen on erect views when absent lung markings are seen lateral to a well-defined lung border. However, ventilated patients are often imaged in a supine position; pneumothorax may be easily missed because it may be laying anterior to normal lung, giving the misleading appearance of lung markings on the radiograph. Supine pneumothorax should be considered if the following are seen:
  - Hyperlucent lung field compared with the contralateral side
  - Loss of clarity of the diaphragm outline
  - 'Deep sulcus' sign, giving the appearance of an inverted diaphragm
  - A particular clear part of the cardiac contour
  - A lateral film may help. Tension pneumothorax results in marked mediastinal shift away from the affected side.
  - Ultrasound—may be helpful but is highly operator dependent
  - CT scan—very sensitive and may be useful in difficult situations (e.g., ARDS), and to direct drainage of localized pneumothorax
- Pneumothorax must be distinguished from bullae, especially with longstanding emphysema. Inadvertent drainage of a bulla may cause a bronchopleural fistula. Assistance should be sought from a radiologist.

Management

1. Increase FiO_2 if hypoxemic.
2. If life threatening with circulatory collapse, conduct needle aspiration of pleural space on affected side, followed by formal chest drain insertion.
3. Needle aspiration may be sufficient in spontaneously breathing patients without respiratory failure; however, this is not recommended if the patient is ventilated.
4. Insert chest drain. This may be done under ultrasound or CT guidance, especially if localized as a result of surrounding lung fibrosis.

A small pneumothorax (<10% hemithorax) may be left undrained, but prompt action should be instituted if cardiorespiratory deterioration occurs. Patients should not be transferred between hospitals, particularly by plane, with an undrained pneumothorax. Drains may be removed, after air leaks are no longer detected.

Bronchopleural fistula

A bronchopleural fistula is denoted by continual drainage of air. It usually responds to conservative treatment with continual application of 40 cmH₂O negative pressure; this may take weeks to resolve. For severe leak and/or compromised ventilation, HFJV and/or a double-lumen endo-bronchial tube may be considered. Surgical intervention is rarely necessary.

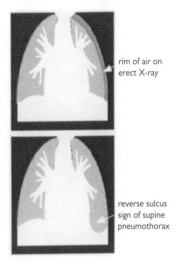

rim of air on erect X-ray

reverse sulcus sign of supine pneumothorax

Fig. 21.1 Chest X-ray appearance.

See also

IPPV—complications of ventilation, p. 14; High-frequency ventilation, p. 20; Chest drain insertion, p. 42; Central venous catheter—insertion, p. 118; Basic resuscitation, p. 268; Respiratory failure, p. 280; Acute respiratory distress syndrome (1), p. 290; Acute respiratory distress syndrome (2), p. 292; Multiple trauma (1), p. 502; Multiple trauma (2), p. 504

Hemothorax

Hemothorax is usually secondary to chest trauma or after a procedure (e.g., cardiac surgery, chest drain insertion, central venous catheter insertion). Spontaneous hemothorax is very rare, even in patients with clotting disorders.

Clinical features
- Dullness to percussion
- Decreased breath sounds
- Hypovolemia and deterioration in gas exchange (if large)

Diagnosis
- Erect CXR—blunting of hemidiaphragm and progressive loss of basal lung field
- Supine CXR—increased opacity of affected hemithorax plus decreased clarity of cardiac contour on that side
- Large-bore needle aspiration to confirm presence of blood. A small-bore needle may be unable to aspirate a hemothorax if it has clotted.

Management
1. If small, observe with serial radiographs and monitor for signs of cardiorespiratory deterioration.
2. Ensure any coagulopathy is corrected by administration of FFP and/or platelets as indicated.
3. Ensure that cross-matched blood is available for urgent transfusion if necessary.
4. If significant in size or patient becomes symptomatic, insert large-bore chest drain (e.g., 28 Fr or larger). The drain should be directed posteroinferiorly toward the dependent area of lung and placed on 40 cmH$_2$O suction.
5. If drainage exceeds 1000 mL or >200 mL/h for 3 to 4 h despite correcting any coagulopathy, contact a thoracic surgeon.
6. Factor VIIa may be considered for intractable bleeding, although only anecdotal reports of benefit exist.
7. Drains inserted for a hemothorax may be removed after 1 to 2 days if no further bleeding occurs.

Perforation of an intercostal vessel during chest drain insertion may cause considerable bleeding into the pleura. If deep tension sutures around the chest drain fail to stem blood loss, remove the chest drain and insert a Foley urethral catheter through the hole. Inflate the balloon and apply traction on the catheter to tamponade the bleeding vessel. If these measures fail, contact a thoracic surgeon.

See also

Chest drain insertion, p. 42; Central venous catheter—insertion, p. 118; Blood transfusion, p. 182; Blood products, p. 250; Coagulants and antifibrinolytics, p. 252; Aprotinin, p. 254; Pneumothorax, p. 298; Bleeding disorders, p. 398

Hemoptysis

- May range from a few specks of blood in expectorated sputum to massive pulmonary hemorrhage
- More likely to disrupt gas exchange before life-threatening hypovolemia ensues
- May be a presenting feature of a patient admitted to intensive care or may result from critical illness and its treatment

Causes

Massive hemoptysis

- Disruption of a bronchial artery by acute inflammation or invasion (e.g., pulmonary neoplasm, trauma, cavitating TB, bronchiectasis, lung abscess, and aspergilloma)
- Rupture of AV malformations and bronchovascular fistulas
- Pulmonary infarction secondary to prolonged pulmonary artery catheter wedging or pulmonary artery rupture

Minor hemoptysis

- Intrapulmonary inflammation or infarction (e.g., pulmonary embolus)
- Endotracheal tube trauma (e.g., mucosal erosion, balloon necrosis, trauma from the tube tip, trauma to a tracheostomy stoma, trauma from suction catheters)
- Tissue breakdown in critically ill patients (e.g., tissue hypoperfusion, coagulopathy, poor nutritional state, sepsis, and hypoxemia)

Investigation and assessment

Urgent assessment of cardiorespiratory function and cardiorespiratory monitoring are required. Massive hemoptysis may require resuscitation and urgent intubation. The diagnosis may be suggested by the history, and a CXR may identify a cavitating lesion. Lower lobe shadowing on a CXR may be the result of overspill of blood from elsewhere in the bronchial tree. Early surgical intervention should be prompted by a changing air–fluid level, persistent opacification of a previous cavity, or a mobile mass. Early bronchoscopy may identify the source of hemoptysis, although only while bleeding is active. Blood in multiple bronchial orifices may be confusing, but saline lavage may leave the source visible. Rigid bronchoscopy is useful in massive hemoptysis, allowing oxygenation and large-bore suction.

Management

- Basic resuscitation (high FiO_2, endotracheal intubation, and blood transfusion) is needed for cardiorespiratory compromise.
- Correction of coagulopathy is a priority.
- Early bronchoscopy is an essential part of management and allows for localization and the direct instillation of 1:200,000 epinephrine if the source of hemorrhage can be found or, alternatively, endobronchial tamponade with a balloon catheter.
- In cases of severe hemorrhage from one lung, a double-lumen endotracheal tube may prevent some overspill to the other lung while definitive treatment is organized.

- Definitive treatment may include radiological bronchial artery embolization or surgical resection.
- Induced hypotension may be useful in bronchial artery hemorrhage.
- In cases of pulmonary artery hemorrhage, PEEP may be used with mechanical ventilation to reduce pulmonary bleeding.
- If possible, position patient with bleeding side down.

See also

Oxygen therapy, p. 2; Ventilatory support—indications, p. 4; Positive end-expiratory pressure (1), p. 22; Positive end-expiratory pressure (2), p. 24; Continuous positive airway pressure, p. 26; Endotracheal intubation, p. 36; Fiberoptic bronchoscopy, p. 46; Blood transfusion, p. 182; Blood products, p. 250; Coagulants and antifibrinolytics, p. 252; Basic resuscitation, p. 268; Acute lower respiratory tract infection (1), p. 286; Acute lower respiratory tract infection (2), p. 288; Pulmonary embolus, p. 306; Bleeding disorders, p. 398; Amniotic fluid embolus, p. 546

Inhalation injury

Causes of inhalation injury include smoke, steam, noxious gases, and aspiration of gastric contents.

Clinical features
- Dyspnea, coughing
- Stridor (if upper airway obstruction)
- Bronchospasm
- Signs of lung/lobar collapse (especially with aspiration)
- Signs of respiratory failure
- Cherry-red skin color (carbon monoxide)
- Agitation, coma
- ARDS (late)

General principles of management
- One hundred percent oxygen
- Early intubation if upper airway compromised or threatened
- Early bronchoscopy if inhalation of soot, debris, vomit suspected

Specific conditions
Smoke inhalation
- Smoke rarely causes thermal injury beyond the level of bronchi because it has a low specific heat content. However, soot is a major irritant to the upper airways and can produce very rapid and marked inflammation.
- Urgent laryngoscopy should be performed if soot is present in the nares, mouth, or pharynx.
- If soot is seen or the larynx appears inflamed, perform early endotracheal intubation. Because the upper airway can obstruct within minutes, it is advisable to intubate as a prophylactic measure rather than as an emergency, when it may prove impossible.
- After intubation, perform urgent bronchoscopy with bronchial toilet using warmed 0.9% saline to remove as much soot as possible.
- Effect specific treatment for poisons contained within smoke (e.g., carbon monoxide, cyanide)

Steam inhalation
- Consider early/prophylactic intubation.
- Steam has a much higher heat content than smoke and can cause injury to the whole respiratory tract.
- Consider early bronchoscopy and lavage with cool 0.9% saline.

Aspiration of gastric contents
- Conduct early bronchoscopy and physiotherapy to remove as much particulate and liquid matter as possible.
- Consider antibiotic therapy with either a cephalosporin plus metronidazole, or a penicillin/penicillinase inhibitor (i.e., piperacillin tazobactam, ampicillin–sulbactam, or ticarcillin clavulanate) for 3 to 5 days.
- Steroid therapy has no benefit.

See also

Oxygen therapy, p. 2; Ventilatory support—indications, p. 4; Endotracheal intubation, p. 36; Fiberoptic bronchoscopy, p. 46; Blood gas analysis, p. 102; Antimicrobials, p. 258; Airway obstruction, p. 278; Inhaled poisons, p. 468; Burns—fluid management, p. 512; Burns—general management, p. 514

Pulmonary embolus

Etiology

- Usually arises from DVT in femoral or pelvic veins. The risk increases after prolonged immobilization and with polycythemia or hyperviscosity disorders
- Amniotic fluid embolus
- Fat embolus after pelvic or long-bone trauma
- Right heart source (e.g., mural thrombus)

Clinical features

- Pleuritic-type chest pain, dyspnea, ± hemoptysis
- The patient with a major embolus often prefers to lie flat. Dyspnea improves as a result of increased venous return and right heart loading.
- Deterioration in gas exchange—may find a low PaO_2, low or high $PaCO_2$, and metabolic acidosis. However, these findings are inconsistent and nondiagnostic.
- Cardiovascular features (e.g., tachycardia, low/high blood pressure and collapse)
- CXR—may be normal but a massive embolus may produce fewer vascular markings (pulmonary oligemia) in a hemithorax ± a bulging pulmonary hilum. A wedge-shaped peripheral pulmonary infarct may be seen a few days later after a smaller embolus.
- ECG—acute right ventricular strain (i.e., $S_1Q_3T_3$, tachycardia, right-axis deviation, RBBB, P pulmonale)
- Echocardiogram—may reveal evidence of pulmonary hypertension and acute right ventricular strain
- D-dimers—although an increased level is nondiagnostic, a normal value carries a high probability of exclusion of a pulmonary embolus.

Definitive diagnosis

- CT scan with contrast—the investigation of choice for major embolus
- Pulmonary angiography
- Ventilation–perfusion scan—Degree of certainty is reduced if area of nonperfused lung corresponds to any CXR abnormality.
- Fat globules or fetal cells in pulmonary artery blood may be found in fat and amniotic fluid embolus respectively.

General management

- FiO_2 0.6 to 1.0 to maintain SaO_2 ≥90% to 95%
- Lay patient flat; improvement often follows increased venous return.
- Fluid challenge to optimize right heart filling
- Epinephrine infusion if circulation still compromised
- Mechanical ventilation may be needed if the patient tires or cannot maintain adequate oxygenation. Gas exchange may worsen because of loss of preferential shunting and decreases in cardiac output.

Management of blood clot embolus

Start anticoagulation with low-molecular weight heparin or an unfractionated heparin infusion adjusted for weight. Consider thrombolysis if there is a major embolus and cardiovascular compromise, and embolectomy if the patient remains moribund. Otherwise, at 24 to 48 h commence warfarin but continue heparin for another 2 to 3 days after adequate oral dosing.

Management of fat embolus

Other than general measures including oxygenation, fluid resuscitation, and right heart loading, treatment remains controversial. Various authorities advocate steroids, heparinization, or no specific therapy.

Low-molecular weight heparin regimen

SC low-molecular weight heparin is given until oral anticoagulant therapy is fully established.

Enoxaparin

1 mg/kg/dose q12h or 1.5 mg/kg once daily

Tinzaparin

175 U/kg body weight anti-Xa once daily

Unfractionated heparin regimen

IV heparin is given until oral anticoagulant therapy is fully established. Administer 80-U/kg bolus (do not exceed 8,000 U initial bolus) followed by an 18-U/kg/h drip (not to exceed 1,800 U/h initial drip) and titrated to achieve PTT two to three times normal.

Thrombolytic regimens

rt-PA (100 mg over 120 min) should be given followed by a heparin infusion to maintain the PTT at two to three times normal. This is the treatment of choice if surgery or angiography is contemplated.

Streptokinase (500,000 U) should be given as a loading dose over 30 min followed by an infusion (100,000 U/h for 24 h).

NB: Central venous catheters should ideally be inserted pre-thrombolysis by an experienced operator to minimize the risk of bleeding/hematoma.

Key trial

Konstantinides S, for the Management Strategies and Prognosis of Pulmonary Embolism-3 Trial Investigators. Heparin plus alteplase compared with heparin alone in patients with submassive pulmonary embolism. *N Engl J Med* 2002; **347**:1143–50.

Cardiovascular disorders

Hypotension

The overall principle in the management of hypotension is to maintain the minimum MAP that will ensure adequate tissue perfusion. A normal blood pressure does not guarantee an adequate cardiac output, and circulatory support should aim to achieve adequate blood flow as well. In extremis, the first-line treatment options should include external cardiac massage and epinephrine 0.05 to 0.2 mg IV boluses (1 mg in cardiac arrest).

Assessment of hypotension

Hypotension requires treatment if the mean blood pressure is <60 mmHg (higher if the patient was previously hypertensive) with signs of poor tissue perfusion (e.g., oliguria, confusion, altered consciousness, cool peripheries, metabolic acidosis). Specific treatment should be considered for hemorrhage, AMI, arrhythmias, pulmonary embolus, cardiac tamponade, pneumothorax, anaphylaxis, diarrhea and vomiting, ketoacidosis, hypoadrenalism, hypopituitarism, and poisoning.

Initial treatment of hypotension

Most cases of hypotension require fluid as first-line management to confirm an adequate circulating volume. Exceptions may include acute heart failure, arrhythmias, cardiac tamponade, and pneumothorax. In cases of life-threatening hemorrhage, group-specific (if available) or O-negative blood should be used urgently.

Pharmacological treatment

If hypotension persists after circulating volume, rate, and rhythm have been restored, the appropriate choice of drug treatment depends on whether there is myocardial failure (signs of low output or measured low stroke volume) or peripheral vascular failure (warm, vasodilated periphery or measured normal stroke volume). A low stroke volume should be treated with an inotrope (e.g., epinephrine, dobutamine), and peripheral vascular failure should be treated with a vasopressor (e.g., norepinephrine).

Inotropic support

Epinephrine (started at 0.2 µg/kg/min), or dopamine or dobutamine (started at 5 µg/kg/min) should be titrated against stroke volume. Most hypotensive patients requiring inotropes should have a pulmonary artery catheter inserted, or some other method of monitoring cardiac output should be used. The alternative is to titrate against blood pressure, but there is a danger of producing inappropriate vasoconstriction. Dobutamine is safer in this respect but has the disadvantage of producing excessive vasodilatation in some patients.

Vasopressors

After stroke volume has been optimized, norepinephrine (started at 0.05 µg/kg/min) should be titrated against mean blood pressure. In most patients with previously normal blood pressure, 60 mmHg is an adequate target, but may need to be higher to ensure organ perfusion in the elderly and in those with previous hypertension. Norepinephrine may reduce cardiac output in individual patients, but can also result in modest increases in cardiac output resulting from its β agonist effect. This effect should be monitored and corrected by adjustment of dose.

Vasopressin (0.01–0.04 U/min) is increasingly used for high output and catecholamine-resistant vasodilatory shock. Care should be taken to avoid excessive peripheral constriction or impairment of organ perfusion.

See also

Hypertension

Hypertension is often defined in adult patients as a diastolic pressure >95 mmHg and a systolic pressure >180 mmHg.

Common causes in intensive care

- Idiopathic/essential
- Agitation/pain, especially when muscle relaxants are used
- Excessive vasoconstriction (e.g., cold, vasopressor drugs)
- Head injury, CVAs
- Drug related
- Dissecting aneurysm, aortic coarctation
- Vasculitis, TTP
- (Pre-)eclampsia
- Aortic coarctation (may present acutely in adulthood)
- Endocrine (e.g., pheochromocytoma [rare])
- Renal failure, renal artery stenosis (rare)
- Spurious—underdamped transducer system

Indications for acute treatment

Hypertensive encephalopathy, heart failure, eclampsia, and acute dissecting aneurysm are the prime indications for rapid and aggressive, albeit controlled, reduction of blood pressure.

In other conditions, especially chronic hypertension and after acute neurological events such as head injury and CVAs, a precipitate reduction in blood pressure may adversely affect perfusion, leading to further deterioration. Hypertension after a cerebral event is not usually treated unless very high (e.g., mean blood pressure >140–150 mmHg, systolic blood pressure >220–230 mmHg. In this instance, controlled and partial reduction is mandatory (e.g., using sodium nitroprusside infusion with continuous invasive monitoring). In the presence of increased ICP, a CPP of ≥60 to 70 mmHg is usually targeted.

Hypertensive crisis

A hypertensive crisis occurs when the patient becomes symptomatic (increasing drowsiness, seizures, papilledema, retinopathy) in the presence of elevated systemic pressures. The diastolic blood pressure usually exceeds 120 to 130 mmHg and the mean blood pressure is >140–150 mmHg, although encephalopathy can occur at lower pressures.

Principles of management

1. Provide adequate monitoring (invasive blood pressure, ECG, central venous pressure, cardiac output, urine output).
2. Consider pain, hypovolemia, hypothermia, and agitation, especially if paralyzed.
3. Consider specific treatment for, for example, pheochromocytoma, thyroid crisis, aortic dissection, and inflammatory vasculitis.
4. Initiate a slow IV infusion of nitrate or nitroprusside. Other options include labetalol or esmolol infusions, and hydralazine (IV or IM) (see Table 22.1). To avoid precipitate decreases in blood pressure, use these agents cautiously and start with low doses.

5. Aim to reduce to mildly hypertensive levels unless a dissecting aneurysm is present, when systolic blood pressure should be lowered to <100 to 110 mmHg. After certain types of surgery (e.g. cardiac, aortic), control of systolic blood pressure <100 to 120 mmHg may be requested to reduce risk of bleeding.
6. Longer term treatment (e.g., an oral ACE inhibitor) should be instituted with caution, starting at low doses.

Table 22.1 Drug doses

Drug	Dose
Sodium nitroprusside	0.5–1.5 µg/kg/min, increased slowly to 0.5–8.0 g/kg/min
Labetalol	10–50 mg IV over 1 min repeated every 5 min to maximum 200 mg; can be followed by a drip between 0.5–2 mg/min
Esmolol	50–200 µg/kg/min
Hydralazine	5–10 mg slow IV followed by 50–150 µg/min

See also

IPPV—failure to tolerate ventilation, p. 12; Blood pressure monitoring, p. 112; Intracranial pressure monitoring, p. 134; Vasodilators, p. 198; Hypotensive agents, p. 202; Opioid analgesics, p. 232; Nonopioid analgesics, p. 234; Sedatives, p. 236; Intracranial hemorrhage, p. 378; Subarachnoid hemorrhage, p. 380; Increased ICP, p. 384; Pain, p. 534; Preeclampsia and eclampsia, p. 540; HELLP syndrome, p. 542

Tachyarrhythmias

If pulses are not palpable or there is severe hypotension, a tachyarrhythmia requires cardiac massage and urgent DC cardioversion. Otherwise, the initial treatment prior to diagnosis includes correction of hypoxemia, potassium (to ensure a plasma K^+ >4.5 mmol/L), and magnesium (often to levels of 4–5 mg/dL).

Causes of tachyarrhythmias

When possible, the cause of a tachyarrhythmia should be treated. Common causes for which specific treatment may be required include hypovolemia, hypotension (may also be the result of the arrhythmia), AMI, pain, anemia, hypercapnia, fever, anxiety, thyrotoxicosis, and digoxin toxicity.

Diagnosis of tachyarrhythmias

Broad-complex tachycardia

Regular complexes with AV dissociation (fusion beats, capture beats, QRS >140 ms, axis <−30°, concordance) suggest VT. If there is no AV dissociation, the arrhythmia is probably supraventricular with aberrant conduction; adenosine may be used as a diagnostic test because SVT may respond and VT will not. Irregular broad complexes are probably atrial fibrillation with aberration. Torsades de pointes is a form of VT with a shifting or 'turning' axis.

Narrow-complex tachycardia

The absence of P waves suggests atrial fibrillation. A P-wave rate of >150 is suggestive of SVT, whereas slower P-wave rates may represent a sinus tachycardia or atrial flutter with block. The P waves are abnormal (flutter waves) in atrial flutter, and QRS complexes may be irregular if the block is variable. Extremely fast SVT may be the result of a reentry pathway with retrograde conduction and premature ectopic atrial excitation. In Wolff–Parkinson–White syndrome, the reentry pathway inserts below the His bundle, allowing rapid AV conduction and reentry tachyarrhythmias. This may be diagnosed by a short PR interval and a delta wave.

Treatment of tachyarrhythmias

VT

Lidocaine (often ineffective), amiodarone, or magnesium form the mainstay of drug treatment (see Table 22.2). Overdrive pacing may be used if a pacing wire is in situ, capturing the ventricle at a pacing rate higher than the arrhythmia and gradually reducing the pacing rate. Torsades de pointes may be exacerbated by antiarrhythmics, so magnesium or overdrive pacing are safest.

SVT and atrial flutter

Carotid sinus massage may be used in patients with no risk of calcified atheromatous carotid deposits. Amiodarone, adenosine, or magnesium are usually the most useful drugs in the critically ill (see Table 22.2). Verapamil may be used if complexes are narrow (no risk of misdiagnosed VT), although it and other AV node blockers must be avoided in reentry tachycardias.

Atrial fibrillation

Acute or paroxysmal atrial fibrillation should be treated as for SVT. Digoxin is more useful for chronic atrial fibrillation and does not prevent paroxysmal episodes.

Table 22.2 Drug dosages and cautions

Adenosine	3 mg IV as a rapid bolus in a large, preferably central, vein; if no response in 1 min give 6 mg followed by 12 mg.
Verapamil	2.5 mg IV slowly; if no response, repeat to a maximum of 20 mg. An IV infusion of 1–10 mg may be used. A total of 10 mL CaCl 10% should be available to treat hypotension associated with verapamil. Verapamil must be avoided in reentry tachyarrhythmias because ventricular response may increase. Life-threatening hypotension may occur in misdiagnosed VT, and life-threatening bradycardia may occur if the patient has been β blocked.
Lidocaine	1 mg/kg IV as a bolus followed by an infusion of 2–4 mg/min. Avoid prolonged use because toxicity may cause seizures.
Amiodarone	For VT, 150–300 mg IV over 10 minutes followed by an infusion at 1 mg/min for 6 hours then 0.5 mg/min for 18 hours. For atrial fibrillation, slower IV loading is advisable. May cause hypotension. Avoid with other class III agents (e.g., sotalol) because QT interval may be severely prolonged.
Magnesium	1–4 g MgSO$_4$ over 20–30 min; in an emergency, 1 g may be given over 2–3 min.

See also

Defibrillation, p. 52; ECG monitoring, p. 110; Antiarrhythmics, p. 204; Basic resuscitation, p. 268; Cardiac arrest, p. 270; Fluid challenge, p. 272; Hypotension, p. 310; Acute coronary syndrome (1), p. 318; Hyperkalemia, p. 422; Hypokalemia, p. 424; Thyroid emergencies, p. 448; Tricyclic antidepressant poisoning, p. 462; Anemia, p. 402; Pyrexia (1), p. 520; Pyrexia (2), p. 522; Pain, p. 534

Bradyarrhythmias

If peripheral pulses are not palpable, a bradyarrhythmia requires external cardiac massage and treatment as for asystole. For asymptomatic brady-cardia, treatment may not be required other than close monitoring and correction of the cause. The exception to this is higher degrees of heart block occurring after an acute anterior MI when pacing may be required prophylactically.

Causes of bradyarrhythmias

When possible, the cause of a bradyarrhythmia should be treated. Common causes for which specific treatment may be required include hypovo-lemia, hypotension (may also be the result of the arrhythmia), AMI, digoxin toxicity, β-blocker toxicity, hyperkalemia, hypothyroidism, hypop-ituitarism, and increased ICP. Digoxin toxicity may require treatment with antidigoxin antibodies.

Diagnosis of bradyarrhythmias

Sinus bradycardia
Sinus bradycardia is defined as a slow ventricular rate with normal P waves, normal PR interval, and 1:1 AV conduction

Heart block
Normal P waves, a prolonged PR interval, and 1:1 AV conduction suggest first-degree heart block. In second-degree heart block, the ventricles fail to respond to atrial contraction intermittently. This may be associated with regular P waves and an increasing PR interval until ventricular depo-larization fails (Mobitz I or Wenckebach) or a normal PR interval with regular failed ventricular depolarization (Mobitz II). In the latter case, the AV conduction ratio may be 2:1 to 5:1. In third-degree heart block, there is complete AV dissociation with a slow idioventricular rate.

Absent P-wave bradycardia
Absent P waves may represent slow atrial fibrillation or sinoatrial dys-function. In the latter case, there will be a slow idioventricular rate.

Treatment of bradyarrhythmias

Hypoxemia must be corrected in all symptomatic bradycardias. First-line drug treatment is usually atropine 0.3 mg or glycopyrrolate 200 µg IV. If the arrhythmia fails to respond, 0.6 mg followed by 1.0 mg atropine may be given. Failure to respond to drugs requires temporary pacing. This may be accomplished rapidly with an external system if there is hemody-namic compromise, or transvenously. Other indications for temporary pacing are listed in the next section. Higher degrees of heart block after an anterior myocardial infarction will usually require permanent pacing.

Indications for temporary pacing
- Persistent symptomatic bradycardia
- Syncope associated with
  - Third-degree heart block
  - Second-degree heart block
  - RBBB and left posterior hemiblock

- Cardiovascular collapse
- Inferior MI with symptomatic third-degree heart block
- Anterior MI with
  - Third-degree heart block
  - RBBB and left posterior hemiblock
  - Alternating RBBB and LBBB

See also

Temporary pacing (1), p. 54; Temporary pacing (2), p. 56; ECG monitoring, p. 110; Chronotropes, p. 206; Basic resuscitation, p. 268; Cardiac arrest, p. 270; Acute coronary syndrome (1), p. 318; Thyroid emergencies, p. 448; Hypothermia, p. 518

Acute coronary syndrome (1)

Principles of management of uncomplicated myocardial infarct

- Oxygen—to maintain SaO_2 ≥98%
- Good venous access
- Continuous ECG monitoring
- Adequate pain relief
- Early thrombolysis plus aspirin (heparin if using rt-PA)
- Early β blockade
- Gradual mobilization

Complications of MI

- Cardiopulmonary arrest
- Continuing chest pain—may be ischemic or pericarditic in origin
- Pump failure
- Hypotension—apart from cardiogenic shock consider hypovolemia (e.g., postdiuretics) and a thrombolytic reaction
- Tachyarrhythmias/bradyarrhythmias
- Valve dysfunction—predominantly mitral
- Pericardial tamponade (rare)
- Ventricular septal defect (unusual, often presents 2 to 5 days after infarct)
- Complications of thrombolytic therapy—arrhythmias, bleeding, anaphylactoid reaction

Management of complicated MI

General

- Oxygen to maintain SaO_2 ≥98%.
- Appropriate and prompt monitoring and investigations as indicated (e.g., echocardiogram, pulmonary artery catheter, angiography, ECG).
- Early thrombolysis. rt-PA followed by heparin should be given in preference to streptokinase if invasive procedures and/or surgery are contemplated (see Table 22.3).
- Arterial or central venous cannulation should not be delayed if clinically indicated. These procedures should be performed by an experienced operator to minimize the risk of bleeding. The subclavian route should be avoided.
- Angioplasty or revascularization surgery is beneficial if performed early. Cardiology consultation should be sought promptly if a patient is admitted in pump failure, continuing pain, or valvular dysfunction.

Specific

- Cardiopulmonary arrest—CPR and consider therapeutic hypothermia
- Continuing chest pain
- If ischemic—IV nitrate and heparin infusions, aspirin, clopidogrel, calcium antagonist and β blocker (unless contraindicated); consider urgent angiography (see Table 22.3)
- If pericarditic—consider nonsteroidal antiinflammatory agent
- Management of heart failure—also consider IABP (intra-aortic balloon pump)

- Tachyarrhythmia—antiarrhythmics, synchronized DC cardioversion
- Bradycardias—chronotrope; consider temporary pacing
- Valve dysfunction—heart failure management; consider surgery
- Pericardial tamponade—pericardial aspiration
- Ventricular septal defect—heart failure management, consider surgery
- Thrombolystic complications

Table 22.3 Drug dosage

Morphine	1–2 mg IV; repeat PRN (consider antiemetic)
Streptokinase	1.5 million U in 100 mL 0.9% saline IV over 1 h
rt-PA (alteplase)	15-mg bolus, then 0.75 mg/kg (max, 50 mg) over 30 min, then 0.5 mg/kg (max, 35 mg) over 60 min
Reteplase	10 U IV and another 10 U IV 30 min later
Aspirin	162–325 mg PO
Clopidogrel	75 mg (consider 300 mg PO × 1 for ACS)
Atenolol	50 mg PO qd (increase to 100 mg qd if not hypotensive and heart rate exceeds 70 bpm) or 5-mg slow IV bolus
Metoprolol	25–50 mg PO bid (titrate to heart rate of 60 bpm)
Isosorbide dinitrate	2–40 mg/h IV
Nitroglycerin	10–200 µg/min IV or 0.5–1 mg SL or paste
Diltiazem	60 mg PO tid
Nifedipine	5–10 mg SL or PO tid
Atropine	0.3 mg IV; repeat to maximum of 2 mg
Lidocaine	1-mg/kg slow IV bolus then 2–4 mg/min
Amiodarone	150–300 mg in 10–20 mL 5% glucose over 3 min then 1mg/min × 6 hours, then 0.5mg/min × 18 hours

Key papers

Task Force for Management of Acute Myocardial Infarction of the European Society of Cardiology. Management of acute myocardial infarction in patients presenting with ST segment elevation. *Eur Heart J* 2003; **24**:28–66.

See also

Acute coronary syndrome (2)

Angina

Angina is ischemic or, rarely, a spasmodic constriction of the coronary arteries resulting in pain, usually precordial, pressing or crushing, and ± radiation to the jaw, neck, or arms. The sedated, ventilated patient will not usually complain of pain, but signs of discomfort may be apparent (e.g., sweating, hypertension, tachycardia). The ECG should be regularly scrutinized for ST-segment and/or T-wave changes.

Unstable angina encompasses a spectrum of syndromes between stable angina and MI. Anginal attacks may be increased in frequency and/or severity, persist longer, respond less to nitrates, and occur at rest or after minimal exertion.

Pathophysiology

- Myocardial oxygen supply–demand imbalance is usually the result of coronary artery atheroma ± disruption of plaque or new nonocclusive thrombus formation. Spasm (Prinzmetal angina) is uncommon.
- Vasopressor drugs may compromise myocardial perfusion by further constricting an already stenosed vessel.
- Vasodilator drugs may also compromise myocardial perfusion by a 'coronary steal' phenomenon during which blood flow is redistributed away from stenosed vessels.

Diagnosis

- Symptoms, especially chest pain but also nonspecific (e.g., sweating)
- ECG changes—ST segment elevation/depression, T-wave inversion
- No increase in cardiac enzymes or troponin above the MI threshold
- Dyskinetic areas of myocardium may be seen on echocardiography or angiography

Treatment

- Ensure adequate oxygenation.
- Correct hypotension and tissue hypoperfusion.
- Consider drug causes (e.g., vasopressors).
- Administer nitroglycerin 0.5 mg SL, or nitrolingual spray (0.4–0.8 mg) repeated as necessary.
- If symptoms are severe and/or persisting, maintain bed rest.
- Administer aspirin 75 mg qd PO (unless contraindicated).

For continuing angina

- IV nitrate infusion (e.g., nitroglycerin, isosorbide trinitrate)
- Consider calcium antagonist (e.g., diltiazem, although not alone)
- Consider β blocker (unless contraindicated; (e.g., propranolol, atenolol)
- Low-molecular weight heparin and clopidogrel (unless contraindicated)
- Consider GP2b3a (glycoprotein 2b3a) inhibitor (IV eptifibatide or tirofiban) in addition to aspirin and clopidogrel if considered at high risk of MI or death
- If symptoms or ST-segment changes persist despite optimal pharmacological intervention, inform cardiologist with a view to angiography and possible angioplasty or surgery

Key trial

Yusuf S, for the Clopidogrel in Unstable Angina to Prevent Recurrent Events Trial Investigators. Effects of clopidogrel in addition to aspirin in patients with acute coronary syndromes without ST-segment elevation. *N Engl J Med* 2001; **345**:494–502.

Heart failure—assessment

Heart failure is the impaired ability of the heart to supply adequate oxygen and nutrients to meet the demands of the body's metabolizing tissues.

Major causes

Investigations used to diagnose heart failure are listed in Table 22.4

- MI/ischemia
- Drugs (e.g., β blockers, cytotoxics)
- Tachy- or bradyarrhythmias
- Valve dysfunction
- Sepsis
- Septal defect
- Cardiomyopathy/myocarditis
- Pericardial tamponade

Clinical features

Decreased forward flow leading to poor tissue perfusion

- Muscle fatigue leading ultimately to hypercapnia and collapse
- Confusion, agitation, drowsiness, coma
- Oliguria
- Increasing metabolic acidosis, arterial hypoxemia, and dyspnea

Increased venous congestion secondary to right heart failure

- Peripheral edema
- Hepatic congestion
- Splanchnic ischemia
- Increased ICP

Increased pulmonary hydrostatic pressure secondary to left heart failure

- Pulmonary edema, dyspnea
- Hypoxemia

Table 22.4 Investigations

Test	Diagnosis
ECG	Myocardial ischemia/MI, arrhythmias
CXR	With left heart failure, pulmonary edema (interstitial perihilar ('bat's wing') shadowing, upper lobe blood diversion, Kerley B lines, pleural effusion) ± cardiomegaly
Pulmonary artery catheter	Low cardiac output and stroke volume, low mixed venous oxygen saturation (<60%), increased PAWP (with left heart failure), increased RAP (right artrial pressure) (with right heart failure), V waves with mitral or tricuspid regurgitation
Blood tests	Low SaO_2, variable $PaCO_2$, base deficit >2 mmol/L; hyperlactatemia; low venous O_2 (mixed or central venous); increased cardiac enzymes, troponin, and BNP; check thyroid function if indicated
Echocardiogram	Poor myocardial contractility, pericardial effusion, valve stenosis/incompetence

Notes

Peripheral edema implies total-body salt and water retention but not necessarily intravascular fluid overload.

See also

Heart failure—management

Basic measures

1. Determine likely cause (see Table 22.4) and treat as appropriate (e.g., antiarrhythmic).
2. Oxygen—to maintain SaO_2 ≥98%
3. Nitroglycerin SL then commence IV nitrate infusion titrated rapidly until good clinical effect. Beware hypotension that, at low dosage, is suggestive of left ventricular underfilling (e.g., hypovolemia, tamponade, mitral stenosis, pulmonary embolus).
4. If patient is agitated or in pain, give morphine IV.
5. Consider early CPAP, BiPAP, and/or IPPV to reduce work of breathing and provide good oxygenation. Cardiac output will often improve. Do not delay until the patient is in extremis.
6. Furosemide is rarely needed as first-line therapy unless intravascular fluid overload is causative. Initial symptomatic relief is provided by its prompt vasodilating action; however, subsequent diuresis may result in marked hypovolemia, leading to compensatory vasoconstriction, increased cardiac work, and worsening myocardial function. Diuretics may be indicated for acute-on-chronic failure, especially if the patient is on long-term diuretic therapy, but should not be used if hypovolemic. If furosemide is required, start at low doses then reassess.

Directed management

1. Adequate monitoring (e.g., pulmonary artery catheterization) and investigation (echocardiography).
2. If evidence exists for hypovolemia, give 100 to 200 mL colloid fluid challenges to achieve optimal stroke volume.
3. If vasoconstriction persists (SVR (systemic vascular resistance) >1400 dyne/s/cm^5) in the face of reduced cardiac output, consider increasing nitrate infusion further to optimize stroke volume and to reduce SVR. If hypovolemia is suspected (i.e., stroke volume decreases), fluid challenges should be given to reoptimize the stroke volume. Within 24 h of nitrate infusion, commence ACE inhibition, initially at low dose but rapidly increase to appropriate long-term doses.
4. Inotropes are indicated if evidence of tissue hypoperfusion, hypotension, or vasoconstriction persists despite optimal fluid loading and nitrate dosing. Consider epinephrine, dobutamine, or milrinone. Although epinephrine may sometimes cause excessive constriction, dobutamine and milrinone may excessively vasodilate. Levosimendan increases cardiac output, although not at the expense of increased cardiac work.
5. Intra-aortic balloon counterpulsation augments cardiac output, reduces cardiac work, and improves coronary artery perfusion.
6. Angioplasty or surgical revascularization are beneficial if performed early after MI. Surgery may also be necessary for mechanical defects (e.g., acute mitral regurgitation).

Treatment end points

1. Blood pressure and cardiac output adequate to maintain organ perfusion (e.g., no oliguria, confusion, dyspnea, or metabolic acidosis).

A mean blood pressure of 60 mmHg is usually sufficient but may need to be higher, especially if premorbid blood pressures are high.

2. A mixed venous oxygen saturation ≥60%. Excessive inotropes should be avoided as myocardial oxygen demand is increased.

3. Symptomatic relief.

Table 22.5 Drug dose

Nitroglycerin	2–40 mg/h IV or 0.5–1 mg SL
Isosorbide dinitrate	2–40 mg/h IV
Nesiritide	2-µg/kg bolus followed by infusion of 0.01–0.03 µg/kg/min
Sodium nitroprusside	20–400 µg/min IV
Captopril	6.25-mg PO test dose increasing to 25 mg tid
Enalapril	2.5-mg PO test dose increasing to 40 mg qd
Lisinopril	2.5-mg PO test dose increasing to 40 mg qd
Epinephrine	Infusion starting from 0.05 µg/kg/min
Dobutamine	2.5–25 µg/kg/min IV
Dopamine	2.5–25 µg/kg/min IV
Milrinone	Loading dose (if needed) of 50 µg/kg IV over 10 min followed by infusion from 0.375–0.75 µg/kg/min
Morphine	1–2 mg IV, repeat every 5 min as necessary
Furosemide	10–40-mg IV bolus, repeat or increase as necessary

Key trials

Cotter G, et al. Randomised trial of high-dose isosorbide dinitrate plus low-dose furosemide versus high-dose furosemide plus low-dose isosorbide dinitrate in severe pulmonary oedema. Lancet 1998; **351**:389–93.

Cuffe MS, et al. Rationale and design of the OPTIME CHF trial: Outcomes of a prospective trial of intravenous milrinone for exacerbations of chronic heart failure. Am Heart J 2000; **139**:15–22.

Follath F, et al. Efficacy and safety of intravenous levosimendan compared with dobutamine in severe low-output heart failure (the LIDO study): A randomised double-blind trial. Lancet 2002; **360**:196–202.

See also

Oxygen therapy, p. 2; Ventilatory support—indications, p4; Positive end expiratory pressure (1), p. 22; Positive end expiratory pressure (2), p. 24; Continuous positive airway pressure, p. 26; Inotropes, p. 196; Vasodilators, p. 198; Vasopressors, p. 200; Antiarrhythmics, p. 204; Chronotropes, p. 206; Basic resuscitation, p. 268; Fluid challenge, p. 272; Heart failure—assessment, p. 322

Renal disorders

Oliguria

A number of definitions for oliguria can be found in the literature, in general ranging from a urine output of <200 to 500 mL in 24 h. To standardize the use of the term across different studies and populations, the Acute Dialysis Quality Initiative (ADQI) has recently adopted a definition of oliguria as urine out <0.3 mL/kg/h for at least 24 h (www.ADQI.net).

- Postrenal—urinary tract obstruction (e.g., blocked catheter, ureteric trauma, prostatism, increased intra-abdominal pressure, blood clot, bladder tumor
- Renal—established acute renal failure, acute tubular necrosis, glomerulonephritis
- Prerenal—hypovolemia, low cardiac output, hypotension, inadequate renal blood flow

Obstruction and prerenal causes of oliguria must be excluded before diagnosing renal failure (see Table 23.1).

Urinary tract obstruction

A full bladder should be excluded by palpation. Ensure a patent catheter is present. If obstruction is the result of blood clot, the bladder should be irrigated. If obstruction is suspected higher in the renal tract, an ultrasound scan is required for diagnosis and possible urological intervention (e.g., nephrostomy). Increased intra-abdominal pressure (abdominal compartment syndrome) may cause oliguria by impeding renal venous drainage (particularly if >20 mmHg). Relief of the high pressure often promotes diuresis.

Hypovolemia

After renal tract obstruction is excluded, it is mandatory to correct hypovolemia by fluid challenge. Oliguria in hypovolemic patients may be a physiological response or the result of reduced renal blood flow.

Inadequate renal blood flow and/or pressure

If cardiac output remains low despite correction of hypovolemia, correction with vasodilators (afterload reduction) and/or inotropes will be necessary. If the blood pressure remains low after improving the cardiac output, vasopressors may be needed to achieve a mean blood pressure of at least 60 mmHg. In elderly patients and others with preexisting hypertension, a higher mean blood pressure may be necessary to maintain renal perfusion and urine output.

Volume overload

Attempts to increase urine output with diuretics should only be directed toward treatment of volume overload or hyperkalemia, not oliguria per se. Large observation studies have failed to show benefit from diuretics in critically ill patients with oliguria, and some studies have shown harm. Diuretics should never be used until after the previous measures have been tried. A loop diuretic such as furosemide is given in a dose of 20–40 mg IV. If this dose is ineffective, a higher dose can be tried in 30 to 60 min. Higher doses may be needed if the patient has previously received diuretic therapy. If bolus doses of 80 mg every 6 h are infective, an infusion may be started (1–5 mg/h IV). A thiazide diuretic such as chlorothiazide (250–500 mg IV) or metolazone (10–20 mg PO) can be used in conjunction with a loop diuretic to improve diuresis (see Table 23.2). Failure to reestablish urine output may require renal support in the form of dialysis or hemofiltration. There is no point in continuing diuretic therapy if it is not effective; loop diuretics in particular may be nephrotoxic. Indications for renal support include fluid overload, hyperkalemia, metabolic acidosis, creation of space for nutrition or drugs, persistent renal failure with increasing urea and creatinine, and symptomatic uremia.

Table 23.1 Biochemical assessment

	Prerenal cause	Renal cause
Urine osmolality (mOsmol/kg)	>500	<400
Urine Na (mmol/L)	<20	>40
Urine-to-plasma creatinine	>40	<20
Fractional Na excretion*	<1	>2

$$*\ \ \frac{100\ \text{Urine-to-plasma}\ [Na^+]}{\text{Urine-to-plasma}\ [\text{Creatinine}]}$$

Table 23.2 Drug dosage

	Oral	IV	Infusion
Metolazone	10–20 mg qd		
Chlorothiazide		250–500 mg IV	
Furosemide	20–40 mg q 6–24 h	5–80 mg q 6–24 h	1–10 mg/h
Torsemide	5–20 mg q 6–24 h	5–20 mg q 6–24 h	1–5 mg/h
Bumetanide	0.5–1 mg q 6–24 h	0.5–2 mg q 6–24 h	1–5 mg/h

See also

Acute renal failure—diagnosis

Renal failure is defined as renal function inadequate to clear the waste products of metabolism despite the absence of or correction of hemodynamic or mechanical causes. Clinical manifestations of renal failure include

- Uremic symptoms (drowsiness, nausea, hiccough, twitching)
- Increased plasma creatinine
- Hyperkalemia
- Hyponatremia
- Metabolic acidosis

For research purposes, international consensus criteria for acute renal failure have been purposed. The acronym RIFLE is used to describe three levels of renal impairment (risk, injury, failure) and two clinical outcomes (loss and end-stage kidney disease). The classification system includes separate criteria for serum creatinine and urine output. The criteria, which lead to the worst possible classification, should be used. Note that RIFLE-F is present even if the increase in serum creatinine is more than three fold, as long as the new serum creatinine level is <4.0 mg/dL in the setting of an acute increase of at least 0.5 mg/dL.

Persistent oliguria may be a feature of acute renal failure but nonoliguric renal failure is not uncommon. Two to 3 L of poor-quality urine per day may occur despite an inadequate glomerular filtration rate. The prognosis is better if urine output is maintained. Clinical features may suggest the cause of renal failure and dictate further investigation. Acute tubular necrosis is a common etiology in the critically ill (e.g., after hypovolemia, extensive burns), but other causes must be borne in mind. In sepsis, the kidney often has a normal histological appearance.

Postoperative renal failure

Risk factors for postoperative renal failure include hypovolemia, hemodynamic instability (particularly hypotension), major abdominal surgery, and sepsis. Surgical procedures (particularly gynecological) may be complicated by damage to the lower urinary tract with an obstructive nephropathy. Abdominal aortic aneurysm surgery may be associated with renal arterial disruption.

Other causes

- Nephrotoxins—may cause renal failure via acute tubular necrosis, interstitial nephritis, or renal tubular obstruction. All potential nephro-toxins should be withdrawn.
- Rhabdomyolysis—suggested by myoglobinuria and increased CPK (creatine phosphokinase) in patients who have sustained a crush injury, coma, or seizures
- Glomerular disease—red cell casts, hematuria, proteinuria, and systemic features (e.g., hypertension, purpura, arthralgia, vasculitis) are all suggestive of glomerular disease. Renal biopsy or specific blood tests (e.g., Goodpasture's syndrome, vasculitis) are required to confirm diagnosis and appropriate treatment.
- Hemolytic uremic syndrome—suggested by hemolysis, uremia, thrombocytopenia, and neurological abnormalities

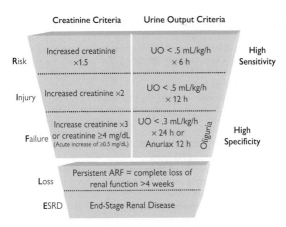

	Creatinine Criteria	Urine Output Criteria	
Risk	Increased creatinine ×1.5	UO < .5 mL/kg/h × 6 h	High Sensitivity
Injury	Increased creatinine ×2	UO < .5 mL/kg/h × 12 h	
Failure	Increase creatinine ×3 or creatinine ≥4 mg/dL (Acute increase of ≥0.5 mg/dL)	UO < .3 mL/kg/h × 24 h or Anuriax 12 h	High Specificity
Loss	Persistent ARF = complete loss of renal function >4 weeks		
ESRD	End-Stage Renal Disease		

Fig. 23.1 RIFLE criteria for acute renal failure Uo, urine output; ARF, acute renal failure.

- Crystal nephropathy—suggested by the presence of crystals in the urinary sediment. Microscopic examination of the crystals confirms the diagnosis (e.g., urate, oxalate). Release of purines and urate are responsible for acute renal failure in tumor lysis syndrome.
- Renovascular disorders—Loss of vascular supply may be diagnosed by renography. Complete loss of arterial supply may occur in abdominal trauma or aortic disease (particularly dissection). More commonly, the arterial supply is partially compromised (e.g., renal artery stenosis) and blood flow is further reduced by hemodynamic instability or locally via drug therapy (e.g., NSAIDs, ACE inhibitors). Renal vein obstruction may be to the result of thrombosis or external compression (e.g., increased intra-abdominal pressure).

Nephrotoxins

The following are some common nephrotoxins:

Allopurinol	Aminoglycosides
Amphotericin	Furosemide
Dextran 40	Herbal medicines
Heavy metals	NSAIDs
Organic solvents	Paraquat
Sulfonamides	Pentamidine
Thiazides	Radiographic contrast

See also

Urinalysis, p. 166; Fluid challenge, p. 272; Hypotension, p. 310; Oliguria, p. 328; Acute renal failure—management, p. 332; Bowel perforation and obstruction, p. 346; Abdominal sepsis, p. 348; Pancreatitis, p. 354; Acute liver failure, p. 360; Hemolysis, p. 406; Platelet disorders, p. 408; Sepsis and septic shock—treatment, p. 488; Malaria, p. 494; Rheumatic disorders, p. 496; Vasculitides, p. 498; Multiple trauma (1), p. 502; Multiple trauma (2), p. 504; Burns—fluid management, p. 512; Burns —general management, p. 514; Postoperative intensive care, p. 536

Acute renal failure—management

Identification and correction of reversible causes of renal failure are crucial. All cases require careful attention to fluid management and nutritional support. Dialysis and/or filtration techniques will make space for adequate fluid and nutritional intake.

Urinary tract obstruction

Lower tract obstruction requires the insertion of a catheter (suprapubic if there is urethral disruption) to allow decompression. Ureteric obstruction requires urinary tract decompression by nephrostomy or stent. A massive diuresis is common after decompression, so it is important to ensure adequate circulating volume to prevent secondary prerenal failure.

Hemodynamic management

Prerenal failure is reversible before it becomes established. Careful fluid management to ensure an adequate circulating volume and any necessary inotrope or vasopressor support may establish a diuresis.

Metabolic management

Hyperkalemia may be life threatening (>6.5 mmol/L or ECG changes) and may be prevented by potassium restriction, early dialysis, or hemofiltration. Hypocalcemia and hyponatremia are best treated with dialysis and/or hemofiltration, although calcium supplementation may be necessary. Hyponatremia is usually the result of water excess, although salt-losing nephropathies (acute tubular necrosis, other renal tubular disorders) may also occur. Hyperphosphatemia may be treated with dialysis, filtration or oral phosphate binding agents. Metabolic acidosis (not the result of tissue hypoperfusion) may be corrected with dialysis, filtration. Oral sodium bicarbonate supplementation may be used particularly in more chronic cases.

Nephrotoxins and crystal nephropathies

All nephrotoxic agents should be withheld if possible. All necessary drugs should have their dosage modified according to the glomerular filtration rate. Dialysis may also be useful.

Glomerular disease

Immunosuppressive therapy may be useful after diagnosis has been confirmed. Dialysis is often required for the more severe forms of glomerulonephritis despite steroid responsiveness.

Urgent treatment of hyperkalemia

- 10–20 mL calcium chloride 10% by slow IV injection
- 100 mL 8.4% sodium bicarbonate IV
- Glucose 50 g and insulin 10 to 20 U IV with careful blood glucose monitoring and urgent hemodialysis

Renal replacement therapy

Continuous hemofiltration forms the mainstay of replacement therapy in critically ill patients who often cannot tolerate hemodialysis because of hemodynamic instability. Peritoneal dialysis is not commonly used today and usually is insufficient. Mortality in the setting of acute renal failure in the critically ill is high (50% to 60%), but it usually recovers within 1 to 6 weeks in surviving patients. Permanent renal failure is rare.

General indications for dialysis or CRRT

- Fluid excess (e.g., pulmonary edema)
- Hyperkalemia (>6.0 mmol/L)
- Metabolic acidosis (pH <7.2) resulting from renal failure
- Clearance of dialyzable nephrotoxins and other drugs
- Uremic symptoms
- To create space for nutrition or drugs

See also

Continuous renal replacement therapy (1), p. 62; Continuous renal replacement therapy (2), p. 66; Peritoneal dialysis, p. 68; Crystalloids, p. 176; Colloids, p. 180; Diuretics, p. 212; Dopamine, p. 214; Basic resuscitation, p. 268; Fluid challenge, p. 272; Oliguria, p. 328; Acute renal failure—diagnosis, p. 330; Hyperkalemia, p. 422; Hyponatremia, p.420; Hypocalcemia, p.430; Metabolic acidosis, p.436

Gastrointestinal disorders

Vomiting/gastric stasis

Although vomiting per se is relatively rare in the ICU patient, large-volume gastric aspirates are commonplace and probably represent the major reason for failure of enteral nutrition.

Ileus

Ileus affects the stomach more frequently than the rest of the gastro intestinal tract. Abdominal surgery, drugs (particularly opiates), gut dysfunction as a component of multiorgan dysfunction, hypoperfusion, and prolonged starvation may all contribute to gastric ileus. Early and continued use of the bowel for feeding appears to maintain forward propulsive action. Management consists of treating the cause when possible, the use of motility stimulants such as metoclopramide or erythromycin and, in resistant cases, bypassing the stomach with a nasoduodenal/nasojejunal tube or a jejunostomy.

Upper bowel obstruction

Upper bowel obstruction is relatively unusual. Apart from primary surgical causes such as neoplasm or adhesions, the predominant cause in the ICU is gastric outlet obstruction. This may be related to long-standing peptic ulcer disease or may occur in the short term from pyloric and/or duodenal swelling consequent to gastritis or duodenitis. This can be diagnosed endoscopically and treated by bowel rest plus an H_2 antagonist, proton pump inhibitor, or sucralfate.

Gastric irritation

Drugs or chemicals—either accidental or adverse reaction (e.g., steroids, aspirin), intentional (e.g., alcohol, bleach), or therapeutic (e.g., syrup of ipecac)—may induce vomiting. Treatment, when appropriate, may comprise removal of the cause, dilution with copious amounts of fluid, neutralization with alkali and/or H_2 antagonist or proton pump inhibitor, and administration of antiemetic (e.g., metoclopramide).

Neurological

Stimulation of the emetic center may follow any neurological event (e.g., trauma, CVA), drug therapy (e.g., chemotherapy), pain, and metabolic disturbances. Management is by treating the cause when possible and by judicious use of antiemetics, initially metoclopramide or prochlorperazine. Consider ondansetron or granisetron if these are unsuccessful.

See also

Diarrhea

The definition of diarrhea in the ICU patient is problematic because the amount of stool passed daily is difficult to measure. Frequency and consistency may also vary significantly. Loose/watery and frequent (four or more times a day) stool will often require investigation and/or treatment.

Common ICU causes

- Infection—*Clostridium difficile*, gastroenteritis (e.g., *Salmonella, Shigella*), rarer tropical causes (e.g., cholera, dysentery, giardiasis, tropical sprue)
- Drugs (e.g., antibiotics, laxatives)
- Gastrointestinal—feed (e.g., lactose intolerance), celiac disease, other malabsorption syndromes, inflammatory bowel disease, diverticulitis, pelvic abscess, bowel obstruction with overflow. Enteral feed is often implicated, but rarely causative
- For bloody diarrhea—infection, ischemic, or inflammatory bowel disease

Diagnosis

- Rectal examination to rule out impaction with overflow. Consider sigmoidoscopy if colitis or *C. difficile* suspected (pseudomembrane seen).
- Stool sent to laboratory for MC&S, *C. difficile* toxin.
- Fat estimation (malabsorption) is rarely necessary in the ICU patient.
- If ischemic or inflammatory bowel disease suspected, perform a supine abdominal radiograph and inspect for dilated loops of bowel (NB: toxic megacolon), thickened walls (increased separation between loops), and 'thumbprinting' (suggestive of mucosal edema). Fluid levels seen on erect or lateral abdominal radiograph may be seen in diarrhea or paralytic ileus and do not necessarily indicate obstruction. Diarrhea is often but not always bloody.
- If abscess suspected, perform ultrasonography or CT scan.

Management

1. Treat cause when possible (e.g., for *C. difficile*, metronidazole ± a probiotic agent).
2. Consider temporary (12–24 h) cessation of enteral feed if very severe. Consider change in feed if appropriate (e.g., celiac disease, lactose intolerance).
3. Consider stopping antibiotics.
4. Give antidiarrheal if infection excluded.
5. Pay careful attention to fluid and electrolyte balance (in particular, Na^+, K^+, Mg^{2+}).
6. Request surgical opinion if infarcted or inflamed bowel or abscess suspected.

See also

Enteral nutrition, p. 82; Antidiarrheals, p. 226; Antimicrobials, p. 258; Abdominal sepsis, p. 348; Infection—diagnosis, p. 482

Failure to open bowels

Common ICU causes

- Prolonged ileus/decreased gut motility (e.g., opiates, postsurgery)
- Lack of enteral nutrition
- Bowel obstruction—relatively uncommon secondary event, mainly seen postoperatively, either after a curative procedure or with development of adhesions

Management

1. Clinically exclude obstruction and confirm presence of stool PR.
2. Ensure adequate hydration.
3. Consider reducing/stopping dose of opiate if possible.
4. Anticonstipation therapy may be given, usually starting with laxatives (e.g., lactulose or, for more urgent response, magnesium citrate), then proceeding to suppositories and, finally, enemata if gentler measures prove unsuccessful.

See also

Anticonstipation agents, p. 228; Opioid analgesics, p. 232; Bowel perforations and obstruction, p. 346; Abdominal sepsis, p. 348

Upper gastrointestinal hemorrhage

Causes
- Peptic ulceration
- Esophagitis/gastritis/duodenitis
- Varices
- Mallory–Weiss lower esophageal tear
- Neoplasms

Pathophysiology
Peptic ulceration is related to protective barrier loss leading to acid or biliary damage of the underlying mucosa and submucosa. Barrier loss occurs secondary to critical illness, alcohol, drugs (e.g., nonsteroidals), and poisons (including corrosives). Direct damage, especially at the lower esophagus, may occur from feeding tubes. Mucosal damage ('stress ulcers') may also occur as a consequence of tissue hypoperfusion. Gastric hypersecretion is uncommon in critically ill patients; indeed, gastric acid content and secretion is often reduced.

Prophylaxis
- Small-bore feeding tubes
- Enteral nutrition
- Adequate tissue perfusion (flow and pressure)
- Patients at highest risk for stress ulcers are those requiring prolonged mechanical ventilation or those with a concurrent coagulopathy. Proton pump inhibitors have no role in the prophylaxis of stress ulcers.

Treatment of major hemorrhage
- Fluid resuscitation with volume expanders and blood with blood products as appropriate to correct any coagulopathy. Maintain Hb between 7 to 10 g/dL and have adequate cross-matched blood available should further large hemorrhages occur.
- If possible, discontinue any ongoing anticoagulation (e.g., heparin).
- Urgent diagnostic endoscopy. Local injection of epinephrine or a sclerosant into (or thermal sealing of) a bleeding peptic ulcer base may halt further bleeding. Likewise, banding or sclerosant injection may arrest bleeding varices.
- If esophageal varices are known or highly suspected, start octreotide (IV bolus of 50 µg followed by continuous infusion of 50 µg/h). Consider placing a balloon tamponade tube for severe hemorrhage, either as a bridge to endoscopy or if banding/injection is unsuccessful (should not be attempted by inexperienced personnel). Remember that sources of bleeding other than varices may be present (e.g., peptic ulcer).
- For peptic ulceration and generalized inflammation, commence a proton pump inhibitor. Give IV to ensure effect. Enteral antacid may also be beneficial.
- Surgery is rarely necessary but should be considered if bleeding continues (e.g., >6–10 U transfusion required). Inform a surgeon promptly of any patient with major bleeding.

See also

Bleeding varices

Varices develop after a prolonged period of portal hypertension, usually related to liver cirrhosis. Approximately one third will bleed. They are commonly found in the lower esophagus, but occasionally in the stomach or duodenum. Torrential hemorrhage may occur. Approximately 50% of patients die within 6 weeks of presentation of their first bleed; each subsequent bleed carries a 30% mortality.

Management

1. If airway and/or breathing are compromised, perform early endotracheal intubation and institute mechanical ventilation. This facilitates endoscopy or balloon tamponade tube placement but may be associated with severe hypotension secondary to covert hypovolemia. If possible, ensure adequate intravascular filling before intubation.

2. Fluid resuscitation with colloid (consider albumin) and blood with blood products as appropriate to correct any coagulopathy. Ensure good venous access (at least two 14-G cannulas). Group-specific or O-negative blood may be needed for emergency use. Maintain Hb approximately 7 to 10 g/dL and have at least 4 U of cross-matched blood available for urgent transfusion. There is a theoretical risk that overtransfusion may precipitate further bleeding by increasing portal venous pressure. Cardiac output monitoring should be considered if the patient remains hemodynamically unstable or there is a history of heart disease.

3. If bleeding is torrential, insert a balloon tamponade tube and commence administration of IV octreotide.

4. Gentle placement of a large-bore nasogastric tube is a reasonably safe procedure that facilitates drainage of blood, lessens the risk of aspiration, and can be used to assess continuing blood loss.

5. Perform urgent fiberoptic endoscopy to exclude other sources of bleeding. This also permits variceal banding or local injection of a sclerosing agent. Bleeding is arrested in up to 90% of cases. Endoscopy may be impossible in the short term if bleeding is too severe. It may have to be delayed for 6 to 24 h until a period of tamponade by the balloon tamponade tube ± octreotide has enabled some control of the bleeding.

6. Either octreotide or vasopressin can be administered for severe bleeding, or prophylaxis against fresh bleeding (see Table 24.1). Vasopressin controls bleeding in approximately 60% of cases, and its efficacy and safety may be enhanced by concurrent nitroglycerin. Octreotide is the preferred agent. It is a somatostatin analogue but is longer acting than its parent compound. Like somatostatin, it is as effective as vasopressin but without the side effects.

7. If bleeding continues after balloon tamponade and repeated endoscopy, consider transjugular intrahepatic portosystemic stented shunt. This can be performed quickly and carries a relatively low mortality comp-ared with surgery, although the risk of encephalopathy is increased.

8. Spontaneous bacterial peritonitis should be considered in the setting of variceal bleeding, and should be treated with the addition of a third-generation cephalosporin until the ascitic fluid can be analyzed.

Table 24.1 Drug dosages

Octreotide	50 μg bolus then 50 μg/h infusion
Vasopressin	20 U over 20 min then 0.4 U/min infusion; also give nitro-glycerin 2–20 mg/h to counteract myocardial and mesenteric ischemia

See also

Endotracheal intubation, p. 36; Balloon tamponade tube, p. 74; Upper gastrointestinal endoscopy, p. 76; Coagulation monitoring, p. 156; Colloids, p. 180; Blood transfusion, p. 182; Basic resuscitation, p. 268; Fluid challenge, p. 272; Upper gastrointestinal hemorrhage, p. 342; Acute liver failure, p. 360; Chronic liver failure, p.364

Bowel perforation and obstruction

Patients with bowel perforation or obstruction may be admitted to the ICU after surgery, for preoperative resuscitation and cardiorespiratory optimization, or for conservative management. Although rarely occurring de novo in the ICU patient, these conditions may be difficult to diagnose because of sedation ± muscle relaxation. Consider when there is

- Abdominal pain, tenderness, peritonitis
- Abdominal distension
- Agitation
- Increased nasogastric aspirates, vomiting
- Increasing metabolic acidosis
- Signs of hypovolemia or sepsis

A firm diagnosis is often not made until laparotomy, although supine and either erect or lateral abdominal radiographs may reveal either free gas in the peritoneum (perforation) or dilated bowel loops with multiple fluid levels (obstruction). Abdominal CT may provide more information. Ultrasound is usually unhelpful, although fecal fluid may occasionally be aspirated from the peritoneum after perforation.

It may be difficult to distinguish bowel obstruction from a paralytic ileus because (1) bowel sounds may be present or absent in either and (2) X-ray appearances may be similar.

Management

1. Correct fluid and electrolyte abnormalities. Resuscitation should be prompt and aggressive and usually consists of colloid replacement plus blood to maintain Hb at >7g/dL. Inotropes or vasopressors may be required to restore an adequate circulation, particularly after perforation. Adjunctive tools to assess the adequacy of resuscitation should be considered if the circulatory status remains unstable or vasoactive drugs are required.
2. The surgeon should be informed early. A conservative approach may be adopted (e.g., with upper small bowel perforation); however, surgery is usually required for large bowel perforation. Small or large bowel obstruction may sometimes be managed conservatively because spontaneous resolution may occur (e.g., adhesions). Prompt exploration should be encouraged if the patient shows signs of systemic toxicity.
3. Both conservative and postoperative management of perforation and obstruction usually require continuous nasogastric drainage to decompress the stomach, nil by mouth The timing of and site for (proximal vs. distal) feeding after surgical repair of perforation remain controversial.
4. Pain relief should not be withheld.
5. Broad-spectrum antibiotic therapy should be commenced for bowel perforation after appropriate specimens have been taken for laboratory analysis. Therapy usually comprises aerobic and anaerobic Gram-negative coverage (e.g., second- or third-generation cephalosporin, quinolone or carbapenem, plus metronidazole ± aminoglycoside).

6. Postoperative management of bowel perforation may involve repeated laparotomies to exclude collections of pus and bowel ischemia/infarction. Surgery should be expedited if the patient's condition deteriorates. Alternatively, regular imaging ± drainage of collections may be needed.

See also

Parenteral nutrition, p. 84; Failure to open bowels, p. 340; Abdominal sepsis, p. 348; Pancreatitis, p. 354; Metabolic acidosis, p. 436; Systemic inflammation/multiorgan failure, p. 486; Postoperative intensive care, p. 536

Lower intestinal bleeding and colitis

Causes of lower gastrointestinal bleeding

- Bowel ischemia/infarction
- Inflammatory bowel disease (ulcerative colitis, Crohn's disease)
- Infection (e.g., *Shigella*, *Campylobacter*, amebic dysentery)
- Upper gastrointestinal source (e.g., peptic ulceration)
- Angiodysplasia
- Neoplasm

Although relatively rare, massive lower gastrointestinal hemorrhage can be life threatening.

Ischemic/infarcted bowel

Ischemic/infarcted bowel can occur after prolonged hypoperfusion or, occasionally, secondary to a mesenteric embolus. It usually presents with severe abdominal pain, bloody diarrhea, and signs of systemic toxicity including rapidly increasing metabolic acidosis. Plasma phosphate levels may also be elevated. X-ray appearances of thickened, edematous bowel loops ('thumbprinting') with an increased distance between bowel loops are suggestive. Treatment is by restoration of tissue perfusion, blood transfusion to maintain Hb >7 g/dL, and, if clinical features fail to settle promptly, laparotomy with a view to bowel excision.

Inflammatory bowel disease

Inflammatory bowel disease presents with weight loss, abdominal pain, and diarrhea that usually contains blood. Complications of ulcerative colitis include perforation and toxic megacolon, whereas complications of Crohn's disease include fistulas, abscesses, and perforations.

Management involves

1. Fluid and electrolyte replacement
2. Blood transfusion to maintain hemoglobin >7 g/dL
3. High-dose steroids IV and, if distal bowel involvement, by enema
4. Nutrition (occasionally parenteral)
5. Regular surgical review. Surgery may be indicated if symptoms fail to settle after 5 to 7 days for toxic megacolon, perforation, abscesses, or obstruction.
6. Antidiarrheal drugs should be avoided.

Angiodysplasia

Angiodysplasia usually presents as fresh bleeding PR, and it may be considerable. It is the result of an AV malformation and is more common in the elderly. Localization and embolization by angiography may be curative during active bleeding, Surgery may be required if bleeding fails to settle on conservative management and, occasionally, 'blind' laparoscopic embolization of a mesenteric vessel. However, localization of the lesion may be difficult at laparotomy, necessitating extensive bowel resection.

See also

Colloids, p. 180; Blood transfusion, p. 182; Coagulants and antifibrinolytics, p. 252; Basic resuscitation, p. 268; Fluid challenge, p. 272; Bowel perforation and obstruction, p. 346; Bleeding disorders, p. 398

Abdominal sepsis

Abdominal sepsis is a common but difficult-to-diagnose condition in intensive care patients. A proportion of such patients are admitted after laparotomy, but others may develop abdominal sepsis de novo or as a secondary complication after abdominal surgery—in particular, after bowel resection. Sepsis may either be localized to an organ (e.g., cholecystitis) or the peritoneal cavity (abscess). Alternatively, there may be a generalized peritonitis. Nonbowel infection or inflammation can present in a similar manner (e.g., pancreatitis, cholecystitis, gynecological infection, pyelonephritis).

Clinical features

- Nonspecific signs including pyrexia, neutrophilia, decreasing platelet count, increasing metabolic acidosis, circulatory instability
- Abdominal distension ± localized discomfort, peritonitis
- Abdominal mass (e.g., gall bladder, pseudocyst, abscess)
- Failure to tolerate enteral feed/large nasogastric aspirates
- Pleural effusion (if subdiaphragmatic sepsis)
- Diarrhea (if pelvic sepsis)

Diagnosis

- History and physical examination
- Ultrasound
- CT scan
- Laparotomy

Samples should be taken for microbiological analysis from blood, urine, stool, abdominal drain fluid, and vaginal discharge if present. A sample of pus is preferred to a swab. Hyperamylasemia may suggest pancreatitis, although amylase levels can also be elevated with other intra-abdominal pathologies.

Treatment

- Antibiotic therapy providing Gram-negative and anaerobic coverage (e.g., second- or third-generation cephalosporin, quinolone or carbapenem, plus metronidazole ± aminoglycoside). Treatment can be amended depending on culture results and patient response.
- Ultrasonic or CT-guided drainage of pus
- Laparotomy with removal of pus, peritoneal lavage, and so on

A negative laparotomy should be viewed as a useful means of excluding intra-abdominal sepsis rather than an unnecessary procedure. Laparotomy should be encouraged if the patient deteriorates and a high suspicion of abdominal pathology persists.

Cholecystitis, with or without (acalculous) gallstones, may present with signs of infection. There is a characteristic ultrasound appearance of an enlarged organ with a thickened, edematous wall surrounded by fluid. Treatment is often conservative with antibiotics (as mentioned earlier) and percutaneous, ultrasound-guided drainage via a pigtail catheter. Cholecystectomy is rarely necessary in the acute situation unless the gall bladder has perforated, although some authorities argue that this is the treatment of choice for acalculous cholecystitis.

See also

Parenteral nutrition, p. 84; Bacteriology, p. 158; Colloids, p. 180; Inotropes, p. 196; Vasopressors, p. 200; Antimicrobials, p. 258; Basic resuscitation, p. 268; Fluid challenge, p. 272; Bowel perforation and obstruction, p. 346; Pancreatitis, p. 354; Infection—diagnosis, p. 482; Infection—treatment, p. 484; Systemic inflammation/multiorgan failure, p. 486; Sepsis and septic shock treatment, p. 552; Pain, p. 534; Postoperative intensive care, p. 536

Pancreatitis

Pancreatitis is defined as inflammation of the pancreas and surrounding retroperitoneal tissues. The appearance of the pancreas may range from mildly edematous to hemorrhagic and necrotizing. A pseudocyst may develop that can become infected, and the bile duct may be obstructed, causing biliary obstruction and jaundice. Although mortality is quoted at 5% to 10%, it is much higher (approximately 40%) in those with severe pancreatitis requiring intensive care.

Causes
- Alcohol
- Gallstones
- Miscellaneous (e.g., ischemia, trauma, viral, hyperlipidemia)
- Part of the multiple-organ failure syndrome

Diagnosis
- Nonspecific features include central, severe abdominal pain; pyrexia; hemodynamic instability; vomiting; ileus. Discoloration around the umbilicus (Cullen's sign) or flanks (Grey Turner's sign) is rarely seen.
- Plasma enzymes—elevated levels of amylase (usually >1000 IU/mL) and pancreatic lipase are suggestive but nonspecific. Levels may be normal, even in severe pancreatitis.
- Ultrasound
- CT scan
- Laparotomy

Complications
- Multiorgan dysfunction syndrome
- Infection/abscess formation
- Hypocalcemia
- Diabetes mellitus
- Bleeding

Management
- General measures including aggressive fluid resuscitation, respiratory support, analgesia, and antiemetics. Adequate monitoring should be instituted if cardiorespiratory instability is present.
- Although some authors recommend empiric treatment with carbapenem, recent meta-analysis shows that prophylactic antibiotics do not prevent infected necrosis or death in acute necrotizing pancreatitis.
- The patient is conventionally kept nil by mouth with continuous nasogastric drainage, and parenteral nutrition. However, recent studies show safety and efficacy of distal nasojejunal feeding.
- Gallstone obstruction should be relieved either endoscopically or surgically.
- Hypocalcemia, if symptomatic, should be treated by intermittent, slow IV injection (or, occasionally, infusion) of 10% calcium chloride.
- Hyperglycemia should be controlled by a continuous insulin infusion.

- No specific treatment is routinely used.
- The role and extent of surgery remains controversial. Some advocate percutaneous drainage of infected and/or necrotic debris whereas surgery frequently consists of regular laparotomy with debridement of necrotic tissue and peritoneal lavage. Pseudocysts may resolve or require drainage either percutaneously or into the bowel.

Ranson's signs of severity in acute pancreatitis
On hospital admission
- Age >55 years
- Blood glucose >200 mg/dL
- Serum LDH >300 U/L
- Serum AST >250 U/L
- White blood count >16×10^9 /L

At 48 h after admission
- Hematocrit decrease >10%
- BUN increase ≥5 mg/dL
- Serum calcium <8 mg/dL
- PaO_2 <60 mmHg
- Arterial base deficit >4 mmol/L
- Estimated fluid sequestration >6000 mL

Pancreatitis is severe if more than two criteria are met within 48 h of admission.

CT severity index
CT scanning is probably the most helpful means to assess the severity of acute pancreatitis, particularly when results are combined with the Ranson score. (See Table 24.2).

Table 24.2 CT severity index (Balthazar score) in acute pancreatitis

Element	Finding	Score
Grade of acute pancreatitis	Normal pancreas	0
	Pancreatic enlargement	1
	Inflammation involving pancreas and peripancreatic fat	2
	Single fluid collection or phlegmon	3
	Two or more fluid collections or phlegmons	4
Degree of pancreatic necrosis	No necrosis	0
	Necrosis of one third of pancreas	2
	Necrosis of one half of pancreas	4
	Necrosis of more than one half of pancreas	6

CT severity index = (points for grade of acute pancreatitis) + (points for degree of pancreatic necrosis). Minimum score 0; maximum score, 10.

Severity index	Mortality (%)	Complications (%)
0–1	0	0
2–3	3	8
4–6	6	35
7–10	17	92

Key articles

Balthazar EJ, Robinson DL, *et al.* Acute pancreatitis: Value of CT in establishing prognosis. *Radiology* 1990; **174**:331–6.
Mazaki T, Ishii Y, Takayama T. Meta-analysis of prophylactic antibiotic use in acute necrotizing pancreatitis. *Br J Surg* 2006; **93**:674–84.

See also

Ventilatory support—indications, p. 4; Enteral nutrition, p. 82; Parenteral nutrition, p. 84; Basic resuscitation, p. 268; Fluid challenge, p. 272; Respiratory failure, p. 280; Acute respiratory distress syndrome (1), p. 290; Acute respiratory distress syndrome (2), p. 292; Hypotension, p. 310; Oliguria, p. 328; Abdominal sepsis, p. 348; Metabolic acidosis, p. 436; Systemic inflammation/multiorgan failure, p. 486; Sepsis and septic shock—treatment, .p. 488; Pain, p. 534

Hepatic disorders

Jaundice

Jaundice is a clinical diagnosis of yellow pigmentation of sclera and skin resulting from increased plasma bilirubin. It is usually visible when the plasma bilirubin exceeds 2 mg/dL.

Common causes seen in the ICU

- Prehepatic—intravascular hemolysis (e.g., drugs, malaria, hemolytic uremic syndrome), Gilbert's syndrome
- Hepatocellular—critical illness, viral (e.g., hepatitis A, B, C, Epstein–Barr), alcohol, drugs (e.g., acetaminophen, halothane), toxoplasmosis, leptospirosis
- Cholestatic—critical illness, intrahepatic causes (e.g., drugs such as chlorpromazine, erythromycin, and isoniazid; primary biliary cirrhosis), extrahepatic causes (e.g., biliary obstruction by gallstones, neoplasm, pancreatitis)

Diagnosis

- Urinalysis—unconjugated bilirubin does not appear in the urine
- Measurement of conjugated and unconjugated bilirubin. Conjugated bilirubin predominates in cholestatic jaundice, unconjugated bilirubin in prehepatic jaundice, and a mixed picture is often seen in hepatocellular jaundice.
- Plasma alkaline phosphatase is usually markedly elevated in obstructive jaundice whereas PTs, aspartate transaminase, and ALT are elevated in hepatocellular jaundice.
- Ultrasound or CT scan will diagnose extrahepatic biliary obstruction.

Management

1. Identify and treat cause. When possible, discontinue any drug that could be implicated. If extrahepatic, consider percutaneous transhepatic drainage, bile duct stenting, or, rarely, surgery.
2. Liver biopsy is rarely necessary in a jaundiced ICU patient unless the diagnosis is unknown and the possibility exists of liver involvement in the underlying pathology, (e.g., malignancy).
3. Nonobstructive jaundice usually settles with conservative management as the patient recovers.
4. An antihistamine and topical medications may provide symptomatic relief for pruritus if troublesome. Cholestyramine 4 g tid PO may be helpful in obstructive jaundice.

See also
Liver function tests, p. 152; Acute liver failure, p. 360; Chronic liver failure, p. 364; Hemolysis, p. 406; Infection control—general principles, p. 478; Infection—diagnosis, p. 482; Infection—treatment, p. 484; Systemic inflammation/multiorgan failure, p. 486; HELLP syndrome, p. 542

Acute liver failure

Acute liver failure results from massive necrosis of liver cells leading to severe liver dysfunction and encephalopathy. Survival rates for liver failure with grade 3 or 4 hepatic encephalopathy vary from 10% to 40% on medical therapy alone, to 60% to 80% with orthotopic liver transplantation.

Major causes

- Alcohol
- Drugs, particularly acetaminophen overdose
- Viral hepatitis, particularly hepatitis B, hepatitis C
- Poisons (e.g., carbon tetrachloride)
- Acute decompensation of chronic disease (e.g., after infection or surgery)

Diagnosis

- Should be considered in any patient presenting with jaundice, generalized bleeding, encephalopathy, or unexplained hypoglycemia
- Abnormal liver function tests, in particular, prolonged PT or INR and hyperbilirubinemia. In severe liver failure, plasma enzyme levels may not be elevated.

Management

- General measures include fluid resuscitation and blood transfusion to keep Hb at 7 to 10 g/dL. The circulation is usually hyperdynamic and dilated; vasopressors may be needed to maintain an adequate blood pressure.
- Correction of coagulopathy is often withheld because this provides a good guide to recovery or the need for transplantation. Use of FFP is restricted to patients who are bleeding or are about to undergo an invasive procedure.
- Adequate monitoring should be instituted if cardiorespiratory instability is present.
- Mechanical ventilation may be necessary if the airway is unprotected or respiratory failure develops. Lung shunts are frequently present, causing hypoxemia.
- Infection is commonplace and is frequently either Gram positive or fungal. Clinical signs are often absent. Samples of blood, sputum, urine, wound sites, drain fluid, intravascular catheter sites and ascites should be sent for regular microbiological surveillance. Systemic antimicrobial therapy, with or without selective gut decontamination, has been shown to reduce the infection rate. Fungal infections are also well recognized. Some liver units give prophylactic antifungal therapy.
- Hypoglycemia is a common occurrence. It should be frequently monitored and treated with either enteral (or parenteral) nutrition, or a 10% to 20% glucose infusion to maintain normoglycemia.
- Renal failure occurs in 30% to 70% of cases and may necessitate renal replacement therapy. The incidence may be reduced by careful maintenance of intravascular volume. Vasopressin/terlipressin has been reported for hepatorenal syndrome, but evidence of effectiveness in improving outcomes is lacking.

- Upper gastrointestinal bleeding is more common because of the associated coagulopathy. Prophylactic H_2 blockers or proton pump inhibitors should be used.
- N-acetylcysteine should be used until acetaminophen toxicity can be excluded.
- Corticosteroids, PGE, and charcoal hemoperfusion have not been shown to have any outcome benefit.

See also

Ventilatory support—indications, p. 4; Liver function tests, p. 152; Coagulation monitoring, p. 156; Hepatic encephalopathy, p. 362; Paracetamol poisoning, p. 458

Hepatic encephalopathy

Grading
- Grade 1—confused, altered mood
- Grade 2—inappropriate, drowsy
- Grade 3—stuporose but can be roused, very confused, agitated
- Grade 4—coma, unresponsive to painful stimuli

The risk of cerebral edema is far higher at grades 3 and 4 (50%–85%) and is the leading cause of death. Suggestive signs include systemic hypertension, progressive heart rate slowing, and increasing muscle rigidity. These occur at ICPs >30 mmHg.

Management of encephalopathy
- Correct/avoid potential aggravating factors (e.g., gastrointestinal tract hemorrhage, oversedation, hypoxia, hypoglycemia, infection, electrolyte imbalance).
- Maintain patient in slight head-up position (30°).
- Administer lactulose (e.g., 20–30 mL qid PO) to achieve four to six bowel motions per day.
- Dietary restriction of protein is now not encouraged because this promotes endogenous protein utilization.

Management of intracranial hypertension
- Consider early ICP monitoring. CT and clinical features correlate poorly with ICP, although no controlled studies have yet been performed to show outcome benefit from ICP monitoring, which carries its own complication rate (bleeding, infection).
- Hyperventilation to achieve a $PaCO_2$ of approximately 30 mmHg can be useful, but should be used only in conjunction with cerebral vascular monitoring (e.g., jugular bulb catheter) because it may also compromise CBF.
- Administer mannitol (0.5–1 mg/kg over 20 to 30 min) if serum osmolality is <320 mOsmol/kg. If severe renal dysfunction is present, use renal replacement therapy in conjunction with mannitol.
- If no response to previous management, consider barbiturate administration (e.g., thiopental infusion at 1–5 mg/kg/h), ideally with ICP monitoring.
- If still no response, consider urgent liver transplantation.
- Exercise caution with concomitant drug usage.

Identification of patients unlikely to survive without transplantation
- PT >100 s

Or any three of the following:
- Age <10 years or >40 years
- Etiology is hepatitis C, halothane, or other drug reaction except acetaminophen
- Duration of jaundice preencephalopathy >2 days
- PT >50 s
- Serum bilirubin >12 mg/dL

If acetaminophen induced
- pH <7.3 or PT >100 s and creatinine >200 µmol/L plus grade 3 or 4 encephalopathy

Because only 50% to 85% of patients identified as requiring transplantation will survive long enough to receive one, a transplantation center should be informed soon after diagnosis of all possible candidates.

See also

Ventilatory support—indications, p. 4; ICP monitoring, p. 134; Liver function tests, p. 152; Coagulation monitoring, p. 156; Sedatives, p. 236; Jaundice, p. 358; Chronic liver failure, p. 364; Paracetamol poisoning, p. 458

Chronic liver failure

Patients admitted to intensive care with chronic liver failure may develop specific associated problems:

- Acute decompensation—may be secondary to infection, sedation, hypovolemia, hypotension, diuretics, gastrointestinal hemorrhage, excess dietary protein, and electrolyte imbalance.
- Infection—The patient may transmit infection (e.g., hepatitis A, B, or C) and, by being immunosuppressed, is also more prone to acquiring infections such as TB and fungi.
- Drug metabolism—Because many drugs are all or partly metabolized by the liver and/or excreted into the bile, the drug action may be prolonged or slowed depending on whether the metabolites are active. In particular, sedatives may have a greatly prolonged duration of action.
- Portal hypertension—results in ascites, varices, and splenomegaly. Ascites may produce diaphragmatic splinting and is at risk of becoming infected. However, routine drainage may cause considerable protein loss. Varices may bleed whereas splenomegaly may result in thrombocytopenia. Renal failure is also seen as a result of high intra-abdominal pressures and hepatorenal syndrome.
- Bleeding—An increased risk is present because of decreased production of clotting factors (II, VII, IX, X), varices, and splenomegaly related thrombocytopenia.
- Alcohol—the most frequent cause of cirrhosis in the Western world. Acute withdrawal may lead to delirium tremens with severe agitation, hallucinations, seizures, and cardiovascular disturbances.
- Second-degree hyperaldosteronism—results in oliguria, and salt and water retention
- Increased tendency to jaundice, especially during critical illness.

Management

1. Ascites
   - Take specimens for microbiological analysis (including TB), protein and cytology. If white blood cell count >250 cells/high-power field, IV antibiotics should be instituted. Effective regimens for empiric therapy include cefotaxime 2 g q12h, ceftriaxone 2 g qd, or amoxicillin/clavulanic acid 1.2 g q8h.
   - If present in large quantity, (1) decrease sodium and water intake, and (2) commence spironolactone PO ± furosemide. Paracentesis ± colloid replacement should be performed, particularly for tense ascites.
2. Coagulopathy
   - Vitamin K 10 mg/day slow IV bolus for 2 to 3 days
   - FFP, platelets as necessary
3. Hypoglycemia—Should be prevented by adequate nutrition or a 10% or 20% glucose infusion
4. Adequate nutrition and vitamin supplementation
5. Acute decompensation—Avoid any precipitating causes (e.g., infection, sedation, hypovolemia, electrolyte imbalance).
6. Drug administration—Review type and dose regularly.

See also
Liver function tests, p. 152; Sedatives, p. 236; Jaundice, p. 358; Acute liver failure, p. 360

Neurological disorders

Acute weakness

Severe acute weakness may require urgent intubation and mechanical ventilation if the FVC is <1 L or gas exchange deteriorates acutely.

Investigation

- Metabolic myopathies—Exclude and treat hypophosphatemia, hypokalemia, hypocalcemia, and hypomagnesemia.
- Prolonged effects of muscle relaxants—A prolonged effect of succinyl-choline will usually be clinically obvious and should prompt assessment of pseudocholinesterase levels. Succinylcholine effects will also be prolonged in myasthenics. Prolonged effects of non depolarizing muscle relaxants are suggested by a response to an anticholinesterase (neostigmine 0.5 mg by slow IV bolus with an anticholinergic). This should not be attempted if paralysis is complete. Patients with myasthenia gravis will also respond.
- Guillain–Barré syndrome—A lumbar puncture should be performed to confirm increased CSF protein with normal cells. If these features are not found but suspicion is strong, nerve conduction studies may demonstrate segmental demyelination with slow conduction velocities.
- Myasthenia gravis—Fatiguing weakness or ptosis suggests myasthenia gravis; response to IV edrophonium (Tensilon test) and a strongly positive acetylcholine receptor antibody titer confirm this diagnosis. A myasthenic syndrome associated with malignancy (Eaton–Lambert syndrome) involves pelvic and thigh muscles predominantly, tending to spare the ocular muscles.
- Other diagnoses are made largely on the basis of clinical suspicion and specific specialized tests.

General management

- FVC should be monitored every 2 to 4h, and intubation and mechanical ventilation should follow if FVC is <1 L. Other indices of respiratory function are less sensitive. In particular, arterial blood gases may be maintained up to the point of respiratory arrest.
- Weak respiratory muscles lead to progressive basal atelectasis and sputum retention. Chest infection is a significant risk. Regular chest physiotherapy with intermittent positive-pressure breathing are required for prevention when mechanical ventilation is not necessary.
- Patients who are immobile are at risk of venous stasis and DVT. Prophylaxis with SC heparin is reasonable. Immobile patients also require attention to posture to prevent pressure sores and contractures.
- Weak bulbar muscles may compromise swallowing, with consequent malnutrition or pulmonary aspiration. Enteral nutritional support via a nasoenteric tube is necessary.
- In cases with coexisting autonomic neuropathy, enteral nutrition may be difficult, necessitating supplemental parenteral nutritional support. These patients may also sustain arrhythmias and hypotension requiring appropriate support.

Causes of severe weakness

Common in ICU
- Metabolic myopathies
- Prolonged effects of muscle relaxants
- Critical illness neuropathy or myopathy
- Guillain–Barré syndrome
- Myasthenia gravis
- Pontine CVA

Uncommon in ICU
- Substance abuse (especially benzene ring compounds)
- Chronic relapsing polyneuritis
- Endocrine myopathies
- Sarcoid neuropathy
- Poliomyelitis
- Diphtheria
- Carcinomatous neuropathy
- Porphyria
- Botulism
- Familial periodic paralysis
- Multiple sclerosis
- Lead poisoning
- Organophosphorus poisoning

See also

Ventilatory support—indications, p. 4; IPPV—assessment of weaning, p. 18; Enteral nutrition, p. 82; Parenteral nutrition, p. 84; Pulmonary function tests, p. 96; Electrolytes (Na^+, K^+, Cl^-, HCO_3^-), p. 146; Calcium, magnesium, and phosphate, p. 148; Muscle relaxants, p. 238; Respiratory failure, p. 280; Guillain–Barré syndrome, p. 386; Myasthenia gravis, p. 388; ICU neuromuscular disorders, p. 390

Agitation/delirium

In the ICU, agitation and/or confusion are predominantly related to sepsis, cerebral hypoperfusion, drugs, or drug withdrawal. Agitation is a descriptor of behavior and can have multiple causes. Delirium is a sudden onset of disturbed cognition and inattention that fluctuates over time. Delirium may be exacerbated by loss of day–night rhythm and inability to sleep, and is a common occurrence in the patient recovering from severe illness.

Common ICU causes

- Infection—including generalized sepsis, chest, cannula sites, urinary tract. Cerebral infection such as meningitis, encephalitis, and malaria are relatively rare but should always be considered.
- Drug related—adverse reaction, particularly affecting the elderly (e.g., sedatives, analgesics, diuretics); withdrawal (e.g., sedatives, analgesics, ethanol); abuse (e.g., opiates, amphetamines, alcohol, hallucinogens)
- Metabolic—hypo- or hyperglycemia, hypo- or hypernatremia, hypercalcemia, uremia, hepatic encephalopathy, hypo- or hyperthermia, dehydration, and others
- Respiratory—infection, hypoxemia, hypercapnia
- Neurological—infection (meningoencephalitis, malaria), posthead injury, space-occupying lesion (including hematoma), postictal, postcardiac arrest
- Cardiac—low output state, hypotension, endocarditis
- Pain—full bladder (blocked Foley catheter), abdominal pain
- Psychosis—other psychiatric states

Principles of management

1. Examine for signs of (1) infection (e.g., pyrexia, purulent sputum, catheter sites, neutrophilia, decreasing platelet count, CXR, meningism); (2) cardiovascular instability (hypotension, increasing metabolic acidosis, oliguria, arrhythmias); (3) covert pain, particularly abdominal and lower limbs (e.g., compartment syndrome, DVT); (4) focal neurological signs (e.g., meningism, unequal pupils, hemiparesis); (5) respiratory failure (arterial blood gases); and (6) metabolic derangement (bio-chemical screen). If any of these are found, treat as appropriate. Psychosis should not be assumed until treatable causes are excluded.
2. Reassure and calm the patient. Maintain quiet atmosphere and reduce noise levels. Attempt to restore day–night rhythm (e.g., by changing ambient lighting and using oral hypnotic agents).
3. Consider starting, changing, or increasing dose of sedative or major tranquilizer to control the patient (see Table 26.1). If highly agitated and likely to endanger themselves, rapid short-term control can be achieved by a slow IV bolus of sedative. Consider propofol, or pref-erably haloperidol, in the smallest possible dose to achieve the desired effect; observe for hypotension, respiratory depression, arrhythmias, and extrapyramidal effects. Opiates may be needed, especially if pain or withdrawal is a factor. An ethanol infusion can be considered for delirium tremens resulting from alcohol withdrawal.

4. Sedation can be maintained by continuous infusion or intermittent injection, either regularly or as required. The less agitated patient may respond to IM injections of a major tranquilizer, although these should be avoided with concurrent coagulopathy.

Table 26.1 Drug dosages for severe agitation

Haloperidol	2.5 mg by slow IV bolus; repeat, doubling dose, every 10–15 min until effect; for regular prescription, give qid
Midazolam	2–5 mg by slow IV bolus (may worsen delirium)
Lorazepam	1–2 mg by slow IV bolus (may worsen delirium)
Propofol	30–100 mg by slow IV bolus
Morphine	2.5–5 mg by slow IV bolus

Beware of excessive central and respiratory depression with these agents.

See also

IPPV—failure to tolerate ventilation, p. 12; Toxicology, p. 162; Sedatives, p. 236; Acute liver failure, p. 360; Chronic liver failure, p. 364; Thyroid emergencies, p. 448; Poisoning—general principles, p. 454; Amphetamines including Ecstasy, p. 464; Cocaine, p. 466; Infection—diagnosis, p. 482; Systemic inflammation/multiorgan failure, p. 486; Head injury (1), p. 506; Head injury (2), p. 508; Pyrexia (1), p. 520; Pyrexia (2), p. 522; Pain, p. 534

Generalized seizures

Control of seizures is necessary to prevent ischemic brain damage, to reduce cerebral oxygen requirements, and to reduce ICP. When possible, correct the cause and give specific treatment. A CT scan may be necessary to identify structural causes. Common causes include
- Hypoxemia
- Hypoglycemia
- Hypocalcemia
- Space-occupying lesions
- Metabolic and toxic disorders
- Drug withdrawal (e.g., alcohol, benzodiazepines, anticonvulsants)
- Infection, especially meningoencephalitis
- Trauma
- Idiopathic epilepsy

Most seizures are self-limiting, requiring no more than protection from injury (coma position, protect head, do not force anything into the mouth).

Specific treatment
- Hypoxemia should be corrected with oxygen (FiO$_2$, 0.6–1.0).
- Provide intubation and ventilation if the airway is unprotected or SpO$_2$ <90%.
- Blood glucose should be measured urgently and hypoglycemia corrected with IV 50 mL 50% glucose.
- Anticonvulsant levels should be corrected in known epileptics.
- Cerebral edema should be managed with sedation, osmotic diuretics, induced hypothermia, or controlled hyperventilation.
- In patients with a known tumor, arteritis, or parasitic infection, high-dose dexamethasone may be given.
- Thiamine 100 mg IV should be given to alcoholics.
- Consider surgery for space-occupying lesions (e.g., blood clot, tumor).

Status epilepticus
Status epilepticus is a single unremitting seizure lasting >30 min or frequent seizures without an interictal return to baseline. Four main classes of drugs are useful in terminating status epilepticus (see Table 26.2):
1. Benzodiazepines (e.g., lorazepam, diazepam, or midazolam) are the usual first line-treatment.
2. Phenytoin—A loading dose should be given IV if the patient has not previously received phenytoin. Phenytoin may not provide immediate control of seizures within the first 24 h. Phenytoin's main advantage is its efficacy in preventing the recurrence of status epilepticus for extended periods of time.
3. Barbiturates (e.g., phenobarbital or pentobarbital) provide excellent seizure control but may necessitate mechanical ventilation and may cause hypotension.
4. Propofol is chemically unrelated to any other anticonvulsant. It rapidly terminates seizure activity but causes hypotension and respiratory depression.

Other supportive treatment

Continuous EEG monitoring is ideal in the setting of status epilepticus to judge seizure control.

With all anticonvulsants, care should be taken to avoid hypoventilation and respiratory failure. However, mechanical ventilation to maintain airway oxygenation will be required if barbiturates or propofol are used in cases of continued seizures.

The addition of barbiturates or propofol to terminate seizures in the face of preexisting benzodiazepine ± phenytoin loading frequently requires volume loading or pressors for maintenance of blood pressure. Correction of circulatory disturbance is required to maintain optimal CBF.

Muscle relaxants prevent muscular contraction during seizures but will not prevent continued seizures.

Table 26.2 Drug dosages

Lorazepam	2–8 mg IV
Diazepam	Initially 2.5–5 mg IV or PR; additional increments as necessary to a maximum of 20 mg
Midazolam	Initially 2.5–5 mg IV; additional increments as necessary to a maximum of 20 mg
Phenytoin	Loading dose of 18 mg/kg IV at a rate <50 mg/min with continuous ECG monitoring; maintenance at 300–400 mg/day IV or PO adjusted according to levels
Phenobarbital	20 mg/kg infused at a rate of 30 to 50 mg/min followed by lowest dose to maintain control
Pentobarbital	10 mg/kg IV followed by lowest dose to maintain control
Propofol	0.5–2 mg/kg IV followed by 1–3 mg/kg/h

Key trial

Treiman VA, for the Veterans Affairs Status Epilepticus Cooperative Study Group. A comparison of four treatments for generalized convulsive status epilepticus. *N Engl J Med* 1998; **339**:792–8.

Meningitis

Meningitis is a life-threatening condition demanding prompt treatment. Because the classic presentation of meningism may be absent, suspect in those presenting with obtundation, agitation, seizures, or focal neurology. Signs may be subtle or present insidiously in neutropenics and the elderly. Meningococcemia presents with a prominent rash in 30% of cases whereas *Listeria monocytogenes* may cause early seizures and focal neurological defects.

Diagnosis

- Bacterial meningitis is primarily diagnosed by CSF examination. This is unnecessary with a classic meningococcal rash in which the organism can often be cultured from skin lesions. Lumbar puncture samples should be sent for urgent microscopy and culture, PCR, antigen virology, and protein and glucose estimation (with concurrent plasma sample). Normal or lymphocytic CSF may be found in early pyogenic meningitis, especially *L. monocytogenes* (see Table 26.3).
- Increased ICP is common; unless confidently excluded, delay lumbar puncture but not antibiotics, until after CT scanning. A normal CT scan does not completely exclude increased ICP.
- Empiric antibiotic therapy with concurrent steroids should be commenced immediately after taking blood cultures. The choice should be based on the patient's age. CSF cultures are positive in 50% if antibiotics are given, compared with 60% to 90% in untreated cases (see Table 26.4).
- CSF bacterial antigen testing is available for most infecting organisms. Sensitivity varies from 50% to 100% whereas specificity is high.

Management

1. Administer antibiotic therapy, usually for ≥10 days, although recent studies suggest equal efficacy with shorter courses.
2. Dexamethasone 10 mg qid for 4 days should be commenced with or just before the first dose of antibiotic, particularly for pneumococcal meningitis.
3. General measures include attention to fluid and electrolyte replacement, adequate gas exchange, nutrition, and skin care.
4. Manage increased ICP if present.
5. Give oral ciprofloxacin (adults only) or rifampicin to family and close social contacts of meningococcal and *Hemophilus* meningitis. The index case should also receive this treatment before discharge home.

Aseptic meningitis

No organisms are identified by routine CSF analysis despite a high neutrophil and/or lymphocyte count. Causes include viruses (e.g., mumps, measles), Lyme disease, fungi, leptospirosis, listeriosis, brucellosis, atypical TB, sarcoidosis, SLE, or primary idiopathic meningitis.

Encephalitis

Presenting features include drowsiness, coma, agitation, pyrexia, seizures, and focal signs. Meningism need not necessarily be present.

Causes
- Bacterial (as for meningitis)
- Viruses (in particular, herpes simplex and postmeasles, chicken pox, mumps infection). Herpes simplex classically affects the temporal lobe and can be suggested by EEG or magnetic resonance imaging (MRI). Give acyclovir 10 mg/kg tid IV for 10 days.

Rarer causes include leptospirosis and brucellosis. The CSF reveals no organisms, but a high lymphocyte count is present. If indicated, send CSF for acid-fast stain (TB) and India ink stain (*Cryptococcus*).

Table 26.3 Typical CSF values in meningitis

	Pyogenic	Viral	TB
Classic appearance	Turbid	Clear	Fibrin web
Predominant cell type	Polymorphs	Lymphocytes	Lymphocytes
Cell count/mm^3	>1000	<500	50–1500
Protein (g/L)	>1	0.5–1	1–5
CSF-to-blood glucose(%)	<60	>60	<60

Table 26.4 Organisms and empiric starting antibiotic therapy

Organism	Patients often affected	Antibiotic and dosage regimen (alternatives in parentheses)
Neisseria meningitidis (meningococcus)	Young adults	Ceftriaxone 2 g IV q12h (cefotaxime 50 mg/kg IV q8h) (penicillin 2–4 million U IV q4 h or 18–24 million U. IV qid as continuous infusion) (chloramphenicol 12.5 mg/kg IV q6h)
Streptococcus pneumoniae (pneumococcus)	Older adults	Ceftriaxone 2 g IV q12h (cefotaxime 50 mg/kg IV q8h) (chloramphenicol 12.5 mg/kg IV q6h)
Haemophilus influenzae	Children	Ceftriaxone 50 mg/kg IV q12h (cefotaxime 50 mg/kg IV q8h) (chloramphenicol 12.5 mg/kg IV q6h)
Listeria monocytogenes	Elderly, immuno-compromised	Ampicillin 1 g IV q4h plus gentamicin 120 mg IV stat, then 80 mg q8–12h (adjust by plasma levels)
Mycobacterium tuberculosis	Children residing in endemic areas	Quadruple therapy (rifampicin, isoniazid, ethambutol, pyrazinamide)
Cryptococcus neoformans	Immuno-compromised	Amphotericin B starting at 250 µg/kg IV qd and flucytosine 50 mg/kg IV q6h
Staphylococcus aureus	Nosocomial	Nafcillin 2 g IV q4 h or 12 g IV qd as continuous infusion

Key papers

de Gans J, et al. Dexamethasone in adults with bacterial meningitis. *N Engl J Med* 2002; **347**:1549–56.
van de Beek D, et al. Corticosteroids in acute bacterial meningitis. *Cochrane Database Syst Rev* 2003; CD004305. [Review].

See also

Intracranial hemorrhage

Epidural hemorrhage

Epidural hemorrhage usually presents acutely after head injury. Characterized by decreasing GCS score progressing to coma, focal signs (lateralizing weakness or anesthesia, pupillary signs), visual disturbances, and seizures. Treatment by random burr holes has been supplanted by directed drainage after CT scan localization.

A conservative approach may be adopted for small hematomata, but increasing size (assessed by regular CT scanning or clinical deterioration) is an indication for surgical drainage.

Subdural hemorrhage

Subdural hemorrhage classically presents days to weeks after head trauma with a fluctuating level of consciousness (35%), agitation, confusion, seizures, signs of increased ICP, localizing signs, or a slowly evolving stroke. Diagnosis is made by CT scan. Treatment is by surgical drainage.

Intracerebral hemorrhage

Causes of intracerebral hemorrhage include hypertension, neoplasm, vasculitis, coagulopathy, and mycotic aneurysms associated with bacterial endocarditis.

Clinical features include sudden-onset coma, drowsiness, and/or neurological deficit. Headache usually occurs only with cortical and intraventricular hemorrhage. The rate of evolution depends on the site and size of the bleed. The area affected is the putamen (55%), thalamus (10%), cerebral cortex (15%), pons (10%), and cerebellum (10%).

Diagnosis

CT scan is the definitive test. A coagulation and vasculitis blood screen may be indicated. Angiography is indicated if surgical repair is contemplated although not for drainage of blood clot.

Treatment

- Bed rest
- Supportive (e.g., hydration, nutrition, analgesia, ventilatory support)
- Physiotherapy
- Blood pressure control remains controversial, but maintenance of systolic blood pressure <220 mmHg is generally accepted.
- Correct any coagulopathy.
- Control increased ICP.
- Surgery—contact a neurosurgeon (e.g., for evacuation of hematoma, repair/clipping of aneurysm).
- Steroid therapy is ineffective.

See also

Ventilatory support—indications, p. 4; Blood pressure monitoring, p. 112; ICP monitoring, p. 134; Coagulation monitoring, p. 156; Neuroprotective agents, p. 242; Basic resuscitation, p. 268; Hypertension, p. 314; Generalized seizures, p. 372; Subarachnoid hemorrhage, p. 380; Increased ICP, p. 384; Bleeding disorders, p. 398; Vasculitides, p. 498; Head injury (1), p. 506; Head injury (2), p. 508; Brainstem death, p. 550; Withdrawal and withholding treatment, p. 552; Care of the potential organ donor, p. 554

Subarachnoid hemorrhage

Pathology

- In 15% no cause is found; most are caused by ruptured aneurysms. Other causes include trauma, AV malformation, vasculitides, dissection, bleeding diatheses, or illicit drug use.
- The anterior part of the circle of Willis is affected in 85%–90% of cases, whereas 10%–15% affect the vertebrobasilar system.
- There is a 30% risk of rebleeding for which the mortality is 40%. Those surviving a month have a 90% chance of surviving a year.
- Cerebral vasospasm occurs in 30% to 40% of patients at 4 to 12 days after the bleed. This is the most important cause of morbidity and mortality.
- Hydrocephalus, seizures, hyponatremia, and inappropriate ADH (anti diuretic hormone) secretion are recognized complications.

Clinical features

- Subarachnoid hemorrhage may be preceded by a prodrome of head-ache, dizziness, and vague neurological symptoms.
- Often there is rapid-onset (minutes to hours) presentation including collapse, severe 'thunderclap' headache, and meningism.
- Cranial nerve palsies, drowsiness, and hemiplegia may also occur.

Diagnosis

Diagnosis is usually made by CT scan. If there is no evidence of increased ICP, a lumbar puncture may be performed revealing blood-stained CSF with xanthochromia. Lumbar puncture is essential if there is a strong clinical suspicion of subarachnoid hemorrhage in the face of a normal CT scan.

Management

- Bed rest
- Maintain adequate hydration, nutrition, analgesia, sedation.
- Cerebral vasospasm is prevented by nimodipine and maintenance of intravascular volume.
- In the absence of ICP monitoring, systemic hypertension should only be treated if severe (e.g., systolic pressure >220–230 mmHg) and prolonged.
- Surgery—timing is controversial, with either early or delayed (7–10 days) intervention being advocated. The neurosurgical consultation is essential for optimal management.
- Antifibrinolytic therapy (e.g., tranexamic acid) reduces the incidence of rebleeding but has no beneficial effect on outcome.

Key trial

Allen GS, *et al.* Cerebral arterial spasm: A controlled trial of nimodipine in patients with subarachnoid hemorrhage. *N Engl J Med* 1983; **308**:619–24.

See also

Stroke

Pathology
- Hemorrhage, embolus, or thrombosis
- 'Secondary' stroke may occur with meningitis, bacterial endocarditis, subarachnoid hemorrhage, and vasculitis.
- Dissection and cerebral venous thrombosis need to be considered, because anticoagulation is indicated for both (unless a large infarct is established, because there is an increased risk of bleeding). Dissection should be suspected in younger patients, often presenting with severe headache or neck pain, Horner's syndrome, or seizures after trauma or neck manipulation. Cerebral venous thrombosis may mimic stroke, tumor, subarachnoid hemorrhage, or meningoencephalitis, and may present with headache, seizures, focal signs, or obtundation.

Urgent CT scan
An urgent CT scan should be obtained as part of the initial evaluation to rule out subarachnoid hemorrhage, hydrocephalus, or trauma, or for patients who are anticoagulated or who have a bleeding tendency. CT should be repeated for continuing deterioration.

Goals of treatment
- To protect the penumbra with close attention to oxygenation, hydration, glycemic control, and avoidance of pyrexia.
- Blood pressure control is needed for severe hypertension (e.g., >200/120 mmHg) and hypotension.
- Early IV thrombolytic therapy with rt-PA remains controversial. The success of the NINDS Trial, which tested rt-PA in the setting of acute ischemic stroke, probably reflects its strict exclusion criteria and the institution of thrombolytics within 3 h of the onset of symptoms. Three-month mortality was not different between the two groups, despite a 10-fold increase in symptomatic intracerebral hemorrhage in the rt-PA group (6% vs. 0.6%). However, patients who received rt-PA were at least 30% more likely to have minimal or no disability at 1 year.
- For thrombolysis, the extent of reperfusion depends on the etiology with basilar >MCA >internal carotid, and embolic >thrombotic. Pooled studies with rt-PA 0.9 mg/kg given within 3 h of stroke onset (and tight blood pressure control) showed a favorable outcome. However, there was a sixfold increase in hemorrhage (to 5.9%), of whom 60% died. This was more common in the elderly and in those with more severe stroke.
- Neurosurgical intervention may be considered for cerebellar hematoma, cerebellar infarction, and the malignant MCA syndrome (for massive infarction on the nondominant side).

Key papers

Hacke W, *et al.* Association of outcome with early stroke treatment: Pooled analysis of ATLANTIS, ECASS, and NINDS rt-PA stroke trials. *Lancet* 2004; **363**:768–74.
The National Institute of Neurological Disorders and Stroke (NINDS) rt-PA Stroke Study Group. Tissue plasminogen activator for acute ischemic stroke. *N Engl J Med* 1995; **333**:1581–7.

See also

Ventilatory support—indications, p. 4; Blood pressure monitoring, p. 112; Neuroprotective agents, p. 242; Basic resuscitation, p. 268; Hypertension, p. 312; Generalized seizures, p. 372; Intracranial hemorrhage, p. 378; Subarachnoid hemorrhage, p. 380; Increased ICP, p. 384

Increased ICP

Clinical features

- Headache, vomiting, dizziness, visual disturbance
- Seizures, focal neurology, papilledema
- Increasing blood pressure, bradycardia (late responses)
- Agitation, increasing drowsiness, coma
- Slow, deep breaths; Cheyne–Stokes breathing; apnea
- Ipsilateral progressing to bilateral pupillary dilatation
- Decorticate progressing to decerebrate posturing

Diagnosis

- CT or MRI
- ICP measurement >20 mmHg

Lumbar puncture should be avoided because of the risk of coning. Neither CT nor absence of papilledema will exclude increased ICP.

Causes

- Space-occupying lesion (e.g., neoplasm, blood clot, abscess)
- Increased capillary permeability (e.g., trauma, infection, encephalopathy)
- Cell death (e.g., postarrest hypoxia)
- Obstruction (e.g., hydrocephalus)

Management

1. Bed rest, 20 to 30° head-up tilt, sedation, quiet environment, minimal suction and noise. Sedation is often necessary to overcome a hyperadrenergic state but sedative-induced hypotension should be avoided. Head positioning and endotracheal tube fixation should not occlude jugular venous drainage.
2. Ventilate if GCS score is ≤8 points, airway unprotected, or patient is excessively agitated.
3. Maintain $PaCO_2$ at 35 to 40 mmHg and avoid rapid increases. CSF bicarbonate levels reequilibrate within 4 ot 6 h, negating any benefit from hyperventilation.
4. Monitor ICP. Aim to maintain ICP at <20 mmHg and CPP (CPP = MAP–ICP) at ≥70 mmHg. Vasopressors may be needed. Do not treat systemic hypertension unless very high (e.g., systolic, 220–230 mmHg).
5. SjO_2 and lactate may be useful monitoring techniques, although they do not detect regional ischemia. Brain tissue PO_2 monitoring may be useful.
6. Give mannitol 0.5 mg/kg over 15 min. Repeat every 4 h depending on CPP measurements and/or clinical signs of deterioration. Stop when plasma osmolality reaches 310 to 320 mOsmol/kg. Hypertonic saline solution is probably as effective as mannitol in this situation.
7. Avoid severe alkalosis because cerebral vascular resistance increases and cerebral ischemia increases.
8. Consider specific treatment (e.g., for meningoencephalitis, malaria, hepatic encephalopathy, surgery). Some neurosurgeons decompress the cranium for generalized edema by removing a skull flap. Seek local advice. Dexamethasone 4 to 16 mg qid IV is beneficial for edema surrounding a tumor or abscess and for herpes simplex encephalitis.

Acute deterioration/risk of imminent coning

1. Mechanically ventilate to $PaCO_2$ 25 to 30 mmHg for 10 to 20 min.
2. Give mannitol 0.5 g/kg IV over 15 min. Repeat every 4 h as necessary while plasma osmolality is <310 to 320 mOsmol/kg. Consider hypertonic saline or therapeutic hypothermia.
3. If no response in ICP, CPP, and/or clinical features, give thiopental (successful in 50% of resistant cases).
4. Consider repeat CT scan and refer for urgent surgery if a surgically amenable space-occupying lesion is diagnosed.

See also

Ventilatory support—indications, p. 4; Blood pressure monitoring, p. 112; ICP monitoring, p. 134; Diuretics, p. 212; Neuroprotective agents, p. 242; Basic resuscitation, p. 268; Hypertension, p. 312; Generalized seizures, p. 372; Intracranial hemorrhage, p. 378; Subarachnoid hemorrhage, p. 380; Stroke, p. 382; Head injury (1), p. 506; Head injury (2), p. 508; Brain stem death, p. 550; Withdrawal and with holding treatment, p. 552; Care of the potential organ donor, p. 554

Guillain–Barré syndrome

Guillain–Barré syndrome is an immunologically-mediated, acute demyelinating polyradiculopathy. Viral infections and immunizations are common antecedents. The syndrome includes a progressive, areflexic motor weakness (often symmetrical, ascending and involving cranial nerves including facial, bulbar, and extraocular) with progression over days to weeks. There are often minor sensory disturbances (e.g. paraesthesias). Autonomic dysfunction is not unusual. There is no increase in cell count on CSF examination, but protein levels usually increase progressively. Nerve conduction studies show slow conduction velocities with prolonged F waves. Other features include muscle tenderness and back pain. The major contributors to morbidity and mortality are respiratory muscle weakness and autonomic dysfunction (hypotension, hypertension, arrhythmias, ileus, and urinary retention).

Differential diagnosis

Other causes of acute weakness must be excluded before a diagnosis of Guillain–Barré syndrome can be made.

Specific treatment

- IV gammaglobulin (0.4 g/kg/day for 5 days) or plasma exchange (five 50-ml/kg exchanges over 8–13 days) is effective if started within 14 days of onset of symptoms.
- Steroids have not been shown to be beneficial.

Supportive treatment

Respiratory care

Regular chest physiotherapy and spirometry are required. Mechanical ventilation is needed if FVC is < 1L or $PaCO_2$ is increased. An early tracheostomy is useful because mechanical ventilation is likely to continue for several weeks. Patients with bulbar involvement or inadequate cough should undergo tracheotomy, even if spontaneous breathing continues.

Cardiovascular care

Continuous cardiovascular monitoring is required because of the effects of autonomic involvement. Arrhythmias are particularly likely with anesthesia (especially with succinylcholine). Hypertensive and hypotensive responses are generally exaggerated with vasoactive drugs.

Nutritional support

Parenteral nutrition may required in cases in which there is ileus. Enteral nutrition is preferred, if possible, even though energy and fluid requirements are reduced in Guillain–Barré syndrome.

Analgesia

Analgesia is required for muscle, abdominal, and back pain. Although NSAIDs may be useful, opiates are often required.

Other support

Particular attention is required to pressure areas and DVT prophylaxis.

Key trials

Plasma Exchange/Sandoglobulin Guillain–Barre Syndrome Trial Group. Randomised trial of plasma exchange, intravenous immunoglobulin, and combined treatments in Guillain–Barré syndrome. *Lancet* 1997; **349**:225–30.

van Koningsveld R, for the Dutch GBS study group. Effect of methylpred-nisolone when added to standard treatment with intravenous immunoglobulin for Guillain–Barre syndrome: Randomised trial. *Lancet* 2004; **363**:192–6.

See also

Ventilatory support—indications, p. 4; Blood pressure monitoring, p. 112; Neuroprotective agents, p. 242; Basic resuscitation, p. 268; Hypertension, p. 312; Generalized seizures, p. 372; Intracranial hemorrhage, p. 378; Subarachnoid hemorrhage, p. 380; Increased ICP, p. 384

Myasthenia gravis

Myasthenia gravis is associated with painless weakness that is worse after exertion, with deterioration during stress, infection, or trauma.

Tendon reflexes are normal. It is an autoimmune disease associated with acetylcholine receptor and, rarely, antistriated muscle antibodies.

There is also an association with other autoimmune diseases (e.g., thyroid disease, SLE, rheumatoid arthritis).

Age <45 years, and predominantly female patients may have a thymoma that, if resected, may provide remission.

Severe weakness may be the result of a myasthenic or cholinergic (e.g., sweating, salivation, lacrimation, colic, fasciculation, confusion, ataxia, small pupils, bradycardia, hypertension, seizures) crisis.

Diagnosis of myasthenia

Edrophonium is a short-acting anticholinesterase used in the diagnosis of myasthenia in patients with no previous history of myasthenia gravis. In myasthenic patients with an acute deterioration, the test may distinguish a myasthenic crisis from a cholinergic crisis.

In cholinergic crisis there is a possibility of further deterioration, and atropine and facilities for urgent intubation and ventilation should be available.

To minimize the risk of an adverse reaction, a test dose of 1 mg edrophonium is administered. If no adverse events are noted after 1 min, an additional 4 mg may be given, and, if no change in the examination is apparent in 1 min, another 5 mg may be administered. A positive test is judged by improvement of weakness within 3 min of injection. The test may be combined with objective assessment of respiratory function by measuring the FVC response or by assessing the response to repetitive stimulation with an electromyogram.

Maintenance treatment

Anticholinesterase drugs provide the mainstay of symptomatic treatment, but steroids, immunosuppressives, and plasma exchange may provide pharmacological remission.

Myasthenic crisis

New myasthenics may present in crisis, and treatment should be started with steroids, azathioprine, and pyridostigmine (see Table 26.5). Plasma exchange may be useful to reduce the antibody load. In known myasthenics, an increased dose of pyridostigmine and steroids will be required. If the condition deteriorates, drug therapy should be stopped; plasma exchange may be life saving. Anticholinesterases may produce improvement in some muscle groups and cholinergic deterioration in others as a result of differential sensitivity. As with any case of acute weakness, mechanical ventilatory support is required if FVC is <1 L or $PaCO_2$ is increased.

Cholinergic crisis

Cholinergic symptoms are usually at their most severe 2 h after the last dose of anticholinesterase. It is common to give atropine prophylactically in the treatment of myasthenia, which may mask some of the cholinergic symptoms. If a deterioration of myasthenia fails to respond to edrophonium, all drugs should be stopped and atropine given (1 mg IV every 30 min to a maximum of 8 mg) (see Table 26.5). The edrophonium test should be repeated every 2 h and anticholinesterases reintroduced when the test is positive. Mechanical ventilation is required if FVC <1 L or $PaCO_2$ is increased.

Table 26.5 Drug dosages

Prednisolone	80 mg/day PO
Azathioprine	2.5 mg/kg/day PO
Pyridostigmine	60–180 mg q6h PO
Atropine	0.6 mg q6h PO

Drugs causing deterioration in myasthenia

- Aminoglycosides
- Streptomycin
- Tetracyclines
- Local anesthetics
- Muscle relaxants
- Opiates

See also

Ventilatory support—indications, p. 4; Endotracheal intubation, p. 36; Special support surfaces, p. 88; Plasma exchange, p. 70; Pulmonary function tests, p. 96; Steroids, p. 260; Respiratory failure, p. 280; Hypotension, p. 310; Tachyarrhythmias, p. 314; Bradyarrhythmias, p. 316; Acute weakness, p. 368

ICU neuromuscular disorders

Neuromuscular disorders in the critically ill have long been recognized, particularly in those being mechanically ventilated. First, suspicions are often raised when patients fail to wean from mechanical ventilation or limb weakness is noted on stopping sedation. Disuse atrophy, catabolic states, and drug therapy (e.g., high-dose steroids, muscle relaxants) are probably responsible for some cases but do not explain all. A neuromyopathic component of multiorgan dysfunction syndrome may be implicated.

Critical illness neuropathy

Neurophysiological studies have demonstrated an acute idiopathic axonal degeneration in patients with a flaccid weakness after a prolonged period of intensive care. Nerve conduction velocities are normal, indicating no demyelination. CSF is normal, unlike Guillain–Barré syndrome. The neuropathy is self-limiting, but prolongs the recovery phase of critical illness. Recovery may take weeks to years. Pyridoxine (100–150 mg daily PO) has been used in the treatment.

Critical illness myopathy

Drug-induced myopathy is not uncommon in critically ill patients. Steroid-induced myopathy is less common because the indications for high-dose steroids have been reduced. Muscle relaxants may have a prolonged effect and may be potentiated by β_2 agonists. Muscle histological studies have demonstrated abnormalities (fiber atrophy, mitochondrial defects, myopathy, and necrosis) that could not be associated with steroid or muscle relaxant therapy. Myopathy may cause renal damage via myoglobinuria. Critical illness myopathy is associated with various forms of muscle degeneration but is usually self-limiting. Recovery may take weeks to years.

See also

Ventilatory support—indications, p. 4; IPPV—assessment of weaning, p. 18; Special support surfaces, p. 88; Pulmonary function tests, p. 96; Respiratory failure, p. 280; Acute weakness, p. 368; Guillain–Barré syndrome, p. 386

Tetanus

The clinical syndrome of tetanus is caused by the exotoxin tetanospasmin from the anaerobe *Clostridium tetani* in contaminated or devitalized wounds. Tetanospasmin ascends intra-axonally in motor and autonomic nerves, blocking the release of inhibitory neurotransmitters. The disease may be modified by previous immunization, thus milder or localized symptoms occur with heavier toxin loads.

Clinical features

- Gradual onset of stiffness, dysphagia, muscle pain, hypertonia, rigidity, and muscle spasm
- Laryngospasm often follows dysphagia.
- Muscle spasm is often provoked by a minor disturbance (e.g., laryngospasm may be provoked by swallowing).
- Onset of symptoms within 5 days of injury implies a heavy toxin load and severe disease.
- The disease is self-limiting, so treatment is supportive but may need to continue for several weeks.

Management of the wound

If a contaminated wound is present, it should be debrided surgically to remove the source of the toxin.

Antimicrobial therapy

Metronidazole 7.5 mg/kg every 6 h IV (not greater than 4 g/day) or alternatively penicillin G (1–10 million U daily IV) may be used.

Neutralization of unbound toxin

Human tetanus immunoglobulin 500 to 1000 U IM may shorten the course of the disease by removing circulating toxin and should be given when considering the diagnosis.

Active immunization

Tetanus does not confer immunity after illness. Patients with tetanus should receive active immunization according to Table 26.6, with a total of three doses of tetanus and diphtheria toxoid, commencing immediately upon diagnosis, with the second dose in 1 month and the third dose in 1 year.

Table 26.6 Wound management

	≥3 doses of Td	<3 doses/unknown
Clean, minor wound	Td if last dose >10 years	Primary series (Td × 3)
Any other wound	Td if last dose > 5 years	Tetanus immunoglobin and primary series

Td, tetanus and diphtheria toxoid

Mild tetanus

Patients with mild symptoms, no respiratory distress, and a delayed onset of symptoms should be nursed in a quiet environment with mild sedation to prevent tetanic spasms.

Severe tetanus

- Intubate and ventilate because asphyxia may occur as a result of prolonged respiratory muscle spasm.
- Sedation may be achieved with diazepam (20 mg every 4–6h via nasogastric tube and 5 mg IV as necessary).
- Muscle rigidity is best treated with magnesium sulfate or benzodiazapines with the addition of muscle relaxants if necessary.
- Autonomic hyperreactivity is a feature (arrhythmias, hypotension, hypertension, and myocardial ischemia). It is minimized by sedation, anesthesia, and analgesia. It may be treated with atropine, labetalol, or magnesium sulfate.

See also

Ventilatory support —indications, p. 4; Sedatives, p. 236; Muscle relaxants, p. 238; Antimicrobials, p. 258; Respiratory failure, p. 280; Hypotension, p. 310; Hypertension, p. 312; Tachyarrhythmias, p. 314; Bradyarrhythmias, p. 316

Botulism

Botulism is an uncommon, lethal disease caused by the exotoxins of the anaerobe *Clostridium botulinum*. Botulism is most commonly a food-borne disease especially associated with canned foods. It may be contracted by wound contamination with aquatic soils. The toxin is carried in the blood to cholinergic neuromuscular junctions, where it binds irreversibly. Symptoms begin between 6 h to 8 days after contamination and are more severe with earlier onset. Botulism is diagnosed by isolating *C. botulinum* from the stool or by mouse bioassay (survival of immunized mice and death of nonimmunized mice when infected serum is injected).

Clinical features
- Symptoms include gastrointestinal disturbance, sore throat, fatigue, dizziness, paraesthesias, cranial involvement, and a progressive, descending flaccid weakness.
- Parasympathetic symptoms are common.
- The disease is usually self-limiting within several weeks.

Respiratory care
Provide regular spirometry and mechanical ventilation if FVC is <1 L. Patients with bulbar palsy need intubation for airway protection.

Toxin removal
If there is no ileus, the use of nonmagnesium-containing cathartics may remove the toxin load. Magnesium may enhance the effect of the toxin.

Antitoxin
Antitoxin therapy with equine serum trivalent botulism antitoxin (A, B, E) is available in the United States through state health departments. Regional poison centers can contact the on-call health department worker after hours. Antitoxin therapy may shorten the course of the disease if given early, although there is a risk of anaphylactoid reactions.

Wound botulism
Surgical debridement and penicillin G (3 million U IV every 4 h) or metronidazole (500 mg IV every 8 h) are the mainstays of treatment for contaminated wounds.

See also

Ventilatory support—indications, p. 4; Antimicrobials, p. 258; Respiratory failure, p. 280; Brady-arrhythmias, p. 316

Hematological disorders

Bleeding disorders

A common problem in the critically ill, bleeding disorders may be the result of (1) large-vessel bleeding usually 'surgical' or after a procedure (e.g., chest drain, tracheostomy, accidental arterial puncture, removal of IV or intra-arterial catheter), upper or lower gastrointestinal bleeding; (2) around vascular catheter sites or from intubated/instrumented lumens and orifices, usually related to severe multisystem illness or excess anticoagulant therapy, including thrombolytics; and (3) small-vessel bleeding (e.g., skin petechia, gastric erosions), usually related to anticoagulation or severe generalized illness including disseminated intravascular coagulation.

A decreasing platelet count is often an early sign of sepsis and critical illness. Recovery of the count usually coincides with overall patient recovery.

Common ICU causes
- Decreased platelet production (e.g., sepsis or drug induced)
- Decreased production of coagulation factors (e.g., liver failure)
- Increased consumption (e.g., DIC, major trauma, bleeding, heparin-induced thrombocytopenia, antiplatelet antibodies, extracorporeal circuits)
- Impaired or deranged platelet function (e.g., renal failure)
- Drugs (e.g., heparin, aspirin)
- Decreased protease inhibitors (e.g., antithrombin III, protein S and protein C deficiency [after sepsis])

Principles of management
1. An INR between 1.5 to 2.5 and/or platelet count of 20 to 40×10^9/L do not usually require correction if the patient is not bleeding or at high risk (e.g., active peptic ulcer, recent cerebral hemorrhage, undergoing an invasive procedure). 6 to 12 U of platelets will increase the count by only 20 to 40×10^9/L. The effect is often transient (<24 h) and the increment reduces with repetitive dosing. Treatment of symptomatic thrombocytopenia aims to increase the count to >50 $\times 10^9$/L. A target INR of <1.5 is acceptable. Vitamin K is given for liver failure and is considered for warfarin overdosage. Vitamin K 1 mg will reverse warfarin effects within 12 h whereas 10 mg will saturate liver stores, preventing warfarin activity for some weeks. FFP is given for short-term control.
2. If bleeding, and INR is 1.5 to 2, give 2 to 3 U FFP. If INR is >2, give 4 to 6 U FFP. If not bleeding (or high risk), generally only correct if INR is >2.5 to 3. Repeat clotting screen 30 to 60 min after FFP is infused. Give more FFP if bleeding continues and/or INR is >3.
3. For bleeding related to thrombolysis, (1) stop the drug infusion; (2) give either aprotinin 500,000 U over 10 min, then 200,000 U over 4 h or tranexamic acid 10 mg/kg repeated every 6 to 8 h; and (3) give 4 U FFP.

4. Cryoprecipitate is rarely needed. Consider when the TT is elevated (e.g., with DIC). Similarly, factor VIII is generally used for hemophiliacs only.
5. If aspirin has been taken within the past 1 to 2 weeks, platelet function may be negatively affected. Consider giving fresh platelets, even though count may be adequate.
6. Factor VIIa may be useful for severe, intractable bleeding, but more studies are needed to confirm its efficacy and cost–effectiveness.

Management of major bleeding

1. If external, direct occlusion/deep suture
2. Urgent expert opinion (e.g., for surgery, endoscopy + injection)
3. Correction of coagulopathy

Management of vascular catheter or percutaneous drain site bleeding

1. Direct pressure/occlusive dressing
2. Correction of coagulopathy. Consider use of aprotinin or tranexamic acid.
3. Surgical intervention is rarely necessary, although perforation/laceration of local artery/vein should be considered if bleeding fails to stop or becomes significant.

See also

Coagulation monitoring, p. 156; Blood transfusion, p. 182; Blood products, p. 250; Coagulants and antifibrinolytics, p. 252; Aprotinin, p. 254; Hemoptysis, p. 302; Upper gastrointestinal hemorrhage, p. 342; Lower intestinal bleeding and colitis, p. 346; Acute liver failure, p. 360; Chronic liver failure, p. 364; Platelet disorders, p. 408; Systemic inflammation/multiorgan failure, p. 486; Postoperative intensive care, p. 536

Clotting disorders

The risk of major venous thrombosis increases with long-term immobility and paralysis, and in specific prothrombotic conditions such as pregnancy, TTP, SLE (lupus anticoagulant), sickle cell crisis, and hyperosmolar diabetic coma.

DIC is associated with microvascular clotting, a consumption coagulopathy, and increased fibrinolysis.

Clotting of extracorporeal circuits (e.g., for renal replacement therapy) may be the result of mechanical obstruction to flow (e.g., kinked catheter), inadequate anticoagulation, or, in severe illness, a decrease in endogenous anticoagulants (e.g., antithrombin III), which may result in circuit blockage despite a coexisting thrombocytopenia and/or coagulopathy.

Axillary vein or subclavian vein thrombosis may result from indwelling IV catheters.

Management

Prophylactic low-dose unfractionated heparin (5000 IU SC every 8–12 h) or low molecular weight heparin should be given for long-term immobility/paralysis and to high-risk patients (e.g., previous DVT, femoral fractures).

For treatment of pulmonary embolism or DVT, IV heparin (unfractionated) is generally preferred and adjusted to maintain PTT at approximately two or three times normal. However, low-molecular weight heparin may be as effective and safe as dose-adjusted IV heparin for the initial treatment of nonmassive pulmonary embolism. Monitoring is not necessary for low-molecular weight heparin, although antifactor Xa levels can be used.

Intra-arterial clot can be treated with local infusion of thrombolytics, usually followed by heparinization. Seek vascular surgical advice.

Axillary vein or subclavian vein thrombosis should be managed by elevation of the affected arm (e.g., in a Bradford sling), and heparinization.

Specific conditions may require specific therapies (e.g., plasma exchange for SLE and TTP, whole blood exchange for sickle cell crisis).

Warfarin is generally avoided until shortly before ICU discharge because of the risk of continued bleeding after routine invasive procedures such as central venous catheterization.

Key study

Quinlan DJ, McQuillan A, Eikelboom JW. Low-molecular-weight heparin compared with intravenous unfractionated heparin for treatment of pulmonary embolism: a meta-analysis of randomized, controlled trials. *Ann Intern Med* 2004; **140**:175–83.

See also

Coagulation monitoring, p. 156; Anticoagulants, p. 246; Thrombolytics, p. 248; Blood products, p. 250; Pulmonary embolus, p. 306

Anemia

Anemia is defined as a low Hb level resulting from a decreased red cell mass. It may also be 'physiological', resulting from dilution from an increased plasma volume (e.g., pregnancy, vasodilated states).

Major causes in the ICU patient

- Blood loss (e.g., hemorrhage, regular blood sampling)
- Severe illness—analogous to the 'anemia of chronic disease'. There is decreased marrow production and, possibly, a decreased red cell lifespan.

Rarer causes

- Microcytic anemia—predominantly iron deficiency
- Chronic disease
- Bone marrow failure (idiopathic, drugs, neoplasm, radiation)
- Hemolysis
- Renal failure
- Macrocytic—vitamin B12 and folate deficiency, alcoholism, cirrhosis, sideroblastic anemia, hypothyroidism
- Congenital diseases—sickle cell, thalassemia

Management

1. Treatment of the cause when possible
2. Blood transfusion
   - The ideal Hb level for optimal oxygen carriage and viscosity remains contentious. A recent multicenter trial showed improved outcomes if a trigger of 7 g/dL was used. A higher transfusion threshold (e.g., 9–10 g/dL) may be needed in those with cardiorespiratory disease.
   - Transfusion is usually given as packed cells with or without a small dose of furosemide to maintain fluid balance. This may need to be given rapidly during active blood loss, or slowly for correction of a gradually decreasing Hb level.
   - Rarely, patients admitted with chronically low Hb (e.g., <4–5 g/dL, which often follows long-term malnutrition or vitamin deficiency, will need a much slower elevation in Hb level to avoid precipitating acute heart failure. An initial target of 7–8 g/dL is often acceptable. Obviously, this may need to be altered in the light of any concurrent acute illness when elevation of oxygen delivery is deemed necessary.
   - Erythropoietin slightly reduces the need for blood transfusion in long-term ICU patients and may be useful in those with multiple antibodies or in those who decline transfusion for religious reasons.

Key trial

Hebert PC, *et al.*, for the Transfusion Requirements in Critical Care Invesigators, Canadian Critical Care Trials Group. A multicenter, randomized, controlled clinical trial of transfusion requirements in critical care. *N Engl J Med* 1999; **340**:409–17.

Sickle cell disease

Sickle cell disease is a chronic, hereditary disease almost entirely confined to the black population in which the gene for Hb S is inherited from each parent. The red blood cells lack Hb A. When deprived of oxygen, these cells assume sickle and other bizarre shapes, resulting in erythrostasis, occlusion of blood vessels, thrombosis, and tissue infarction. After stasis, cells released back into the circulation are more fragile and prone to hemolysis. Occasionally, there may be bone marrow failure.

Chronic features

Patients with sickle cell disease are chronically anemic (7–8 g/dL) with a hyperdynamic circulation. Splenomegaly is common in youth but, with progressive episodes of infarction, splenic atrophy occurs, leading to an increased risk of infection, particularly pneumococcal.

Chronic features include skin ulcers, renal failure, avascular bone necrosis (± supervening osteomyelitis, especially *Salmonella*), hepatomegaly, jaundice, and cardiomyopathy. Sudden cardiac death is not uncommon, usually before the age of 30.

Sickle cell crises

Crises are precipitated by various triggers, such as hypoxemia (e.g., air travel, anesthesia), infection, cold, dehydration, and emotional stress.

Thrombotic crisis

Thrombotic crisis occurs most frequently in bones or joints, but also affects the chest and abdomen, giving rise to severe pain. Neurological symptoms (e.g., seizures, focal signs), hematuria, or priapism may be present. Pulmonary crises are the most common reason for ICU admission. Secondary chest infection or ARDS may supervene, worsening hypoxemia and further exacerbating the crisis.

Aplastic crisis

Related to parvovirus infection, aplastic crisis is suggested by worsening anemia and a reduction in the normally elevated reticulocyte count (10–20%).

Hemolytic crisis

In hemolytic crisis, intravascular hemolysis with hemoglobinuria, jaundice, and renal failure sometimes occurs.

Sequestration crisis

Sequestration crisis is rapid hepatic and splenic enlargement resulting from red cell trapping with severe anemia. This condition is particularly serious.

Management

Prophylaxis against crises includes avoidance of hypoxemia and other known precipitating factors, prophylactic penicillin and pneumococcal vaccine, and exchange transfusions.

1. Painful crises usually require prompt opiate infusions. Although psychological dependence is high, analgesia should not be withheld.

2. Give oxygen to maintain SaO_2 at 100%.
3. Rehydrate with IV fluids and keep warm.
4. If infection is suspected, antibiotics should be given as indicated.
5. Transfuse blood if Hb level drops or CNS or lung complications present.
6. Lower proportion of sickle cells to <30% by exchange transfusion.
7. Mechanical ventilation may be necessary for chest crises.

See also

Oxygen therapy, p. 2; Pulse oximetry, p. 92; Full blood count, p. 154; Bacteriology, p. 158; Acute chest infection (1), p. 286; Acute chest infection (2), p. 288; Acute renal failure—diagnosis, p. 330; Acute renal failure—management, p. 332; Jaundice, p. 358; Anemia, p. 402; Hemolysis, p. 406

Hemolysis

Hemolysis is the shortening of erythrocyte life span below the expected 120 days. Marked intravascular hemolysis may lead to jaundice and hemoglobinuria.

Causes

- Blood transfusion reactions
- HUS (microangiopathic hemolytic anemia)
- Trauma (e.g., cardiac valve prosthesis)
- Malaria
- Sickle cell hemolytic crisis
- Drugs (e.g., high-dose penicillin, methyldopa)
- Autoimmune (cold or warm antibody mediated)—may be idiopathic or secondary (e.g., lymphoma, SLE, mycoplasma)
- Glucose-6-phosphate dehydrogenase deficiency—Oxidative crises occur after ingestion of fava beans, primaquine, and sulfonamides, leading to rapid-onset anemia and jaundice.

Diagnosis

- Unconjugated hyperbilirubinemia, increased urinary urobilinogen (increased red blood cell breakdown)
- Reticulocytosis (increased red blood cell production)
- Splenic hypertrophy (extravascular hemolysis)
- Methemoglobinemia, hemoglobinuria, free plasma Hb (intravascular hemolysis), reduced serum haptoglobins
- Red blood cell fragmentation (microangiopathic hemolytic anemia)
- Coombs' test (immune-mediated hemolysis)
- Other (including Hb electrophoresis, bone marrow biopsy)

Management

1. Identification and specific treatment of the cause when possible.
2. Blood transfusion to maintain Hb >7 g/dL.
3. Massive intravascular hemolysis may lead to acute renal failure. Maintain a good diuresis and CRRT if necessary.

See also

Platelet disorders

Thrombocytopenia

Thrombocytopenia is rarely symptomatic until the platelet count is $<50 \times 10^9$/L. Spontaneous bleeding is more likely at $<20 \times 10^9$/L. Although bleeding is often minor (e.g., skin petechiae, oozing at intravascular catheter sites), it may be massive or life threatening (e.g., hemoptysis, intracranial hemorrhage).

Causes

- Sepsis—In the ICU, this is the most common cause of a low platelet count. It often provides a good barometer of recovery or deterioration.
- DIC
- Drugs
  - Related to antiplatelet antibody production, such as heparin (HITS), sulfonamides, quinine
  - Resulting in bone marrow suppression (e.g., chemotherapy agents)
  - Others (e.g., aspirin, chlorpromazine, prochlorperazine, digoxin)
- After massive bleeding and multiple blood transfusions
- Bone marrow failure (e.g., tumor infiltration, drugs)
- Splenomegaly
- TTP, HUS
- ITP
- Specific infections (e.g., measles, infectious mononucleosis, typhus)
- Collagen vascular diseases (e.g., SLE)

Management

1. Directed at the cause (e.g., antibiotics for sepsis, stopping offending drugs, plasma exchange for TTP, splenectomy and steroids for ITP)
2. Platelet support
   - Given routinely (e.g., 6–12 U/day) when counts are <10 to 20×10^9/L
   - 6 to 12 U given if $<50 \times 10^9$/L and either symptomatic or the result of surgery or another invasive procedure
3. Unless actively bleeding, avoid platelet transfusions in TTP or HUS.

Deranged platelet function

Function may be deranged, albeit with normal counts (e.g., after ingesting aspirin within the past 1 to 2 weeks, epoprostenol, uremia). Fresh platelets may be required if the patient is symptomatic. In uremia, one dose of vasopressin (20 µg IV over 30 min) may be useful to reverse platelet dysfunction.

Thrombocythemia

Thrombocythemia is rare in ICU patients. Platelet counts can exceed 800×10^9/L.

Causes

Causes include prolonged low-level bleeding, postsplenectomy, and myeloproliferative disorders. Essential (idiopathic) thrombocythemia is unusual.

Management
Because the major risk is thrombosis, management is based on mobilizing the patient and administering either prophylactic aspirin (150 mg bid PO) or heparin (5000 IU SC every 8h). Dipyridamole (300–600 mg tid PO) is occasionally used.

See also

Neutropenia

Neutropenia is defined as a neutrophil count of $<2 \times 10^9$/L. Life-threatening infections may develop at $<1 \times 10^9$/L, and more commonly at $<0.5 \times 10^9$/L. Absolute numbers of neutrophils are more relevant than percentages because the total white cell count may be either decreased, normal, or increased.

Clinical features
- Usually asymptomatic until infection supervenes

Causes
- Systemic inflammation results in margination and aggregation of neutrophils in organs (e.g., lung, liver, gut). Predominantly seen in the first 24 h after severe infection or trauma, it is often a precursor of multiple-organ dysfunction.
- Hemopoietic diseases (e.g., leukemia, lymphoma, myeloma, or as a consequence of chemotherapy or radiation)
- Nutritional deficiencies (e.g., folate, vitamin B12, malnutrition)
- Adverse drug reaction (e.g., carbimazole, sulfonamides)
- Part of aplastic anemia (e.g., idiopathic, drugs, infection)
- Specific infections (e.g., brucellosis, typhoid, viral, protozoal)
- Hypersplenism
- Antineutrophil antibodies (e.g., SLE)

Infections
- Initial infections are with common organisms such as pneumococci, staphylococci, and coliforms.
- With recurrent infections or after repeated courses of antibiotics, more unusual and/or antibiotic-resistant organisms may be responsible (e.g., *Pseudomonas*, fungi [particularly *Candida* and *Aspergillus* spp.], *Pneumocystis*, CMV, TB).

Management
1. If no diagnosis has been made, urgent investigations including a bone marrow aspiration are indicated.
2. Any implicated drugs should be immediately discontinued.
3. If the neutrophil count decreases to $<1 \times 10^9$/L, the patient should be protectively isolated in a cubicle with strict infection control procedures. Consider laminar flow air-conditioning if available.
4. Minimize invasive procedures.
5. Maintain good oral hygiene. Apply topical treatment as necessary (e.g., nystatin mouthwashes for oral fungal infection).
6. Apply clotrimazole cream for fungal skin infection.
7. Institute antibiotic therapy.
   - For suspected infection use aggressive, parenteral antibiotics (broad spectrum if no organism has been isolated).
   - Have a high index of suspicion for atypical infections such as fungi.

- Although prophylactic broad-spectrum antibiotics are often prescribed, this encourages antibiotic resistance. Another alternative is to maintain strict infection control with regular surveillance and to treat infections aggressively as indicated by likely sites and lab results. Avoid uncooked foods such as salads (Pseudomonas risk) and bottled pepper (Aspergillus).
8. Granulocyte-colony stimulating factor is frequently given to stimulate a bone marrow response.

See also

Full blood count, p. 154; Bacteriology, p. 158; Antimicrobials, p. 258; Infection control—general principles, p. 478; Infection—diagnosis, p. 482; Infection—treatment, p. 484

Leukemia

Patients with leukemia may present acutely to an ICU with complications arising from either the disease or the therapy.

Complications arising from the disease

- Decreased resistance to infection
- Hyperviscosity syndrome—drowsiness, coma, focal neurological defects
- CNS involvement
- Anemia, thrombocytopenia, bleeding tendency, DIC

Complications arising from the therapy

- Tumor lysis syndrome—Hyperkalemia, hyperuricemia, and acute renal failure may follow rapid destruction of a large white cell mass.
- Neutropenia and immune compromise with an increased risk of infection
- Anemia
- Thrombocytopenia leading to spontaneous bleeding, usually from intravascular catheter sites, skin, lung, gut, and brain
- Lung fibrosis (e.g., after radiotherapy, bleomycin)
- Myocardial failure (e.g., after mitoxantrone)
- Graft versus host disease (GVHD)—Features include mucositis, hepatitis, jaundice, diarrhea, abdominal pain, rash, and pneumonitis

Management

1. Tumor lysis syndrome can be prevented by adequate hydration, maintaining a good diuresis, and administering allopurinol. Once established, hemofiltration and other measures to lower serum potassium levels may be necessary.
2. The increased white cell mass may be reduced by leukophoresis.
3. Frequent blood transfusions to maintain Hb levels at >7 g/dL.
4. Platelet transfusions are required if counts remain <10 to 20×10^9/L, or if $<50 \times 10^9$/L and remaining symptomatic or undergoing an invasive procedure.
5. Give FFP and other blood products as needed.
6. Neutropenia management, including protective isolation, appropriate antibiotic therapy, ± granulocyte-colony stimulating factor.
7. GVHD is managed by supportive treatment and parenteral nutrition. PGE1 and immunosuppression may be helpful.
8. Psychological support for both patient and family is vital.

Respiratory failure

1. Maintain gas exchange. Mortality is high (>60%) if mechanical ventilation is necessary. Noninvasive techniques including CPAP and BiPAP can prove highly effective in avoiding the need for intubation.
2. When possible, treat the cause. Infection (including atypical organisms), fluid overload, ARDS, and a pneumonitis/fibrosis secondary to chemo- or radiotherapy should be considered.

See also

Metabolic disorders

Electrolyte management

A balance must be achieved between electrolyte intake and output.

Consider
- Altered intake
- Impaired renal excretion
- Increased body losses
- Body compartment redistribution (e.g., increased capillary leak, secondary hyperaldosteronism)

In addition Na^+ and K^+, consider Mg^{2+}, Ca^{2+}, Cl^-, and PO_4^{3-} balance.

Plasma electrolyte values are poorly reflective of whole-body stores; however, excessively high or low plasma levels may induce symptoms and deleterious physiological and metabolic sequelae.

Water balance must also be taken into account. Depletion or excess repletion may respectively concentrate or dilute electrolyte levels.

The usual daily requirements of Na^+ and K^+ are 60 to 80 mmol.

Gravitational peripheral edema implies increased total-body Na^+ and water, although intravascular salt and water depletion may coexist.

Electrolyte losses

Large nasogastric aspirate, vomiting	Na^+, Cl^-
Sweating	Na^+, Cl^-
Polyuria	Na^+, Cl^-, K^+, Mg^{2+}
Diarrhea	Na^+, Cl^-, K^+, Mg^{2+}
Ascitic drainage	Na^+, Cl^-, K^+

Principles of management

1. Establish sources and degree of fluid and electrolyte losses.
2. Assess patient for signs of (1) intravascular fluid depletionhypotension (e.g., after changes in posture, PEEP, vasodilating drugs) oliguria, increasing metabolic acidosis, and thirst; and (2) total-body NaCl and water overload (i.e., edema).
3. Measure BUN, creatinine, osmolality, and electrolyte content of plasma and urine.
4. As appropriate, either replace estimated fluid and electrolyte deficit or increase excretion (with diuretics, hemofiltration). For rate of fluid and specific electrolyte replacement, see individual sections.

See also

Hypernatremia

Clinical features

Hypernatremia can be caused by excessive loss of water or retention of Na (see Table 28.1). Clinical features of hypernatremia include thirst, lethargy, coma, seizures, muscular tremor and rigidity, and an increased risk of intracranial hemorrhage. Thirst usually occurs when the plasma sodium level increases 3 to 4 mmol/L above normal. Lack of thirst is associated with CNS disease.

Treatment

Treatment depends on the cause and whether total-body sodium stores are normal, low, or elevated, and body water is normal or low.

Rate of correction

- If hyperacute (<12 h), correction can be rapid.
- Otherwise, aim for gradual correction of plasma sodium levels (over 1–3 days), particularly in chronic cases (>2 days' duration), to avoid cerebral edema through sudden lowering of osmolality. A rate of plasma sodium lowering <0.7 mmol/h has been suggested.

Hypovolemia

- If hypovolemia is accompanied by hemodynamic alterations, use colloid initially to restore the circulation; otherwise, use isotonic saline.

Normal total-body Na (water loss)

- Water replacement either PO (addition to enteral feed) or as 5% glucose IV. Up to 5 L/day may be necessary.
- If central diabetes insipidus (CDI), restrict salt and give thiazide diuretics. Complete CDI will require desmopressin (10 μg bid intranasally or 1–2 μg bid IV), whereas partial CDI may require desmopressin but often responds to drugs that increase the rate of ADH secretion or end-organ responsiveness to ADH (e.g., chlorpropamide, hydrochlorothiazide).
- If nephrogenic diabetes insipidus, manage by a low-salt diet and thiazides. High-dose desmopressin may be effective. Consider removal of causative agents (e.g., lithium).

Low total-body Na (Na and water losses)

- Treat hyperosmolar nonketotic diabetic crisis, uremia as appropriate.
- Otherwise, consider 0.9% saline or hypotonic (0.45%) saline.

Increased total-body Na (Na gain)

- Water replacement either PO (addition to enteral feed) or as 5% glucose IV
- In addition, furosemide 10 to 20 mg IV PRN may be necessary.

Table 28.1 Causes of hypernatremia

Type	Etiology	Urine
Low total-body Na	Renal losses: diuretic excess, osmotic diuresis (glucose, urea, mannitol)	[Na$^+$] >20 mmol/L iso- or hypotonic
	Extrarenal losses: excess sweating	[Na$^+$] <10 mmol/L hypertonic
Normal total-body Na	Renal losses: diabetes insipidus	[Na$^+$] variable hypo-, iso-, or hypertonic
	Extrarenal losses: respiratory and renal insensible losses	[Na$^+$] variable hypertonic
Increased total-body Na	Conn's syndrome, Cushing's syndrome, excess NaCl, hypertonic NaHCO$_3$	[Na$^+$] >20 mmol/L iso- or hypertonic

See also

Continuous renal replacement therapy (1), p. 62; Continuous renal replacement therapy (2), p. 66; Enteral nutrition, p. 82; Parenteral nutrition, p. 84; Electrolytes (Na$^+$, K$^+$, Cl$^-$, HCO$_3^-$), p. 146; Urinalysis, p. 166; Crystalloids, p. 176; Colloids, p. 180; Diuretics, p. 212; Electrolyte management, p. 416; Diabetic ketoacidosis, p. 444; Hyperosmolar diabetic emergencies, p. 446

Hyponatremia

Clinical features

Hyponatremia can best be diagnosed by assessing ECF (see Table 28.2). Clinical features of hyponatremia include nausea, vomiting, headache, fatigue, weakness, muscular twitching, obtundation, psychosis, seizures, and coma. Symptoms depend on the rate as well as the magnitude of the decrease in plasma [Na^+].

Treatment

Rate and degree of correction

- Rate and degree of correction depend on how rapidly the condition has developed and whether the patient is symptomatic. Hyponatremia that has developed over more than 48 h is considered 'chronic.'
- In chronic asymptomatic hyponatremia, correction should not exceed 4 mmol/24 h, and the rate of correction should not exceed 0.3 mmol/L/h.
- In chronic symptomatic (e.g., seizures, coma) hyponatremia, correction should be 1 to 1.5 mmol/L/h until symptoms resolve, then correct as per asymptomatic cases.
- In acute hyponatremia (<48 h) the ideal rate of correction is controversial, although elevations in plasma Na^+ can be faster, but should not exceed <20 mmol/L/day.
- Plasma Na^+ of 125 to 130 mmol/L is a reasonable target for initial correction of both acute and chronic states. Attempts to achieve eunatremia rapidly should be avoided.
- Neurological complications (e.g., central pontine myelinolysis) are related to the degree of correction and (in chronic hyponatremia) the rate. Premenopausal women are at highest risk for this complication.

Extracellular fluid volume excess

- If symptomatic (e.g., seizures, agitation), 100-mL aliquots of hypertonic (1.8%) saline can be given, checking plasma levels every 2 to 3 h.
- If symptomatic and edematous, consider furosemide (10–20-mg IV bolus PRN), in addition to hypertonic saline. Check plasma levels every 2 to 3 h. Hemofiltration or dialysis may be necessary if renal failure is established.
- If not symptomatic, restrict water to 1 to 1.5 L/day. If hyponatremia persists, consider inappropriate ADH (SIADH) secretion.
- If SIADH likely, give isotonic saline and consider demeclocycline.

Extracellular fluid volume depletion

- If symptomatic (e.g., seizures, agitation), give isotonic (0.9%) saline. Consider hypertonic (1.8%) saline initially, especially if acute.
- If asymptomatic, use isotonic (0.9%) saline.

General points

- Equations that calculate excess water are unreliable. It is safer to monitor plasma sodium levels closely.
- Hypertonic saline may be dangerous, especially in the elderly and in those with impaired cardiac function. An alternative is to use furosemide with replacement of urinary sodium (and potassium) losses every 2 to 3 h. Thereafter, simple water restriction is usually sufficient.

- Many patients achieve eunatremia by spontaneous water diuresis.
- Use isotonic solutions for reconstituting drugs, parenteral nutrition, and so forth.
- Hyponatremia may intensify the cardiac effects of hyperkalemia.
- A true hyponatremia may occur with a normal osmolality in the presence of abnormal solutes (e.g., ethanol, ethylene glycol, glucose).

Causes of inappropriate ADH secretion

- Neoplasm (e.g., lung, pancreas, lymphoma)
- Most pulmonary lesions
- Most CNS lesions
- Surgical and emotional stress
- Glucocorticoid and thyroid deficiency
- Idiopathic
- Drugs (e.g., chlorpropamide, carbamazepine, narcotics)

Table 28.2 Causes of hyponatremia

Type	Etiology	Urine [Na$^+$]
ECF volume depletion	Renal losses: diuretic excess, osmotic diuresis (glucose, urea, mannitol), renal tubular acidosis, salt-losing nephritis, mineralocorticoid deficiency	>20 mmol/L
	Extrarenal losses: vomiting, diarrhea, burns, pancreatitis	<10 mmol/L
Modest ECF volume excess (no edema)	Water intoxication (NB: postoperative, TURP syndrome), inappropriate ADH secretion, hypothyroidism, drugs (e.g., carbamazepine, chlorpropamide), glucocorticoid deficiency, pain, stress	>20 mmol/L
	Acute and chronic renal failure	>20 mmol/L
ECF volume excess (edema)	Nephrotic syndrome, cirrhosis, heart failure	<10 mmol/L

ECF, extracellular fluid; TURP, trasnsuretural resection of prostate.

See also

Continuous renal replacement therapy (1), p. 62; Continuous renal replacement therapy (2), p. 66; Enteral nutrition, p. 82; Parenteral nutrition, p. 84; Electrolytes (Na$^+$, K$^+$, Cl$^-$, HCO$_3^-$), p. 146; Urinalysis, p. 166; Crystalloids, p. 176; Colloids, p. 180; Diuretics, p. 212; Acute renal failure—diagnosis, p. 332; Acute renal failure—management, p. 334; Electrolyte management, p. 416; Diabetic ketoacidosis, p. 444; Hyperosmolar diabetic emergencies, p. 446

Hyperkalemia

Plasma potassium depends on the balance between intake, excretion, and the distribution of potassium across cell membranes. Excretion is normally controlled by the kidneys.

Causes

- Reduced renal excretion (e.g., renal failure, adrenal insufficiency, diabetes, potassium-sparing diuretics)
- Intracellular potassium release (e.g., acidosis, rapid transfusion of old blood, cell lysis including rhabdomyolysis, hemolysis, and tumor lysis)
- Potassium poisoning

Clinical features

Hyperkalemia may cause dangerous arrhythmias, including cardiac arrest. Arrhythmias are more closely related to the rate of increase in potassium, rather than the absolute level. Clinical features such as paraesthesia and areflexic weakness are not clearly related to the degree of hyperkalemia but usually occur after ECG changes (tall T waves, flat P waves, prolonged PR interval, and wide QRS).

Management

Potassium restriction is needed for all cases, and dialysis may be needed for resistant cases.

Cardiac arrest associated with hyperkalemia

Sodium bicarbonate (8.4%) 50 to 100 mL should be given in addition to standard CPR and other treatment detailed next.

Potassium >7 mmol/L

Calcium chloride (10%) 10 mL should be given urgently in addition to treatment detailed next. Although calcium chloride does not reduce the plasma potassium, it stabilizes the myocardium against arrhythmias.

Clinical features of hyperkalemia or potassium >6 mmol/L with ECG changes

Glucose (50%) 50 mL and soluble insulin 10 IU should be given IV over 20 min. Blood glucose should be monitored every 15 min and more glucose given if necessary.

See also

Continuous renal replacement therapy (1), p. 62; Continuous renal replacement therapy (2), p. 66; Enteral nutrition, p. 82; Parenteral nutrition, p. 84; Electrolytes (Na^+, K^+, Cl^-, HCO_3), p. 146; Urinalysis, p. 166; Crystalloids, p. 176; Diuretics, p. 212; Cardiac arrest, p. 270; Bradyarrhythmias, p. 316; Acute renal failure—diagnosis, p. 330; Acute renal failure—management, p. 332; Electrolyte management, p. 416; Rhabdomyolysis, p. 530

Hypokalemia

Plasma potassium depends on the balance between intake, excretion, and the distribution of potassium across cell membranes. Excretion is normally controlled by the kidneys.

Causes
- Inadequate intake
- Gastrointestinal losses (e.g., vomiting, diarrhea, fistula losses)
- Renal losses (e.g., diabetic ketoacidosis, Conn's syndrome, secondary hyperaldosteronism, Cushing's syndrome, renal tubular acidosis, metabolic alkalosis, hypomagnesemia, drugs including diuretics, steroids, theophyllines)
- Hemofiltration losses
- Potassium transfer into cells (e.g., acute alkalosis, glucose infusion, insulin treatment, familial periodic paralysis)

Clinical features
- Arrhythmias (SVT, VT, and torsades de pointes)
- ECG changes (ST depression, T- wave flattening, U waves)
- Metabolic alkalosis
- Constipation
- Ileus
- Weakness

Management
- Whenever possible, the cause of potassium loss should be treated.
- Potassium replacement should be IV with ECG monitoring when there is a clinically significant arrhythmia (20 mmol over 30 min, repeated according to levels).
- Slower IV replacement (20 mmol over 1 h) should be used when there are clinical features without arrhythmias.
- Oral supplementation (to a total intake of 80–120 mmol/day, including nutritional input) can be given when there are no clinical features.

See also

Enteral nutrition, p. 82; Parenteral nutrition, p. 84; Electrolytes (Na^+, K^+, Cl^-, HCO_3^-), p. 146; Urinalysis, p. 166; Crystalloids, p. 176; Diuretics, p. 212; Steroids, p. 260; Cardiac arrest, p. 270; Tachyarrhythmias, p. 314; Electrolyte management, p. 416; Metabolic alkalosis, p. 438; Diabetic ketoacidosis, p. 444; Postoperative intensive care, p. 536

Hypomagnesemia

Causes

- Excess loss (e.g., diuretics), other causes of polyuria [including poorly controlled diabetes mellitus], severe diarrhea, prolonged vomiting, large nasogastric aspirates)
- Inadequate intake (e.g., starvation, parenteral nutrition, alcoholism, malabsorption syndromes)

Clinical features

Magnesium is primarily an intracellular ion involved in the production and utilization of energy stores, and in the mediation of nerve transmission. Low plasma levels, which do not necessarily reflect either intracellular or whole-body stores, may thus be associated with features related to the following functions:

- Confusion, irritability
- Seizures
- Muscle weakness, lethargy
- Arrhythmias
- Symptoms related to hypocalcemia and hypokalemia, which are resistant to calcium and potassium supplementation respectively

Normal plasma levels range from 1.7 to 2.4 mg/dL. Severe symptoms do not usually occur until levels decrease to < 1.0 mg/dL.

Management

- When possible, identify and treat the cause.
- For severe, symptomatic hypomagnesemia, 10 mmol magnesium sulfate can be given IV over 3 to 5 min. This can be repeated once or twice as necessary.
- In less acute situations or for asymptomatic hypomagnesemia, 1 to 2 g $MgSO_4$ solution can be given over 1 to 2 h and repeated as necessary, or according to repeat plasma levels.
- A continuous IV infusion can be given; however, this is usually reserved for therapeutic indications when supranormal plasma levels (4–5 mg/dL) of magnesium are sought (e.g., treatment of supraventricular and ventricular arrhythmias, preeclampsia, and eclampsia).
- Oral magnesium sulfate has a laxative effect and may cause severe diarrhea.
- High plasma levels of magnesium may develop in renal failure. Caution should be applied when administering IV magnesium.

See also

Hypercalcemia

Causes

- Malignancy (e.g., myeloma, bony metastatic disease, hypernephroma)
- Hyperparathyroidism
- Sarcoidosis
- TB
- Excess intake of calcium, vitamin A or D
- Drugs (e.g., thiazides, lithium)
- Immobilization
- Rarely, thyrotoxicosis, Addison's disease

Clinical features

Clinical features of hypercalcemia usually become apparent when total (ionized and nonionized) plasma levels are >13 mg/dL (normal range, 8.5–10.5 mg/dL). Symptoms depend on the patient's age, the duration and rate of increase of plasma calcium, and the presence of concurrent medical conditions.

- Nausea, vomiting, weight loss, pruritus
- Muscle weakness, fatigue, lethargy
- Depression, mania, psychosis
- Drowsiness, coma
- Abdominal pain, constipation
- Acute pancreatitis
- Peptic ulceration
- Polyuria, renal calculi, renal failure
- Arrhythmias

Management

1. Identify and treat cause when possible.
2. Carefully monitor hemodynamic variables, urine output, and ECG morphology with frequent estimations of plasma Ca^{2+}, PO_4^{3-}, Mg^{2+}, Na^+, and K^+.
3. Intravascular volume repletion— inhibits proximal tubular reabsorption of calcium and often lowers the plasma calcium by 1 to 2 mg/dL. It should precede diuretics or any other therapy. Either colloid or 0.9% saline should be used, depending on the presence of hypovolemia-related features.
4. Calciuresis—After adequate intravascular volume repletion, a forced diuresis of calcium with furosemide plus 0.9% saline (6–8 L/day) may be attempted. An effect is usually seen within 12 h. Loop diuretics inhibit calcium reabsorption in the ascending limb of the loop of Henle. More aggressive furosemide regimens can be attempted, but can potentially result in complications. Thiazides should not be used because tubular reabsorption may be reduced and hypercalcemia worsened. (See Table 28.3.)
5. Dialysis/hemofiltration may be indicated at an early stage if the patient is in established oliguanuric renal failure ± fluid overloaded.
6. Steroids can be effective for hypercalcemia related to hematological cancers (lymphoma, myeloma), vitamin D overdose, and sarcoidosis.

7. Calcitonin has the most rapid onset of action, with a nadir often reached within 12 to 24 h. Its action is usually shortlived, and rebound hypercalcemia may occur. It generally does not decrease the plasma level more than 2 mg/dL.

8. Biphosphonates (e.g., pamidronate) and IV phosphate should only be given after other measures have failed, in view of their toxicity and potential complications.

Table 28.3 Drug dosage

Diuretics	Furosemide 10–40 mg IV q 2–4 h (may be increased to 80–100 mg IV q 1–2 h)
Steroids	Hydrocortisone 100 mg qid IV or prednisolone 40–60 mg PO for 3–5 days
Pamidronate	15–60 mg slow IV bolus
Calcitonin	3–4 U/kg IV followed by 4 U/kg SC bid

See also

Calcium, magnesium, and phosphate, p. 148; Diuretics, p. 212; Steroids, p. 260; Acute renal failure—diagnosis, p. 330; Acute renal failure—management, p. 332; Pancreatitis, p. 354; Electrolyte management, p. 416; Diabetic ketoacidosis, p. 444; Thyroid emergencies, p. 448; Hypoadrenal crisis, p. 450

Hypocalcemia

Causes
- Associated with hyperphosphatemia
  - Renal failure
  - Rhabdomyolysis
  - Hypoparathyroidism (including surgery), pseudohypoparathyroidism
- Associated with low/normal phosphate
  - Critical illness including sepsis, burns
  - Hypomagnesemia
  - Pancreatitis
  - Osteomalacia
  - Overhydration
- Massive blood transfusion (citrate binding)
- Hyperventilation and the resulting respiratory alkalosis may reduce the ionized plasma calcium fraction and induce clinical features of hypocalcemia.

Clinical features
Clinical features of hypocalcemia these usually appear when total plasma calcium levels are <8 mg/dL and the ionized fraction is <0.8 mmol/L.
- Tetany (including carpopedal spasm)
- Muscular weakness
- Hypotension
- Perioral and peripheral paresthesia
- Chvostek and Trousseau's signs
- Prolonged QT interval
- Seizures

Management
1. If respiratory alkalosis is present, adjust ventilator settings or, if spontaneously hyperventilating and agitated, calm ± sedate. Rebreathing into a bag may be beneficial.
2. If symptomatic, give 5 to 10 mL 10% calcium chloride or 10 to 20 mL 10% calcium gluconate solution over 10 to 15 min. Repeat as necessary.
3. Correct hypomagnesemia or hypokalemia if present.
4. If asymptomatic and in renal failure or hypoparathyroid, consider enteral/parenteral calcium supplementation and vitamin D analogues.
5. If hypotensive or cardiac output is decreased after administration of a calcium antagonist, give 5 to 10 mL 10% calcium chloride solution over 2 to 5 min.

See also

Hypophosphatemia

Causes

- Critical illness
- Inadequate intake
- Loop diuretic therapy (including low-dose dopamine)
- Parenteral nutrition—Levels decrease rapidly during high-dose IV glucose therapy, especially with insulin.
- Alcoholism
- Hyperparathyroidism

Clinical effects

Hypophosphatemia is often asymptomatic even when severe (<1 mg/dL). Symptoms may include muscle weakness (including respiratory muscles, and can be associated with inability to wean from mechanical ventilation), rhabdomyolysis, paresthesias, hemolysis, platelet dysfunction, and cardiac failure.

Treatment

Mild hypophosphatemia may be treated with oral phosphate supplements. In severe and symptomatic cases 20 to 40 mmol $NaPO_4$ (sodium phosphate) or $KaPO_4$ (potassium phosphate) should be given by IV infusion over 6 h and repeated according to the plasma phosphate level.

See also

Enteral nutrition, p. 82; Parenteral nutrition, p. 84; Calcium, magnesium, and phosphate, p. 148; Diuretics, p. 212; Acute weakness, p. 368

General acid–base management

Increased intake, altered production, or impaired/excessive excretion of acid or base leads to derangements in blood pH. With time, respiratory and renal adjustments correct the pH toward normalcy by altering the plasma levels of PCO_2 or strong ions (Na^+, Cl^-).

Increased intake
- Acidosis—chloride administration (e.g., saline), aspirin overdose
- Alkalosis—$NaHCO_3$ administration, antacid abuse, buffered replacement fluid (hemofiltration)

Altered production
- Increased acid production—lactic acidosis, diabetic ketoacidosis

Altered excretion
- Hypercapnic respiratory failure, permissive hypercapnia
- Alkalosis—vomiting, large gastric aspirates, diuretics, hyperaldosteronism, corticosteroids
- Acidosis—diarrhea, small bowel fistula, urethroenterostomy, renal tubular acidosis, renal failure, distal renal tubular acidosis, acetazolamide

Principles of management
- Correct (when possible) the underlying cause (e.g., hypoperfusion).
- NaCl infusion for vomiting-induced alkalosis; insulin, Na^+, and K^+ in diabetic ketoacidosis
- Correct pH in specific circumstances only (e.g., $NaHCO_3$ in renal failure).
- Avoid large-volume saline-based fluids. Consider lactated Ringer's solution or hetastarch in balanced electrolyte solution (Hextend) for fluid resuscitation.

See also

Metabolic acidosis

Metabolic acidosis is reduced arterial blood pH with a reduced strong ion difference and a base deficit >2 mEq/L. Outcome in critically ill patients has been linked to the severity and duration of metabolic acidosis and hyperlactatemia.

Causes of metabolic acidosis

- Lactic acidosis—can be the result of tissue hypoperfusion (e.g., circulatory shock). The anion gap (or SIG) is increased with lactic and other organic acids, and poisons. Anaerobic metabolism contributes in part to metabolic acidosis; however, other cellular mechanisms are involved and may be more important. May be seen with increased muscle activity (e.g., postseizure, respiratory distress). Lung lactate release seen in acute lung injury. High, sustained levels suggest tissue necrosis (e.g., bowel, muscle).
- Hyperchloremia (e.g., excessive saline infusion)
- Ketoacidosis—high levels of β-hydroxybutyrate and acetoacetate related to uncontrolled diabetes mellitus, starvation and alcoholism
- Renal failure—accumulation of organic acids (e.g., sulfuric)
- Drugs—in particular, aspirin (salicylic acid) overdose, acetazolamide (carbonic anhydrase inhibition), ammonium chloride. Vasopressor agents may be implicated, possibly by inducing regional ischemia or, in the case of epinephrine, accelerated glycolysis.
- Ingestion of poisons (e.g., paraldehyde, ethylene glycol, methanol)
- Cation loss (e.g., severe diarrhea, small bowel fistulas, large ileostomy losses)

Causes of lactic acidosis

- Acute infection
- Acute lung injury
- Diabetes mellitus
- Drugs (e.g., phenformin, metformin, alcohols)
- Circulatory shock (e.g., septic shock, hemorrhage, heart failure)
- Glucose-6-phosphatase deficiency
- Hematological malignancy
- Hepatic failure
- Renal failure
- Short bowel syndrome (D-lactate)
- Thiamine deficiency

Clinical features

- Dyspnea
- Hemodynamic instability
- A rapidly increasing metabolic acidosis (over minutes to hours) is not the result of renal failure. Other causes, particularly severe tissue hypoperfusion, sepsis, or tissue necrosis, should be suspected when there is associated systemic deterioration.

Management

1. The underlying cause should be identified and treated when possible, rather than administering alkali or manipulating minute volume to normalize the arterial pH.
2. Urgent dialysis/hemofiltration may be necessary if oliguria persists.
3. Reversal of metabolic acidosis is generally an indication of successful therapy. An increasing base deficit suggests that the therapeutic maneuvers in operation are either inadequate or wrong.
4. The benefits of buffers such as Carbicarb and tris-hydroxymethyl-aminomethane remain unproved.

See also

Continuous renal replacement therapy (1), p. 62; Continuous renal replacement therapy (2), p. 66; Blood gas analysis, p. 102; Sodium bicarbonate, p. 178; Blood transfusion, p. 182; Acute renal failure—diagnosis, p. 330; Acute renal failure—management, p. 332; General acid–base management, p. 434

Metabolic alkalosis

- Metabolic alkalosis is an increased arterial blood pH with an increased strong ion difference and base excess >2 mEq/L caused either by loss of anions or gain of cations. Because the kidney is usually efficient at regulating the strong ion difference, persistence of metabolic alkalosis usually depends on either renal impairment or diminished extracellular fluid volume with severe depletion of K^+, resulting in an inability to reabsorb Cl^- in excess of Na^+.
- The patient is usually asymptomatic, although if breathing spontaneously, will hypoventilate.
- Metabolic alkalosis will cause a left shift of the oxyhemoglobin curve, reducing oxygen availability to the tissues.
- If severe (pH >7.6), it may result in encephalopathy, seizures, altered coronary arterial blood flow, and decreased cardiac inotropy.

Causes

- Loss of total body fluid, Cl^-, usually the result of
  - Diuretics
  - Large nasogastric aspirates, vomiting
- Secondary hyperaldosteronism with KCl depletion
- Use of hemofiltration replacement fluid containing excess buffer (e.g., lactate)
- Renal compensation for chronic hypercapnia, which can develop within 1 to 2 weeks. Although more apparent when the patient hyperventilates, or is hyperventilated to normocapnia, overcompensated metabolic alkalosis can occasionally be seen in the chronic state (i.e., increased pH in an otherwise stable, long-term hypercapnic patient).
- Excess administration of sodium bicarbonate
- Excess administration of sodium citrate (large blood transfusion)
- Drugs, including laxative abuse, corticosteroids
- Rarely, Cushing's, Conn's, and Bartter's syndromes

Management

1. Replacement of fluid, Cl^- (i.e., give 0.9% saline), and K^+ losses are often sufficient to restore acid–base balance.
2. With distal renal causes related to hyperaldosteronism, addition of spironolactone can be considered.
3. Active treatment is rarely necessary. If so, administer 150 mL 1.0 N HCl in 1 L sterile water using a central line. Infuse at a rate not greater than 1 mL/kg/h. Alternatives include ammonium chloride PO or, if volume overloaded with intact renal function, acetazolamide 500 mg IV or PO every 8 h.
4. Compensation for long-standing respiratory acidosis, followed by correction of that acidosis (e.g., with mechanical ventilation), will lead to uncompensated metabolic alkalosis. This usually corrects with time, although treatments such as acetazolamide can be considered. Mechanical 'hypoventilation' (i.e., maintaining hypercapnia) can also be considered.

See also

Continuous renal replacement therapy (1), p. 62; Continuous renal replacement therapy (2), p. 66; Blood gas analysis, p. 102; Sodium bicarbonate, p. 178; Blood transfusion, p. 182; Acute renal failure—diagnosis, p. 330; Acute renal failure—management, p. 332; Vomiting/gastric stasis, p. 336; Hypokalemia, p. 424; General acid–base management, p. 434

Hypoglycemia

Causes

- Inadequate intake of carbohydrate
- Excess insulin or sulfonylurea
- Liver failure with depletion of glycogen stores
- Alcohol
- Hypoadrenalism (including Addison's disease), hypopituitarism
- Quinine, aspirin toxicity

Clinical features

- Nausea, vomiting
- Increased sympathetic activity (e.g., sweating, tachycardia)
- Altered behavior and level of consciousness
- Seizures, focal neurological signs
- Should always be considered in patients found unconscious or having seizures

Management

1. Monitor carefully with regular bedside estimations. The frequency should be increased in conditions known to precipitate hypoglycemia (e.g., insulin infusion, liver failure, quinine treatment of malaria).
2. Administer 50 mL 50% glucose solution if the blood glucose is
   - ≤50 mg/dL
   - ≤80 mg/dL and the patient is symptomatic

   Repeat as necessary every few minutes until symptoms abate and the blood glucose level has normalized.
3. If blood glucose is 50 to 70 mg/dL and the patient is nonsymptomatic, either reduce the rate of insulin infusion (if present) or increase calorie intake (enterally or parenterally). In insulin-dependent diabetes mellitus, the insulin should continue with adequate glucose intake.
4. A continuous parenteral infusion of 10%, 20%, or 50% glucose solution varying from 10 to 100 mL/h may be required, depending on the degree of continuing hypoglycemia and the patient's fluid balance/urine output. Five percent glucose solution only contains 20 KCal/100 mL and should not be used to prevent or treat hypoglycemia.
5. In the rare instance of no venous access, hypoglycemia may be temporarily reversed by glucagon 1 mg given either IM or SC.
6. Continuing hypoglycemia in the face of adequate treatment and lack of symptoms should be confirmed with a formal laboratory blood sugar estimation to exclude malfunction of bedside testing equipment.

See also

Nutrition—use and indications, p. 80; Enteral nutrition, p. 82; Parenteral nutrition, p. 84; Crystalloids, p. 176; Acute liver failure, p. 360; Generalized seizures, p. 372; Hypoadrenal crisis, p. 450; Paracetamol poisoning, p. 458

Hyperglycemia

Causes

- A common occurrence in critically ill patients resulting from a combination of impaired glucose tolerance, insulin resistance, high circulating levels of endogenous catecholamines and corticosteroids, and regular administration of drugs that antagonize the effect of insulin
- Pancreatitis resulting in islet cell damage

Clinical features

In hyperglycemia there are no clinical features in the short term, other than polyuria from osmotic diuresis. The patient may complain of thirst or show signs of hypovolemia if fluid balance is allowed to become too negative.

Metabolic effects

Relative lack of insulin prevents cellular glucose uptake and utilization, resulting in
- Increased lipolysis
- Altered cellular metabolism
- Increased risk of infection (decreased neutrophil function)

Prognostic significance

Strict maintenance of glycemic control (approximately 80–110 mg/dL) resulted in significant outcome improvement in a surgical ICU population. Whether this is related to prevention of hyperglycemia and/or an effect related to additional administration of insulin remains uncertain.

Management

1. Treatment should be given if blood glucose elevations persist (>110–130 mg/dL).
2. A short-acting insulin infusion should be used and titrated to maintain normoglycemia (80–110 mg/dL). Usually 1 to 4 U/h is required, although it may need to be much higher in diabetics who become critically ill. Regular bedside monitoring of blood sugar should be performed; this should be undertaken hourly if unstable.
3. Oral hypoglycemic agents should be generally avoided in the ICU patient because of their prolonged duration of action and unpredictable absorption.

Key trial

Van den Berghe G, *et al.* Intensive insulin therapy in critically ill patients. *N Engl J Med* 2001;
345:1359–67.

Diabetic ketoacidosis

Diabetic ketoacidosis may occur de novo in a previously undiagnosed diabetic patient or after an acute insult (e.g., infection) in a known diabetic patient.

Clinical features

- Excess fat metabolism to fatty acids with ketone production
- Osmotic diuresis with large losses of fluid (up to 6–10 L), sodium (400–800 mmol), potassium (250–800 mmol), and magnesium

Symptoms result from hypovolemia, metabolic acidosis, and electrolyte imbalance with polyuria. Hyperventilation is a prominent feature.

Coma need not necessarily be present for life to be threatened.

Plasma amylase is commonly increased but does not indicate pancreatitis. If suspected, perform an abdominal ultrasound or CT.

Monitoring

Adequate invasive monitoring is essential, particularly if the patient has circulatory instability or cardiac dysfunction. Urine output, blood gases, and plasma electrolytes should also be monitored frequently.

Fluid and electrolyte management

1. Fluid and electrolyte repletion should be tailored to individual needs.
2. Colloid fluid challenges can be given to restore the circulating blood volume in tissue hypoperfusion. However, crystalloids are usually chosen to replace fluid losses.
3. Fluid replacement with 0.9% saline should be given at a rate of 200 mL/h until the salt and water debt has been replenished.
4. Hypotonic (0.45%) saline resuscitation may be appropriate in patients without shock if plasma sodium is increasing rapidly (shift of water and potassium into cells and sodium out).
5. Substitute 5% glucose solution 100 to 200 mL/h after replacing the sodium debt—usually when the blood sugar decreases to <200 mg/dL.
6. Carefully monitor K^+ replacement. Both acidosis and excessive K^+ administration cause hyperkalemia, whereas fluid and insulin will produce hypokalemia. Check levels frequently to maintain normokalemia. KCl infusions are usually needed.
7. Carefully monitor magnesium replacement; 2 to 3 g $MgSO_4$ is usually sufficient.

Hyperglycemia

For hyperglycemia correct slowly at a rate of 40 to 80 mg/dL/h by adjusting the short-acting insulin infusion (usually 1–10 U/h). Monitor blood glucose hourly. Continue IV insulin (with glucose after achieving normoglycemia) until heavy ketonuria has disappeared and the anion gap has normalized.

Other aspects of managing ketoacidosis

1. Seek a precipitating cause and treat as indicated. Approximately 50% of cases are related to underlying disease (e.g., sepsis, MI, stroke, infective gastroenteritis).
2. Only give antibiotics for proved or highly suspected infection.

3. Abdominal pain should not be dismissed as part of the syndrome.
4. A nasogastric tube should be considered, because gastric emptying is often delayed and acute gastric dilatation is common, particularly in older patients.
5. Avoid sodium bicarbonate except in severe acidosis (pH <7.0). It is usually unnecessary and may result in respiratory depression resulting from relative CSF alkalosis. Sodium overload and "overshoot" alkalosis may also occur.
6. Low-molecular weight or unfractionated heparin is indicated in immobile or comatose patients.

See also

Hyperosmolar diabetic emergencies

Hyperosmolar diabetic emergencies are more common in elderly, noninsulin-dependent diabetic patients, although they can present de novo in young adults. Precipitating factors are similar to ketoacidosis (e.g., sepsis, MI).

Clinical features

- Fluid depletion is greater, blood glucose levels are often higher, coma more frequent, and mortality much higher than in diabetic ketoacidosis
- Confusion, agitation, and drowsiness that may persist for 1 to 2 weeks
- Metabolic acidosis may be present, but is not usually profound. Ketoacidosis is not a major feature.
- Hyperosmolality may predispose to thrombotic events. which is the major cause of mortality. Severe hyperosmolality does not always occur.
- Focal neurological signs and DIC are occasionally recognized.

Management

Manage as for diabetic ketoacidosis; however,

1. Unless the patient shows signs of hypovolemia and tissue hypoperfusion, in which case fluid challenges should be given for prompt resuscitation, fluid replacement should be more gradual because the risk of cerebral edema is higher. This can be with either 0.9% saline or, if the plasma sodium is high, 0.45% saline at a rate of 100 to 200 mL/h.
2. Plasma sodium increases with treatment, even with 0.45% saline, and can often increase in the first few days to 160 to 170 mmol/L before gradually declining thereafter. Aim to correct slowly.
3. Serum phosphate and magnesium levels decrease rapidly with this condition. Replacement may be needed, as guided by frequently taken plasma levels.
4. Patients may be hypersensitive to insulin and may require lower doses
5. Low-molecular weight or unfractionated heparin is indicated in immobile or comatose patients

See also

Thyroid emergencies

Thyrotoxic crisis

Thyrotoxic crisis presents as an exacerbation of the clinical features of hyperthyroidism (e.g., pyrexia, hyperdynamic circulation, heart failure, confusion). There is usually a precipitating factor such as infection, surgery, ketoacidosis, MI, or childbirth. It may present with exhaustion in the elderly with few features of hyperthyroidism. The diagnosis is confirmed by standard thyroid function tests.

Management

- Pyrexia should be controlled by surface cooling (avoid aspirin which displaces thyroxine from plasma proteins).
- Catecholamine effects should be reduced by β blockade (e.g., propranolol 1–5 mg IV then 20–80 mg qid PO). These should be used with caution if there is acute heart failure.
- Blockade of thyroxine synthesis is achieved by potassium iodide 200 to 600 mg IV over 2 h then 2 g/day PO and carbimazole 60 to 120 mg/day PO.
- Blockade of peripheral T4-to-T3 conversion is achieved by dexamethasone 2mg q6h IV.
- Careful fluid and electrolyte management is essential.

Myxedema coma

Myxedema coma presents as an exacerbation of the features of hypothyroidism (e.g., hypothermia, coma, bradycardia, metabolic and respiratory acidosis, anemia). There may be a precipitating factor (e.g., cold, infection, surgery, MI, CVA, CNS- depressing drugs). Diagnosis is confirmed by thyroid function tests.

Management

- Treatment of the complications of severe hypothyroidism (e.g., hypotension, heart failure, hypothermia, bradycardia, seizures) is more important than thyroid hormone replacement.
- A single dose of IV levothyroxine (0.2–0.5 mg) should be administered followed by 0.1 mg IV until oral dosing can be started. Doses may need to be reduced if ischemic heart disease is possible.
- Steroids (hydrocortisone 100 mg q6h IV) should be given because coexisting hypoadrenalism is masked by myxedema.

Sick euthyroid/low T3 syndrome

Sick euthyroid/low T3 syndrome is a frequent complication of critical illness with low T3 and T4, and high reverse T3 levels. These correlate with the severity of disease and a poor outcome. There is both reduced thyroid stimulating hormone secretion and altered peripheral thyroid metabolism. A trial of thyroxine administration in critically ill patients produced a negative outcome, although those with sick euthyroid syndrome were not identified. Treatment for this syndrome is thus not recommended.

See also

Hypoadrenal crisis

Clinical features

Primary hypoadrenalism

- Glucocorticoid deficiency (e.g., weakness, vomiting, diarrhea, abdominal pain, hypoglycemia)
- Mineralocorticoid deficiency (e.g., dehydration, hyponatremia, weight loss, postural hypotension, hyperkalemia)
- Skin pigmentation resulting from ACTH excess

Secondary hypoadrenalism

- May be the result of critical illness (e.g., sepsis), steroid withdrawal after 2 weeks of treatment, hypopituitarism, or etomidate use
- No skin pigmentation
- Features of mineralocorticoid deficiency may be absent.

Diagnosis

Diagnosis is confirmed by plasma cortisol, ACTH levels and, ACTH stimulation test, although treatment should begin on clinical suspicion. A dose of ACTH 250 μg IV should produce a >9 μg/dL increase in plasma cortisol by 60 min. In primary hypoadrenalism, levels remain <20 μg/dL. However, baseline levels may be normal or elevated in the relative adrenal insufficiency seen in sepsis and other critical illnesses. Dexamethasone may be used for steroid replacement for 48 h before an ACTH test is performed, because other steroid treatments are detected in the plasma cortisol assay.

Management

- Salt and water deficiency should be corrected urgently. Initial fluid replacement should be with colloid if there is hypotension or evidence of poor tissue perfusion. Otherwise 4 to 5 L/day 0.9% saline will be needed for several days.
- Fluid management should be carefully monitored to ensure adequate replacement without fluid overload.
- Glucocorticoid replacement should be with hydrocortisone 50 to 100 mg q8h IV. Hydrocortisone may be changed to equivalent doses of dexamethasone before the ACTH test has been performed.
- Relative hypoadrenalism related to sepsis can be treated with hydrocortisone 50 mg q6h for 5 to 7 days, and then a reducing dose over the next 5 to 7 days. Fludrocortisone 0.1 mg PO qd can also be used in addition to hydrocortisone for patients with hypotension. Studies have shown more rapid resolution of shock and an improved outcome in those showing a suboptimal response to synthetic ACTH (<9 μg/dL increase), despite increased baseline levels.

See also

Blood pressure monitoring, p. 112; Central venous catheter—use, p. 116; Electrolytes (Na⁺, K⁺, Cl⁻, HCO₃⁻), p. 146; Calcium, magnesium, and phosphate, p. 148; Crystalloids, p. 176; Colloids, p. 180; Steroids, p. 258; Fluid challenge, p. 270; Hypotension, p. 308; Diarrhea, p. 336; Hyponatremia, p. 420; Hypercalcemia, p. 428; Hypoglycemia, p. 440

Poisoning

Poisoning—general principles

Poisoning should be considered in patients presenting with altered consciousness, respiratory or cardiovascular depression, vomiting, hyperthermia, or seizures. The history usually makes diagnosis obvious, although clinical signs may be confused as a result of ingestion of multiple poisons or absent if effects are delayed. It should be remembered that poisons may enter the body via routes other than ingestion (e.g., inhalation or transdermally). Salicylate and acetaminophen are extremely common agents in self-poisoning, and patients often present with no alteration of consciousness.

Investigation

All patients require BUN and electrolyte, blood glucose, and blood gas estimations. Rapid bedside kits detect the presence of common agents such as acetaminophen, aspirin, and several recreational drugs. Urine samples and gastric aspirate should be saved for possible later toxicology analysis. Acetaminophen levels are necessary in every case of suspected self-poisoning because of the common lack of early signs and to allow specific early treatment. Clinically significant salicylate intoxication may be suspected in the setting of an elevated anion gap, especially with mixed metabolic acidosis and respiratory alkalosis. Other drug levels may help in diagnosis, but treatment is often supportive. Early support from the local poison control center should be solicited (800-222-1222).

Supportive treatment

Treatment of cardiovascular and respiratory compromise and neurological disturbance is by standard methods outlined elsewhere in the book. In the unconscious patient, opiates and benzodiazepines may be reversed temporarily to allow assessment of underlying neurological status.

Gastric elimination

Consider gastric emptying if the poison is not a corrosive or hydrocarbon and has been ingested <4 h previously. If salicylates or tricyclics have been ingested, gastric emptying may be useful for 12 h after ingestion. There are no clear advantages for forced emesis (ipecac syrup 30 mL in 200 mL water) or gastric lavage. Forced emesis may be delayed for 30 min and then may be intractable. Aspiration is a serious risk with either form of gastric emptying therapy; the patient should be intubated for airway protection if consciousness is at all impaired.

Activated charcoal

Activated charcoal is probably more effective than gastric emptying to prevent drug absorption. A charcoal-to-poison weight ratio of 10:1 is recommended. Activated charcoal (50–100 g as a single dose) should be given nasogastrically to adsorb poison remaining in the bowel and adsorb any poison back diffusing across the bowel mucosa. A cathartic agent may be given with the charcoal. Multiple doses of activated charcoal are probably not effective. Activated charcoal is particularly useful for benzodiazepines, anticonvulsants, tricyclics, theophylline, phenothiazines, and antihistamines.

Forced diuresis and dialysis

Forced diuresis with appropriate urinary acidification or alkalinization is useful for water-soluble poisons that are distributed predominantly extracellularly. Forced diuresis should not be used if renal function is abnormal. Small molecules may also be removed by hemodialysis (e.g., ethylene glycol, methanol, oxalic acid, formic acid).

Forced alkaline diuresis

- Used for soluble acidic drugs (e.g., salicylates).
- Furosemide or mannitol to maintain urine output >200 mL/h.
- IV crystalloid to prevent hypovolemia.
- Avoid excessive positive fluid balance.
- Use 1.26% bicarbonate to maintain urinary pH >7.
- Stop bicarbonate if arterial pH is >7.5 and use 0.9% saline.
- Alternate bicarbonate/saline with 5% glucose.
- Monitor and replace potassium and magnesium carefully.

Forced acid diuresis

- Used for soluble basic drugs (e.g., amphetamines, quinine, phencyclidine).
- Furosemide or mannitol to maintain urine output >200 mL/h.
- IV crystalloid to prevent hypovolemia.
- Avoid excessive positive fluid balance.
- Use 750 g NH_4Cl in each 500 mL 5% glucose to maintain urinary pH <7.0.
- Alternate 0.9% saline with 5% glucose.
- Monitor and replace potassium and magnesium carefully.

See also

Ventilatory support—indications, p. 4; Endotracheal intubation, p. 36; ECG monitoring, p. 110; Blood pressure monitoring, p. 112; Toxicology, p. 162; Respiratory stimulants, p. 188; Basic resuscitation, p. 268; Respiratory failure, p. 280; Hypotension, p. 310; Tachyarrhythmias, p. 314; Bradyarrhythmias, p. 316; Salicylate poisoning, p. 456; Acetaminophen poisoning, p. 458; Sedative poisoning, p. 460; Tricyclic antidepressant poisoning, p. 462; Amphetamines, including Ecstasy, p. 464; Cocaine, p. 466; Inhaled poisons, p. 468; Household chemicals, p. 470; Methanol and ethylene glycol, p. 472; Organophosphate poisoning, p. 474; Rhabdomyolysis, p. 530

Salicylate poisoning

Serious, life-threatening toxicity is likely after ingestion of >7.5 g salicylate. Aspirin is the most common form ingested, although salicylic acid and methyl salicylate are occasionally implicated.

Loss of consciousness is rare, but metabolic derangements are complex (e.g., respiratory alkalosis resulting from respiratory center stimulation, dehydration resulting from salt and water loss, renal bicarbonate excretion and hyperthermia, hypoklemia, metabolic acidosis resulting from interference with carbohydrate, lipid and amino acid metabolism, hyperthermia resulting from uncoupling of oxidative phosphorylation and increased metabolic rate).

There may also be pulmonary edema resulting from capillary leak, and bleeding resulting from reduced prothrombin levels.

Although gastric erosions are common with aspirin treatment, bleeding from this source is rare in acute poisoning.

Management

Gastric elimination

The use of ipecac syrup is controversial. It should not be administered in conjunction with activated charcoal. Gastric lavage may also be beneficial up to 60 min after salicylate ingestion. Activated charcoal (25–100 g as a single dose) should be given nasogastrically to adsorb salicylate remaining in the bowel and adsorb any salicylate back diffusing across the bowel mucosa. A cathartic agent may be given with the charcoal. Multiple doses of activated charcoal are probably not effective. Insoluble aspirin may form a gastric mass that is difficult to remove by gastric lavage.

Salicylate levels

Repeat salicylate levels at least every 2 h until the salicylate level decrease and the acid–base disturbance improves. Levels taken 12 h after ingestion may underestimate the degree of toxicity because of tissue binding. If salicylate levels are <50 mg/dL after 1 h of ingestion and there is no metabolic derangement, then observation, fluids, and repeat levels are all that are required. Urine alkalinization is required if levels are >50 mg/dL or there is metabolic derangement but no renal failure. Levels >110 mg/dL (or >50 mg/dL with renal failure) require hemodialysis.

Alkaline diuresis

Alkalinization rather than forced diuresis is more important for salicylate excretion. Urinary pH must be >7.0 without arterial alkalosis (pH <7.5). Potassium loss will occur with the bicarbonate infusion, as a result of the diuresis and as a toxic effect of the salicylate. Potassium levels must be monitored and corrected in a closely monitored or ICU environment. Alkalinization, if successful, should continue until salicylate levels are <50 mg/dL. Calcium levels may decrease with prolonged alkalinization.

Hemodialysis

Indications for hemodialysis include salicylate levels at >110 mg/dL or renal failure.

See also

Blood gas analysis, p. 102; Toxicology, p. 162; Hypokalemia, p. 424; Metabolic acidosis, p. 436; Poisoning—general principles, p. 454

Acetaminophen poisoning

Serious, life-threatening toxicity is likely after ingestion of >15 g acetaminophen, particularly with coingestion of enzyme-inducing drugs (e.g., anticonvulsants, anti-TB therapy) and/or alcohol.

Acetaminophen is rapidly absorbed from the stomach and upper small bowel and is metabolized by conjugation in the liver. Hepatic necrosis occurs as a result of the toxicity of an alkylating metabolite that is normally removed by conjugation with glutathione. Glutathione is rapidly depleted with overdose and may already be low in starvation, alcoholism, and possibly, HIV, thus predisposing these groups to an increased risk of toxicity.

Toxicity is usually asymptomatic for 1 to 2 days, although laboratory assessment of liver function may become abnormal after 18 h.

Hepatic failure, if manifest, develops after 2 to 7 days, with an earlier onset being associated with more severe toxicity.

Management

If ingestion has occurred <4 h previously, gastric decontamination with activated charcoal should be used. Acetaminophen levels may be taken to confirm ingestion, but should not be interpreted for toxicity until after 4 h from ingestion. The mainstay of treatment is with N-acetylcysteine to restore hepatic glutathione levels by increasing intracellular cysteine levels.

N-acetylcysteine

N-acetylcysteine has been approved by the Food and Drug Administration for both PO and IV administration. If given PO, dilute in juice or cola to a 5% solution. May be given via nasogastric tube if nausea threatens administration. Repeat dose if vomiting occurs within 1 h of administration. When administered IV, dilute in 5% dextrose solution, infuse per recommended IV protocol. Treatment is most effective if started within 8 h of ingestion but is currently advised for up to 36 h of ingestion. Treatment is required if the acetaminophen levels are in the toxic range (Fig. 29.1), or >15 g acetaminophen has been ingested. It should be continued acetaminophen is not detected in the blood. N-acetylcysteine is given by continuous IV infusion (150 mg/kg loading dose diluted in 200 mL 5% dextrose, infused over 15 min, followed by 50 mg/kg in 500 mL of 5% dextrose infused over 4 h, followed by 100 mg/kg in 1000 mL 5% dextrose infused over 16 h) or PO (140 mg/kg loading dose, followed by 70 mg/kg q4 h for 17 additional doses).

Complications

The major complication is hepatic (± renal) failure. An increase in PT, INR, and bilirubin are early warning signs of significant hepatic damage, and this should prompt early referral to a specialist center capable of managing fulminant hepatic failure.

Guidelines for referral to a specialist liver center

- Arterial pH <7.3
- INR >3 on day 2 or >4 thereafter
- Oliguria and/or increasing creatinine level
- Altered level of consciousness
- Hypoglycemia

Guidelines for liver transplantation

- Arterial pH <7.3

Plus all of the following:
- PT >100, INR >6.5
- Creatinine >300 µmol/L
- Grade 3 to 4 encephalopathy

High lactate levels (>3.5 mmol/L at 4 and 12 h) and low factor V levels are also associated with a poor outcome if not transplanted.

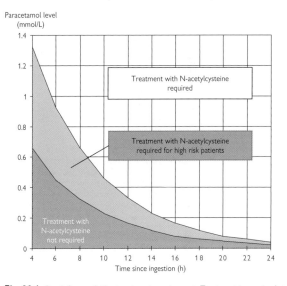

Fig. 29.1 Graph for predicting treatment requirement. Treatment is required at lower levels if the patient is a known alcoholic, protein-depleted, HIV positive, or is taking enzyme-inducing drugs such as phenytoin.

See also

Liver function tests, p. 152; Coagulation monitoring, p. 156; Toxicology, p. 162; Acute renal failure—diagnosis, p. 330; Acute renal failure—management, p. 332; Acute liver failure, p. 360; Hepatic encephalopathy, p. 362; Poisoning—general principles, p. 454

Sedative poisoning

With sedative poisoning, patients present with alteration of consciousness, respiratory failure, and, in some cases, cardiovascular disturbance. After prolonged immobility, the possibility of rhabdomyolysis should be considered. In most cases treatment is supportive.

Benzodiazepine poisoning

- Benzodiazepines are common agents used for self-poisoning, but severe features are uncommon, except at extremes of age.
- Flumazenil may be used as a specific antidote (0.2–1.0 mg IV given in 0.1-mg increments).
- Flumazenil is short acting, so benzodiazepine reversal may be temporary.
- Rapid reversal of benzodiazepines may lead to anxiety attacks or seizures.

Opioid poisoning

- Treatment is supportive, with attention particularly to respiratory depression and cardiovascular disturbance.
- Naloxone may be used as an antidote (0.2–0.4 mg IV), although rapid reversal is not desired in abusers.
- Naloxone is short acting, so reversal may be temporary.
- Consider HIV infection and endocarditis in IV drug abusers.
- In iatrogenic poisoning, naloxone will reverse the pain relief for which opioids were given. In these cases, respiratory depression is better reversed by smaller aliquots of Narcan (0.1 mg IV).

Barbiturates

Treatment of barbiturate poisoning is supportive, with particular attention to respiratory and cardiovascular depression. Vasodilatation may be extreme, requiring fluid support and, in some cases, inotropic support. Hypothermia is also of concern. Gastrointestinal decontamination with activated charcoal is indicated after a secure airway has been established. Phenobarbital and other long-acting barbiturates may be eliminated by forced alkaline diuresis.

See also

Ventilatory support—indications, p. 4; Blood gas analysis, p. 102; Blood pressure monitoring, p. 112; Toxicology, p. 162; Respiratory stimulants, p. 188; Opioid analgesics, p. 232; Sedatives, p. 236; Basic resuscitation, p. 268; Poisoning—general principles, p. 454; Rhabdomyolysis, p. 530

Tricyclic antidepressant poisoning

Tricyclic antidepressant use has declined after the introduction of less toxic selective serotonin reuptake inhibitor antidepressants. However, they are still among the most commonly reported drugs associated with poisoning. They are rapidly absorbed from the gastrointestinal tract, although gastric emptying is delayed.

Clinical features

- Anticholinergic effects (dilated pupils, dry mouth, ileus, retention of urine)
- Arrhythmias (particularly associated with prolonged QT interval and QRS waves)
- Hypotension related to arrhythmias and/or cardiac depression through Na^+ channel blockade
- Hyperreflexia with extensor plantars, visual hallucinations, coma, and seizures; drug levels do not correlate with severity
- Metabolism is usually rapid and improvement can be expected within 24 h.

Management

1. There is no specific treatment for tricyclic antidepressant poisoning.
2. Patients require ECG monitoring during the first 24 h and until ECG changes have disappeared for 12 h.
3. Gastric elimination may be useful for 24 h after ingestion because tricyclics slow gastric emptying.
4. Activated charcoal via a nasogastric tube will adsorb tricyclics remaining in the bowel.
5. Cardiac arrhythmias are more common if there is acidosis. Bicarbonate should be used to achieve an arterial pH of 7.5 urgently. If arrhythmias occur with no acidosis and fail to respond to treatment with amiodarone or phenytoin, bicarbonate (25–50 mL 8.4% IV) may still be useful.
6. Seizures are best managed with benzodiazepines and phenytoin.

See also

Ventilatory support—indications, p. 4; Blood gas analysis, p. 102; ECG monitoring, p. 110; Blood pressure monitoring, p. 112; Toxicology, p. 162; Sodium bicarbonate, p. 178; Basic resuscitation, p. 268; Tachyarrhythmias, p. 314; Generalized seizures, p. 372; Poisoning—general principles, p. 454

Amphetamines, including Ecstasy

Amphetamines, including 3,4-methylenedioxymethamphetamine (MDMA, 'Ecstasy') and 3,4-methylenedioxyethamphetamine ('Eve'), are stimulants taken predominantly for recreational use, or as appetite suppressants. These drugs are hallucinogenic at higher doses. MDMA has been shown to cause rapid decreases in CNS 5-hydroxytryptamine and 5-hydroxyindole-3-acetic acid levels, and increases in dopamine release.

Clinical features of overdose

Clinical features of amphetamine overdose include agitation, hyperactivity, hypertension, hallucinations, and paranoia followed by exhaustion, coma, convulsions, and hyperthermia.

Idiosyncratic responses to Ecstasy and Eve are more common, with numerous reports of mortality and major morbidity after ingestion of just one to two tablets. These appear related to ingestion in hot environments (e.g., nightclubs), and concurrent dehydration. Features include profound hyperthermia (>40°C), agitation, seizures, muscle rigidity, hypertension, tachycardia, sweating, coma, DIC, and rhabdomyolysis. These complications lead to hypovolemia, electrolyte imbalance (particularly hyperkalemia), and metabolic acidosis.

Some patients taking Ecstasy or Eve have been admitted with water intoxication and acute hyponatremia after ingesting large amounts of water.

Management

1. Provide supportive care, including airway protection, fluid resuscitation, electrolyte correction, and, if needed, mechanical ventilation.
2. Early stages of amphetamine poisoning can often be controlled with tepid sponging, benzodiazepines, and β-blockade. Forced acid diuresis to increase urinary excretion is rarely needed.
3. Severe complications should be managed as they arise (e.g., aggressive cooling ± neuromuscular blockade for hyperpyrexia, anticonvulsants for seizures, forced alkaline diuresis ± fasciotomies for rhabdomyolysis, platelet and FFP infusions for coagulopathy).
4. Dantrolene may be given to treat the hyperpyrexia at a dose of 1 mg/kg IV, repeated to a cumulative maximum dose of 10 mg/kg, particularly if the temperature is >40°C.

See also

Cocaine poisoning

Modes of action

- Blocks reuptake of dopamine (causing euphoria, hyperactivity) and noradrenaline (causing vasoconstriction and hypertension)
- Blocks Na^+ channels, resulting in a local anesthetic action and myocardial depression
- Activates platelets.

Complications

- Chest pain related to myocardial ischemia or MI. Local chest pain guidelines should be followed. ECG abnormalities often resolve within 12 h. Arrhythmias should be treated conventionally, although avoiding selective β-blockers.
- Heart failure from myocardial depression or a cardiomyopathy
- Seizures
- CVAs
- Pneumothorax
- Rhabdomyolysis
- Premature labor—abruption
- Agitated delirium, hyperthermia
- Thermal injury from smoke inhalation

Management

1. Oxygen
2. Benzodiazepines for agitation, delirium, chest pain
3. Aspirin for chest pain, CVA
4. Nitrates for chest pain, heart failure
5. Sodium bicarbonate and forced diuresis for rhabdomyolysis
6. Selective β-blockers allow unopposed α-stimulation in the setting of cocaine poisoning and should be avoided.

See also

Oxygen therapy, p. 2; Ventilatory support—indications, p. 4; Blood gas analysis, p. 102; ECG monitoring, p. 110; Blood pressure monitoring, p. 112; Toxicology, p. 162; Basic resuscitation, p. 268; Hypertension, p. 312; Tachyarrhythmias, p. 314; Acute coronary syndrome (1), p. 318; Acute coronary syndrome (2), p. 320; Generalized seizures, p. 372; Stroke, p. 382; Poisoning—general principles, p. 454; Hyperthermia, p. 524; Rhabdomyolysis, p. 530

Inhaled poisons

Carbon monoxide

Carbon monoxide poisoning should be considered in anyone found in a smoke-filled, enclosed space. Carbon monoxide displaces oxygen from Hb, to which it has 200 times greater affinity, and thus prevents oxygen carriage. There is also a direct toxic effect on mitochondrial oxidative phosphorylation as it competes with oxygen for the same binding site on cytochrome oxidase.

Clinical features
- Fatigue, headache, vomiting, dizziness, confusion, dyspnea.
- A cherry-red appearance of the skin and mucosa is classic but not common.
- PaO_2 will be normal unless there is respiratory depression and pulse oximetry is misleading.
- The half-life of carboxyhemoglobin is 4 h when breathing room air and 50 min when breathing 100% oxygen.

Management
- Carboxyhemoglobin levels should be measured by co-oximetry and treatment started immediately with oxygen at the maximum concentration that can be delivered (FiO_2 at 1.0 if ventilated and 0.6–1.0 if self-ventilating).
- Hyperbaric oxygen therapy remains controversial. If carboxyhemoglobin levels are >25% or carbon monoxide poisoning is associated with mental disturbance, hyperbaric oxygen at 3 atm for 30 min, repeated q6h if levels remain at >25%, may be useful. The closest hyperbaric chamber can be located by contacting the Diver's Alert Network at (919) 684-8111. If hyperbaric oxygen is used, prophylactic myringotomy is mandatory for intubated patients, as is chest tube placement for pneumothorax. Consider prophylactic chest tube placement in patients who have experienced chest compressions, or central venous catheterization in the setting of positive-pressure ventilation.
- High-concentration oxygen treatment should continue until carboxyhemoglobin levels are <10%.
- Death is likely with carboxyhemoglobin levels >60%.

Cyanide
- Severe cyanide poisoning has an extremely rapid onset and occurs in some cases of smoke inhalation. Survival may be associated with anoxic brain damage.
- Diagnosis must be made clinically because a blood cyanide level takes >3 h to acquire.

Clinical features
Clinical features include anxiety, agitation, hyperventilation, headache, loss of consciousness, dyspnea, weakness, dizziness, and vomiting. The skin remains pink, and hypotension may be severe. Unexplained lactic acidosis in the setting of normal or reduced $AVDO_2$ is suggestive.

Management

- High-concentration oxygen may be efficacious.
- In mild cases, rapid, natural detoxification reduces cyanide levels by 50% within 1 h, allowing supportive therapy only.
- Sodium thiosulfate (150 mg/kg, IV followed by 30–60 mg/kg/h) converts cyanide to thiocyanate and should be used if there is unconsciousness. It is, however, slowacting.
- Nitrites produce methemoglobinemia and may potentially worsen cyanide toxicity.
- Dicobalt edetate (300 mg IV) is the specific antidote to cyanide but is severely toxic (vomiting, urticaria, tachycardia, hypotension, dyspnea, chest pain) in the absence of cyanide. It is therefore best avoided unless cyanide toxicity is likely.

Key trial

Weaver LK, et al. Hyperbaric oxygen for acute carbon monoxide poisoning. N Engl J Med 2002; **347**:1057–67.

See also

Oxygen therapy, p. 2; Ventilatory support—indications, p. 4; Blood gas analysis, p. 102; ECG monitoring, p. 110; Blood pressure monitoring, p. 112; Toxicology, p. 162; Basic resuscitation, p. 268; Inhalation injury, p. 304; Metabolic acidosis, p. 436; Poisoning—general principles, p. 448

Household chemicals

Corrosives

Strong acids and alkalis are increasingly available in the household, and ingestion may lead to shock and bowel perforation. Gastric elimination techniques must be avoided because aspiration of corrosives may cause severe lung damage. Early surgical repair of perforation may be necessary.

Petroleum

Although not strictly a household chemical, access to petroleum in the home is easy.

Clinical features

Gastrointestinal ingestion and absorption gives clinical features similar to those of alcohol intoxication, with more severe CNS depression.

Management

• Gastric elimination techniques must be avoided because a few drops of petroleum spilling into the lungs can lead to severe pneumonitis. This is a result of the low surface tension and vapor pressure of petroleum that allows rapid spreading through the lungs.
• Treatment involves supportive therapy.

See also
Toxicology, p. 162; Poisoning—general principles, p. 454

Methanol and ethylene glycol

Methanol

Methanol toxicity mainly arises as a result of oxidation of methanol to formic acid and formaldehyde. The oxidative pathway is an enzymatic process involving alcohol dehydrogenase, but it proceeds at 20% of the rate of ethanol oxidation.

Clinical features

Clinical features of poisoning include blindness (because of the concentration of methanol in the vitreous humor), severe metabolic acidosis with increased anion gap and osmolar gap, headache, nausea, vomiting, and abdominal pain.

Management

- Metabolism of methanol is slow, so treatment will need to be prolonged (several days).
- Treatment includes gastric emptying (within 4 h of ingestion), sodium bicarbonate titrated to correct arterial pH, and ethanol to saturate the oxidative pathway.
- On presentation, 1 mL/kg 50% ethanol is given orally followed by 0.5 mL/kg q2h for 5 days.
- Alternatively, metabolism can be blocked by 4-methyl pyrazole (fomepizole), which can be infused or injected q12h.
- If methanol levels are >1000 mg/L, hemodialysis is used until levels are <250 mg/L.

Ethylene glycol

Ethylene glycol is partially metabolized by alcohol dehydrogenase to oxalic acid, which is responsible for a severe metabolic acidosis with increased anion gap and osmolar gap, renal failure, and seizures.

Clinical features

Clinical suspicion is aroused by odorless drunkenness, oxalate crystals in the urine or blood, and severe acidosis. As little as 50 mL can be fatal.

Management

Treatment is as for methanol.

See also

Urinalysis, p. 166; Toxicology, p. 162; Sodium bicarbonate, p. 178; Acute renal failure—management, p. 332; Vomiting/gastric stasis, p. 336; Metabolic acidosis, p. 436; Poisoning—general principles, p. 454

Organophosphate poisoning

Organophosphate pesticides are the major cause of suicidal poisoning in developing countries and are used as nerve agents in terrorist attacks (e.g., Sarin, Tabun, VX, GF). Their mode of action is via cholinergic toxicity.

Cholinergic (anticholinesterase) syndrome

- Salivation, lacrimation
- Vomiting, diarrhea
- Bradycardia
- Bronchospasm
- Meiosis

Management

- Atropine—antagonizes acetylcholine at muscarinic receptors. A dose of 2 mg should be given every 15 min until the mouth is dry. Severe poisonings may require >100 mg atropine.
- Pralidoxime—reactivates inhibited enzymes if given before the agent permanently binds to the enzyme
- Diazepam—neuroprotection

See also

Oxygen therapy, p. 2; Ventilatory support—indications, p. 4; ECG monitoring, p. 110; Toxicology, p. 162; Bronchodilators, p. 186; Chronotropes, p. 206; Bradyarrhythmias, p. 316; Vomiting/gastric stasis, p. 336; Diarrhea, p. 338; Poisoning—general principles, p. 454

Infection and inflammation

Infection control—general principles

Infection acquired within the ICU is a major cause of mortality, morbidity, and increased duration of stay. There are remarkable variations in practice, for which the lack of a good evidence base is chiefly responsible. Examples include different policies with regard to patient isolation, microbiological surveillance, hand-washing procedures, use of impregnated vascular catheters, the duration of indwelling catheters, and frequency of change of disposables such as IV infusion sets and filters. It is nevertheless accepted that adequate hand washing before and after patient contact, and strict aseptic technique when performing procedures are mandatory.

ICU design
- Ample sinks with soap and antiseptic dispensers
- Separate clean treatment and dirty utility areas
- Some isolation cubicles with positive/exhaust airflow facility
- Ample space around bed areas

Staff measures
- Remove watches and jewelry, remove long-sleeve white coats and jackets, roll shirt sleeves up to elbow
- Wash hands and forearms before and after touching patient.
- Wear disposable gloves if in contact with patient, and wear disposable gowns if contact isolation is required.
- Wear gloves and gowns when handling any body fluid, and wear eye protection when there is any danger of fluid or droplet splash.
- Use strict aseptic technique for invasive procedures (e.g., central venous catheter insertion) and clean technique for basic procedures (e.g., endotracheal suction, changing ventilator circuits, drug infusions).
- Have previous immunization against hepatitis B.
- Stethoscopes should be cleaned between patients, and dedicated disposable stethoscopes can be used for patients in contact isolation.
- Clearly post signs noting on cubicle doors noting precautions to be taken.

Visitors
- Non-ICU medical and paramedical staff, relatives, and friends should adhere to the guidelines in force regarding the patient being visited (e.g., hand washing, gowns and gloves as directed).
- Traffic through the ICU should be minimized.

Cross-infection
- Inform the infection control service if cross-infection arises with more than one patient infected by the same strain of bacteria.
- Affected patients should generally be source isolated, especially if the organism is multiresistant; treated with antibiotics and topical antiseptics if necessary; and strict barrier precautions should be enforced.
- If cross-infection persists/spreads, other sources should be sought (e.g., taps, sinks, reusable equipment rebreathing bags, ventilators).

Protective isolation

- Some patients carry potentially contagious or infective organisms and require source isolation (e.g., TB).
- Immunosuppressed patients (e.g., when neutropenic after chemotherapy) are at risk of acquiring infection.

See also

Bacteriology, p. 158; Virology, serology, and assays, p. 160; Antimicrobials, p. 258; Acute chest infection (1), p. 286; Acute chest infection (2), p. 288; Infection—diagnosis, p. 482; Infection—treatment, p. 484; ICU layout, p. 568

Routine changes of disposables

Care of intravascular catheters

- Sites should be covered with transparent semipermeable dressings to allow observation and to prevent secretions from accumulating.
- Routine changes of intravascular catheters are no longer recommended. Because the risk of infection does increase considerably after a week in situ, catheters should be removed as soon as clinically feasible.
- Catheters should be changed to a fresh site if
  - The site appears infected
  - The patient shows signs of infection and the line is a potential source (the longer the line has been in situ, the higher the risk)
  - A positive blood culture is obtained

Table 30.1 Routine changes of disposables

	Frequency
Ventilator circuit (if using bacterial filters)	Between patients unless soiled
Ventilator circuit (if using water bath humidifier)	Daily
Endotracheal tube catheter mount and bacterial filter	Between patients unless soiled
Disposable oxygen masks	Between patients unless soiled
CPAP circuits	Between patients unless soiled
Rebreathing bags and masks	Between patients unless soiled
IV infusion sets	48 h
Parenteral nutrition infusion sets	Daily
Enteral feeding infusion sets	Daily
AV pressure transducer sets	48 h
Wound dressings	Depends on type of dressing
Tracheostomy site	As necessary
Urinary catheter bags	Weekly

Infection—diagnosis

Infection is both a common cause of admission to intensive care and a major secondary complication. Critically ill patients are predisposed to further nosocomial infections because many of their natural barriers and defense mechanisms have been lost, altered, or penetrated. They are often heavily instrumented, sedated, and immobile. They often develop immune hyporesponsiveness as part of their critical disease process, notwithstanding any therapeutic immune suppression they may have received. The high antibiotic load given to these sick patients encourages colonization by pathogenic organisms and subsequent development of infections by multidrug-resistant and/or atypical (e.g., fungi) organisms.

Sepsis is defined as the systemic response to an insult of proved or high likelihood of infection. Although infection can be applied to a localized phenomenon, sepsis initiates a systemic inflammatory response that affects distant organs.

Diagnosis

- Diagnosis often problematic in the critically ill patient because focal signs may be lacking and/or camouflaged by concurrent disease (e.g., ventilator-associated pneumonia on top of ARDS). Symptoms are often not forthcoming because of the patient's mentally incompetent state.
- In addition, all the traditional clinical and biochemical markers of infection are nonspecific. These include pyrexia, neutrophilia, and altered sputum. Furthermore, the frequent presence of colonizing organisms (e.g., MRSA on skin, *P. aeruginosa* in the respiratory tract) does not imply concomitant infection. As a consequence, many patients are overtreated with antibiotics, enhancing the risk of overgrowth of resistant/atypical organisms.
- Markers of inflammation (CRP, procalcitonin) may be useful, although studies have produced conflicting results regarding their specificity/sensitivity in diagnosing underlying infection.
- The value of routine screening (microbiological surveillance) has not been proved, although this may help to identify infecting organisms earlier.
- For cases of suspected infection, appropriate samples should be taken for analysis, including blood, sputum, wound swabs, drainage fluid, aspirated pus, catheter tips, CSF, and so on. These should generally be taken before new antibiotics are commenced.
- Consider less common causes of infection such as endocarditis or osteomyelitis, particularly if the patient fails to improve after a standard course of therapy.

Differential diagnosis of pyrexia

- Infection
- Noninfective causes of inflammation (e.g., trauma, surgery, burns, MI, vasculitis, hepatitis, acalculous cholecystitis, pancreatitis)
- Adverse drug reactions
- Excessive ambient heating
- Miscellaneous causes (e.g., neoplasm, central fever)

Definitions

Infection
Microbial phenomenon characterized by an inflammatory response to the presence of microorganisms or the invasion of normally sterile host tissue by those organisms

Bacteremia
The presence of viable bacteria in the blood

Sepsis
The systemic response to infection

Severe sepsis
Sepsis plus organ failure

Septic shock
Sepsis with hypotension or hypoperfusion not responsive to adequate fluid loading

Table 30.2 Sites of infection before and after admission to an ICU

Organ	Primary site of infection needing admission to ICU	Secondary site of infection acquired while in ICU
Brain	+	+
Sinuses	—	+
Cannula/wound sites	++	+++++
Other skin and soft tissue	++	+
Chest	++++	++++
Urogenital tract	++	+
Abdomen	++++	++
Bone	+	+
Heart valves	+	+

− Negligible
+ Rarely
++ Occasionally
+++ Commonly
++++ Frequently
+++++ Very frequently

Key paper
American College of Chest Physicians/Society of Critical Care Medicine Consensus Conference: Definitions for sepsis and organ failure and guidelines for the use of innovative therapies in sepsis. *Crit Care Med* 1992; **20**:864–74.

See also
Bacteriology, p. 158; Virology, serology, and assays, p. 160; Pyrexia (1), p. 520; Pyrexia (2), p. 522

Infection—treatment

Treatment

- Drain pus.
- Change cannula sites if necessary.
- institute appropriate antibiotic therapy after laboratory specimens taken (although this may not be necessary for mild infections when the cause has been removed, such as an infected catheter).
- Provide radiological and/or surgical intervention if indicated.

Input from microbiological ± infectious disease specialists may be helpful to advise on best options for empiric therapy and for possible modifications based on early communication of laboratory results (including antibiotic sensitivity patterns).

Empiric antibiotic therapy is based on the severity of illness of the patient, likely site of infection, and likely infecting organisms, whether the infection is community acquired or nosocomial (including ICU acquired), patient immunosuppression, and known antibiotic resistance patterns of hospital and local community organisms. In general, critically ill patients should receive parenteral antibiotics at appropriate the dosage, taking into account any impaired hepatic or renal clearance, or concurrent renal replacement therapy. Broad-spectrum therapy may be needed initially, with refinement, cessation, or change after 2 to 3 days, depending on the clinical response and organisms subsequently isolated. The duration of treatment remains highly contentious. Apart from specific conditions such as endocarditis, TB, and meningitis, for which prolonged therapy is probably advisable, it may be sufficient to stop within 3 to 5 days, provided the patient has shown adequate signs of recovery. Alternatively, patients not responding or deteriorating should be considered to be either treatment failures or inappropriately treated (i.e., no infection was present in the first place). As described earlier, commonly accepted markers of infection are poorly specific in the intensive care patient. Indeed, pyrexia may resolve on stopping antibiotic treatment. Cessation or change of antibiotic therapy must be considered on individual merits according to the patient's condition and any subsequent laboratory results. An advantage of ceasing therapy is the ability to take further specimens for culture in an antibiotic-free environment.

It may be necessary to remove indwelling pacemakers, tunneled vascular catheters, prosthetic joints, plates, implants, grafts, and stents if these are the suspected cause of infection. This should be done in consultation with the appropriate specialist, because individual risk and benefit need to be carefully weighed.

Table 30.3 Empiric antibiotic regimens (organism unknown)

Sepsis of unknown origin	Second-/third-generation cephalosporin or quinolone or carbapenem or pip tazobactam + aminoglycoside (if Gram negative suspected) + metronidazole (anaerobic coverage) + vancomycin or linezolid (if MRSA suspected)
Pneumonia, community acquired (ICU admit)	IV beta lactam (cefotaxime or ceftriaxone) + either IV azithromycin or IV fluoroquinolone If risk factors for *Pseudomonas* (e.g., underlying lung disease, steroid use) use antipseudomonal beta lactam (cefepime, imipenem, meropenem, piptazobactam) + ciprofloxacin + consider aminoglycoside
Pneumonia, nosocomial	Third-generation cephalosporin or quinolone or carbapenem or piptazobactam + aminoglycoside (if Gram negative suspected) + vancomycin or linezolid (if MRSA likely)
Skin and soft tissue	Nafcillin or cefazolin (if MRSA likely), vancomycin or linezolid (if MRSA likely), necrotizing fasciitis (surgery usually required): carbapenem or ampicillin–sulbactam or piptazobactam + clindamycin
Abdominal/pelvic	Second-/third- generation cephalosporin or quinolone or, carbapenem or piptazobactam + consider aminoglycoside + consider metronidazole
Nephrourological	Ceftriaxone or quinolone; If enterococcus is suspected, pip tazobactam or ampicillin + gentamicin

The choice of agents should be guided by the susceptibility patterns of microorganisms in the local community and hospital.

See also

Blood pressure monitoring, p. 112; Bacteriology, p. 158; Antimicrobials, p. 258; Acute chest infection (1), p. 286; Acute chest infection (2), p. 288; Hypotension, p. 310; Abdominal sepsis, p. 348; Meningitis, p. 374; Tetanus, p. 392; Botulism, p. 394; Neutropenia, p. 410; Systemic inflammation/multi-organ failure, p. 486; Sepsis and septic shock—treatment, p. 488; HIV-related disease, p. 492; Malaria, p. 494; Pyrexia (1), p. 520; Pyrexia (2), p. 522; Postoperative intensive care, p. 536

Systemic inflammation/multiorgan failure

Exposure to an exogenous insult can result in an exaggerated, generalized, and potentially inappropriate inflammatory response. Stimulation of inflammatory pathways leads to activation of macrophages, endothelium, neutrophils, platelets, coagulation, and fibrinolytic and contact systems with release of inflammatory mediators and effectors (e.g., cytokines, prostanoids, free oxygen radicals, proteases, nitric oxide, endothelin). This may result in microvascular flow abnormalities, blood flow redistribution, interstitial edema and fibrosis, and cellular/mitochondrial dysfunction. The consequences of these effects may be organ dysfunction, varying from 'mild' to severe, and affecting single or multiple organs, resulting in cardiovascular collapse, gastrointestinal failure, renal failure, hepatic failure, encephalopathy, neuropathy, myopathy, and/or disseminated intravascular coagulation. ARDS is the respiratory component of this pathophysiological response.

Causes
- Infection
- Trauma, burns
- Pancreatitis
- Inhalation injuries
- Ischemia/reperfusion
- Massive blood loss/transfusion
- Miscellaneous, including drug related (including overdose), MI, drowning, hyperthermia, pulmonary embolus

Treatment
Treatment is largely supportive, although the cause should be removed/treated if at all possible. Treatment includes antibiotics, drainage of pus, fixation of femoral/pelvic fractures, and debridement of necrotic tissue.

An important facet of organ support is to minimize iatrogenic trauma. It is sufficient to maintain survival with relative homeostasis until recovery takes place, rather than attempting to achieve normal physiological or biochemical target values. An example of this is permissive hypercapnia.

Specific treatment regimens remain contentious because of a lack of adequately powered studies showing optimal hemodynamic goals, inotropic/pressor agents, antibiotic regimens, and so on. Local policies may favor the use of one or more of a range of therapies that may offer a reasonable theoretical basis for administration, or anecdotal success, although these all remain essentially unproved. Examples include antioxidants, protease inhibitors, immunonutrition, plasmapheresis, vasodilators, and immunoglobulins. It is generally agreed that rapid resuscitation and restoration of oxygen delivery, glycemic control, and prompt removal of any treatable cause are desirable in preventing the onset of organ failure.

Because of nonstandardization of definitions, outcome data are conflicting, although single-organ 'failure' carries an approximate 20% to 30%

mortality whereas three or more organ 'failures' lasting ≥3 days carries a mortality in excess of 50%. Recovery is often complete in survivors, although recent studies are revealing long-term physical and psychological sequelae in a significant proportion of patients.

Table 30.4 UPMC (University of Pittsburgh Medical Center) Hospitals principles of management for patients with sepsis and/or organ failure

Respiratory	SaO_2 >90–95% (lower values may be tolerated in severe respiratory failure); mechanical ventilation, 6 mL/kg V_T and maintain peak inspiratory pressure <30 cmH_2O_3; daily weaning trails (when PEEP <8 and FiO_2 <50%) and early tracheostomy; head of the bed elevated at 45°.
Cardiovascular	Maintain cardiac output/oxygen delivery and blood pressure compatible with adequate organ perfusion (typically CI (cardiac index) >2.5, MAP >65 mmHg, SVO_2 (mixed venous oxygen saturation) ≥65)
Renal	Maintain adequate metabolic and fluid homeostasis by intravascular filling, diuretics, and/or hemofiltration
Hematological	Maintain Hb >7 g/dL (>9 g/dL if coronary ischemia), platelets >20–40 × 10^9/L, INR <1.5–2.5
Gastrointestinal	Stress ulcer prophylaxis (H_2 blockers, enteral nutrition)
Infection	Culture-guided antibiotics, abscess drainage, good infection control, bronchoalveolar lavage for diagnosis of ventilator-associated pneumonia
Nutrition	Preferably early and by enteral route, tight glucose control (80–110 mg/dL)
Pressure area/mouth/joint care	Frequent turns, low-pressure support surfaces, nursing care, and physiotherapy
Neuropsychological	Daily interruption of sedation, support to both patient and family

Definition

Multiorgan dysfunction syndrome

The presence of altered organ function in an acutely ill patient such that homeostasis cannot be maintained without intervention; multiple-organ failure has not achieved worldwide uniformity of definition

See also

Ventilatory support—indications, p. 4; Blood pressure monitoring, p. 112; Bacteriology, p. 158; Antimicrobials, p. 258; Acute respiratory distress syndrome (1), p. 290; Acute respiratory distress syndrome (2), p. 292; Inhalation injury, p. 304; Hypotension, p. 310; Abdominal sepsis, p. 348; Pancreatitis, p. 354; Infection control—general principles, p. 478; Sepsis and septic shock—treatment, p. 488; Multiple trauma (1), p. 502; Multiple trauma (2), p. 504; Burns—fluid management, p. 512; Burns—general management, p. 514; Pyrexia (1), p. 520; Pyrexia (2), p. 522

Sepsis and septic shock—treatment

Principles of treatment

As for other causes of multiorgan dysfunction syndrome, outcome in sepsis improves with

- Prompt diagnosis and treatment of the underlying cause
- Early goal-directed resuscitation to prevent prolonged tissue hypoxia
- Good glycemic control
- Strict infection control
- Recognition and appropriate treatment of secondary infections
- Adequate nutrition
- Recognition that 'normal' physiological/biochemical levels do not necessarily need to be attained while the patient is critically ill, provided he or she is not compromised (e.g., a mean blood pressure of 55–60 mmHg is often acceptable unless evidence of poor perfusion or ischemia suggests higher levels should be sought)
- Avoidance of preventable mishaps (e.g., prolonged hypotension, pressure sores, thromboembolism)
- Prevention of contractures, early mobilization, and so on.
- Specific treatments (see next section)

Specific treatments for severe sepsis/septic shock

1. Activated protein C significantly improves outcome in patients with severe sepsis and an APACHE II score ≥25 points.
2. 'Low-dose' hydrocortisone (50 mg qid) given for 7 days improved outcome in patients with septic shock, although only in the subset with an abnormal cortisol response to synthetic ACTH. Our current practice is to start hydrocortisone after performing an ACTH stimulation test and to discontinue this therapy if the test is normal.
3. For norepinephrine-resistant septic shock (i.e., high-output severe hypotension not responding to adequate fluid loading and a norepinephrine dose >0.4 µg/kg/min), we consider careful administration of vasopressin (0.01–0.04 U/min). Until more data are forthcoming, these agents should be viewed as rescue therapies rather than a straight alternative for norepinephrine.
4. We favor early hemofiltration for sepsis-induced acute renal failure and occasionally use plasma exchange for sepsis-induced thrombocytopenia.

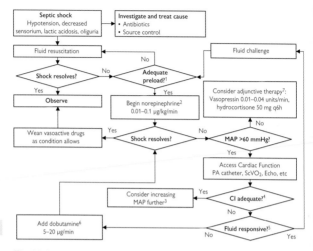

Fig. 30.1 Suggested approach to hemodynamic management for septic shock. MAP: mean arterial pressure; CI: cardiac index; PA: pulmonary artery; ScVO$_2$: central venous oxygen saturation. Notes: 1. Assessment of preload by physical exam is difficult and prone to error. We recommend hemodynamic monitoring for all septic shock patients who do not respond to initial fluid resuscitation. 2. Norepinephrine can be increased above the stated range but we recommend assessment cardiac function and consideration of adjunctive therapy for higher dose requirements or persistent need for norepinephrine. 3. Particularly in patients with long standing hypertension, MAP of 60 mmHg may not be sufficient for perfusion of some vascular beds. 4. What constitutes an adequate cardiac index is a mater of debate. The cardiac index is usually high in resuscitated septic shock but pushing for super normal values in patients does not appear to improve outcome. We recommend maintaining CI > 2.5 L/min/m^2 until shock resolves. However, ongoing evidence of tissue hypoperfusion in a patient with MAP >60 mmHg might indicate need for high CI. 5. Fluid responsiveness can be assessed by an increase in CI with fluid or predicted by technius such as pulse-pressure variation. No right atrial pressure can predict preload responsiveness. 6. Other inotropic agents can be used. For example dopamine can be used as a combination vasopressor and inotrope in place of norepinephrine and dobutamine. Milrinone can be used in place of dobutamine particular in patients with tachycardia or arrythmias. 7. Norepinephrine should be increased and consideration should be given to addition of vasopressin and a trial of hydrocortisone. Epinephrine can be used here as well. High-dose hemofitration can be effective in improving blood pressure but evidence of improved outcomes are lacking.

Key paper

Dellinger RP *et al.* Surviving Sepsis Campaign guidelines. *Crit Care Med* 2004; **32**:858–73.

Key trials

Annane D, *et al.* Effect of treatment with low doses of hydrocortisone and fludrocortisone on mortality in patients with septic shock. *JAMA* 2002; **288**:862–71.

Bernard GR, for the PROWESS Study Group. Efficacy and safety of recombinant human activated protein C for severe sepsis. *N Engl J Med* **344**:699–709.

See also

HIV related disease

Patients affected with HIV-related disease may present electively after diagnostic biopsies of brain or lung, or when elective ventilation is needed postoperatively. Other cases present with complications of HIV-related disease, especially pulmonary infection (e.g., *P. carinii*, CMV) or seizures (e.g., cerebral lymphoma, cerebral abscess, meningitis). HIV-related diseases are now considered to be chronic, manageable conditions with an often good short-term prognosis. It is therefore reasonable that intensive care should be offered.

Infection control

The protection of staff from transmission of HIV follows basic measures. Body fluids should not be handled (wear gloves), and the face and eyes should be protected when there is a risk of splash contamination.

Needles should be disposed of in appropriate bins without resheathing. Any fluid spills should be cleaned up immediately. Robust procedures are adhered to when a patient is known HIV positive; the real risk is in the patient of unknown HIV status. Remember that patients presenting with non-HIV-related illness may be unknown positives. It follows that precautions should be taken for all patients.

P. carinii pneumonia

- *P. carinii* pneumonia is the most common respiratory disorder affecting HIV-positive patients. The majority survive their first attack, but prognosis is not as good in those requiring mechanical ventilation. Intensive, early support with CPAP and appropriate chemotherapy may avert the need for ventilatory support.
- Treatment is usually started without waiting for laboratory confirmation.
- Mild to moderate cases can often be treated with oral therapy. First- line treatment for severe cases is IV TMP-SMX or pentamidine with adjuvant high-dose steroids. TMP-SMX has a faster onset of effect and a broader spectrum of antibacterial activity covering the common secondary pathogens. Pentamidine is usually used when TMP-SMX fails or when patients cannot take TMP-SMX.
- Methylprednisolone is used to suppress peribronchial fibrosis and alveolar infiltrate. It is usual for there to be an initial deterioration on treatment lasting several days.
- Respiratory support is provided with CPAP (5–10 cmH$_2$O) if hypoxemic despite high FiO$_2$. Lower CPAP pressures should be used when possible because these patients are at risk of pneumothorax.
- Mechanical ventilation is reserved for those who have deteriorating gas exchange and fatigue despite CPAP.
- CXR changes respond very slowly.

Lactic acidosis

Nucleoside reverse transcriptase inhibitors are frequently used antiretroviral agents. However, an associated mitochondrial impairment can cause severe lactic acidosis and high mortality. Anecdotal use of L-carnitine is reported to be of benefit.

IV drug abusers

IV drug abusers are at high risk for HIV-related disease, although they present more commonly for other reasons (e.g., drug withdrawal syndromes, overdose, sepsis, endocarditis, hepatitis B or C, rhabdomyolysis).

Table 30.5 Drug dosages

TMP-SMX	15 mg/kg/day in divided doses IV for 10–14 days then PO to complete 21 days
Pentamidine	4 mg/kg/day IV for 21 days
Prednisone	40 mg PO bid for 5 days then taper over next 16 days

See also

Ventilatory support—indications, p. 4; Endotracheal intubation, p. 36; Continuous positive airway pressure, p. 26; Bacteriology, p. 158; Virology, serology, and assays, p. 160; Antimicrobials, p. 258; Steroids, p. 260; Acute chest infection (1), p. 286; Acute chest infection (2), p. 288; Pneumothorax, p. 298; Infection control—general principles, p. 478

Rheumatic disorders

Rheumatoid arthritis

Rheumatoid arthritis is a debilitating arthritis that may present to intensive care through pulmonary involvement or through complications of treatment (e.g., renal failure, immunosuppression, bleeding disorders). Pleuropulmonary involvement may precede the arthritic symptoms and is more common in those with active rheumatoid disease and middle-age men. Care is required when intubating patients with rheumatoid arthritis because the cervical spine may sublux and result in cord injury.

Rheumatoid pleurisy

Rheumatoid pleurisy, often with effusion, is most common and is usually asymptomatic. However, effusions may be recurrent or chronic and may impede respiratory function. The effusion is an exudate, low in glucose and often high in cholesterol.

Rheumatoid lung

Rheumatoid lung is a diffuse interstitial pneumonitis with bibasal fibrotic changes on CXR. The condition may be difficult to distinguish from idiopathic pulmonary fibrosis and it produces a restrictive pulmonary defect. The mainstay of treatment is early systemic steroid therapy, although chronic cases do not respond.

SLE

SLE is nonorgan-specific autoimmune disease characterized by antinuclear antibodies with high titres of antidouble-stranded DNA antibodies. Vasculitis is prominent, although cutaneous and CNS involvement are not vasculitic. SLE may present to intensive care through pulmonary, renal, or CNS involvement.

Renal failure

Renal failure is vasculitic in origin and may progress to end-stage renal failure requiring long-term dialysis. Early treatment with systemic steroids and immunosuppressives may halt disease progress.

Lupus pleuritis and pericarditis

Unlike rheumatoid pleurisy, the pleural involvement in SLE is often painful and associated with large pleural effusions.

Pulmonary hemorrhage

Pulmonary hemorrhage is associated with renal failure and may be life threatening. Plasma exchange may be helpful.

Interstitial pneumonitis

Interstitial pneumonitis is uncommon in SLE. It is more likely that parenchymal infiltrates are infectious in origin secondary to immunosuppressive therapy.

Pulmonary thromboembolic disease

Patients typically have a prolonged APTT as a result of circulating lupus anticoagulant, but are actually more prone to thrombotic episodes. Lupus anticoagulant is associated with anticardiolipin antibodies and a false-positive VDRL (venereal disease research laboratory). Recurrent pulmonary emboli may be associated with chronic pulmonary hypertension. Treatment is long-term anticoagulation.

See also
Endotracheal intubation, p. 36; Plasma exchange, p. 70; Nonopioid analgesics, p. 234; Steroids, p. 260; Hemoptysis, p. 302; Acute renal failure—diagnosis, p. 330; Acute renal failure—management, p. 332; Upper gastrointestinal hemorrhage, p. 342; Vasculitides, p. 498

Vasculitides

Vasculitis should be suspected in any patient with multisystem disease, especially involving the lungs and kidneys.

Wegener's granulomatosis

Wegener's granulomatosis is systemic vasculitis characterized by necrotizing granulomas of the upper and lower respiratory tract, glomerulonephritis, and small-vessel vasculitis. Wegener's granulomatosis is associated with positive core antineutrophil cytoplasmic antibodies, particularly granular with central attenuation on immunofluorescence. Intensive care admission is usually because of renal and/or pulmonary involvement.

Renal failure

Focal necrotizing glomerulonephritis leads to progressive renal failure. Treatment with steroids and cyclophosphamide may give complete remission.

Upper airway disease

Most patients will have nasal symptoms including epistaxis, nasal discharge, and septal perforation. Intensive care admission may be required rarely for severe epistaxis. Ulcerating lesions of the larynx and trachea may cause subglottic stenosis. This is usually insidious, but may present problems on attempted intubation.

Pulmonary involvement

Pulmonary involvement is usually associated with hemoptysis, dyspnea, and cough with rounded opacities on CXR. There may be cavitation. Nodules may be solitary. Alveolar hemorrhage may be life threatening. The mainstay of treatment is steroids and cyclophosphamide, which may produce complete remission. Plasma exchange may be helpful.

Polyarteritis nodosa

Polyarteritis nodosa is a necrotizing vasculitis affecting small and medium-size muscular arteries. Intensive care admission may be provoked by renal failure, ischemic heart disease, hypertensive crisis, and bronchospasm, although true pulmonary involvement is uncommon. Diagnosis may be confirmed by mesenteric angiography or renal biopsy. Treatment involves renal replacement therapy, high-dose steroids, and cyclophosphamide.

Goodpasture's syndrome

Antiglomerular basement membrane antibodies bind at the glomerulus and alveolus. Patients present with a proliferative glomerulonephritis and hemoptysis. Diagnosis is confirmed by positive antiglomerular basement membrane antibodies and renal biopsy. Treatment is with immunosuppressive therapy and plasma exchange.

See also

Plasma exchange, p. 70; Airway obstruction, p. 278; Steroids, p. 260; Hemoptysis, p. 302; Acute renal failure—diagnosis, p. 330; Acute renal failure—management, p. 332; Rheumatic disorders, p. 496

Anaphylactoid reactions

Minor reactions to allergens (itching, urticaria) are common before a severe reaction occurs. Any such history should be taken seriously and potential allergens avoided. Most reactions are acute in onset and clearly related to the causative allergen. However, some complement-mediated reactions may take longer to develop.

Clinical features
- Respiratory—laryngeal edema, bronchospasm, pulmonary edema, pulmonary hypertension
- Cardiovascular—hypotension, tachycardia, generalized edema
- Other—urticaria, angioedema, abdominal cramps, rigors

Management
1. Stop all infusions and blood transfusions and withhold any potential drug or food allergen. Blood and blood products should be returned to the laboratory for analysis.
2. Start oxygen (FiO_2 0.6–1.0). If there is evidence of persistent hypoxemia, consider urgent intubation and mechanical ventilation.
3. If there is laryngeal obstruction, bronchospasm, or facial edema, give IM or nebulizer epinephrine and IV hydrocortisone. If there is not rapid relief of airway obstruction, consider urgent intubation or, in extremis, emergency cricothyroidotomy. Persistent bronchospasm may require an epinephrine infusion or mechanical ventilation.
4. Hypotension should be treated with epinephrine IV/IM and rapid fluid resuscitation. Large volumes of fluid may be required to replace the plasma volume deficit in severe anaphylaxis; colloids (hetastarch) may be more effective.
   - Severe edema may coexist with hypovolemia.
   - Plasma volume has not been adequately replaced if Hb is higher than normal.
5. Persistent hypotension should be treated with further epinephrine, hydrocortisone, and fluids guided by CVP ± cardiac output monitoring. An epinephrine infusion may be required to overcome myocardial depression. The use of norepinephrine should be considered to divert blood centrally and to increase peripheral resistance.
6. Urticaria will usually respond to H_1 receptor antagonists— hydroxyzine or diphenhydramine IV or PO depending on the severity of the reaction. Refractory cases may respond to the addition of H_2 receptor antagonists.
7. After control of the anaphylactoid reaction, advice should be sought from the immunology laboratory and appropriate samples taken for confirmation.
8. Reactions to long-acting drugs or fluids will require continued support (perhaps for many hours).

Table 30.6 Drug dosages for laryngeal edema and bronchospasm

	Initial dose	Continued treatment
Epinephrine	0.3–0.5 mg IM or 0.5 mg nebulized	Start at 0.05 µg/kg/min
Hydrocortisone	200 mg IV	

Table 30.7 Drug dosages for hypotension

	Initial dose	Continued treatment
Epinephrine	0.5–1.0 mg IM or 0.05–0.2 mg IV	Start at 0.05 µg/kg/min
Hetastarch 6%	500 mL	According to response
Hydrocortisone	200 mg IV	100 mg IV q6 h
Diphenhydramine		50mg IV q6 h

Table 30.8 Drug dosages for urticaria

Diphenhydramine or hydroxyzine	25–50 mg IV or PO q6 h
Hydrocortisone	50–100 mg IV q8 h
Prednisolone	20 mg PO qd

See also

Ventilatory support—indications, p. 4; Endotracheal intubation, p. 36; Colloids, p. 180; Blood transfusion, p. 182; Inotropes, p. 196; Blood products, p. 250; Steroids, p. 260; Basic resuscitation, p. 268; Fluid challenge, p. 272

Trauma and burns

Multiple trauma (1)

Patients with multiple trauma are admitted either after surgery or for close observation and medical management. The principles of management are to

- Maintain or restore quickly adequate tissue perfusion and gas exchange
- Control pain
- Secure hemostasis and correct any coagulopathy
- Provide adequate nutrition
- Monitor closely and deal promptly with any complications

Circulatory management

- Patients are often cold and vasoconstricted on admission. This serves to camouflage concurrent hypovolemia and to compromise tissue perfusion.
- Adequate monitoring should be instituted at an early stage.
- Adequate perfusion must be restored promptly by repeated fluid challenges.
- Increasing lactic acidosis should prompt suspicion of inadequate resuscitation, covert hemorrhage, or tissue necrosis. Myocardial depression or failure may also be implicated.
- Neither metabolic acidosis (base deficit) or lactate are specific for tissue hypoperfusion, but both are associated with an increased risk of death. An increased SIG on presentation has also been shown to be highly predictive of adverse outcome in trauma patients.

Respiratory management

- Consider the possibility of an unstable cervical spine, especially in unconscious patients. This should be excluded by appropriate radiology and an expert opinion. Until then, the neck should be immobilized.
- If ventilated, ensure hemodynamic stability, correction of any metabolic acidosis, adequate rewarming, and satisfactory gas exchange before attempting to wean. If the patient remains unstable, it is advisable to delay extubation in case urgent surgery is required.
- If spontaneously breathing, give supplemental oxygen to provide adequate arterial oxygenation, encourage deep breathing to prevent atelectasis and secondary infection, and ensure sufficient analgesia, albeit not too much to suppress ventilatory drive. Epidurals may provide significant analgesia without compromising respiratory drive.

Hematological management

- Maintain Hb at >7 g/dL (more with coronary artery disease) to assist oxygen transport. Cross-matched blood should be readily available for secondary hemorrhage.
- Correct any coagulopathy with FFP, ± platelets, and other blood products (e.g., cryoprecipitate) or activated factor VII.

Peripheries

Injury to the limbs may result in nerve injuries, obstruction of the vascular supply, or muscle damage that may lead to compartment syndrome and rhabdomyolysis. A high level of suspicion should be held and corrective surgery undertaken promptly if necessary.

See also

Multiple trauma (2)

Analgesia

- Adequate analgesia is imperative to avoid circulatory instability and decreased chest wall excursion, especially after chest, abdominal, or spinal trauma.
- Increased use of regional techniques (depending on absence of infection and coagulopathy) and patient-controlled analgesia has facilitated pain relief and weaning.
- Opiates are recommended for initial analgesia. NSAIDs are particularly effective for bone pain, although they may occasionally precipitate coagulopathies, stress ulceration, and renal failure.
- Agitation may be to the result of causes other than pain (e.g., infection, withdrawal, or intracranial lesion).

Nutrition

Early nutrition has been shown to reduce postoperative complications. This should ideally be enteral, an approach that has been demonstrated to be safe, even after abdominal laparotomy for trauma.

Infection

- Depending on the site of trauma, the type of wound (open/closed, clean/dirty), and the need for surgery, prophylactic tetanus and antibiotic coverage varying from one dose to 1 to 2 weeks may be needed.
- The trauma patient is at high risk of developing secondary infection—in particular chest, wound sites, intravascular catheter insertion sites, postabdominal trauma, and intra-abdominal abscesses. Preventive measures and strict infection control should be undertaken.
- Intravascular catheters inserted during emergency resuscitation under nonsterile conditions should be replaced.

Prophylaxis

- Attention should be paid to pressure areas. This may involve the use of specialized mattresses or support beds.
- Clear instructions should be obtained from the surgeon regarding care of the wound and drain sites.
- Especially after orthopedic procedures on the pelvis and lower limbs, or if the patient will remain immobilized, low-molecular weight heparin prophylaxis against DVT should be instituted.

Review

- Regular review of the patient is necessary to ensure complications are detected and dealt with promptly. This may require repeat laparotomy, ultrasound, or CT scanning.
- Later complications include pancreatitis, acalculous cholecystitis, and multiple-organ dysfunction (including ARDS).

See also

Head injury

The head may be injured with or without significant trauma to other parts of the body. Priority in management of the multiply injured patient must be placed on securing adequate gas exchange and circulatory resuscitation, and dealing with any life-threatening chest or abdominal injury before definitive treatment for head injury. Prevention of secondary systemic insults, such as hypotension and hypoxia, are paramount. The patient will usually be admitted to the ICU after CT scanning has identified the extent of injury. The neck should also be imaged by CT, particularly if the patient is ventilated. It is also likely that surgery will have been undertaken for any significant space-occupying lesion or for elevation of a depressed fracture.

General management

- All head-injured patients admitted to an ICU should have neurosurgical input regarding management of increased ICP. Local policy may encourage invasive monitoring (e.g., ICP, SjO_2) or early bone flap decompression.
- ICP monitoring is usually indicated in patients with severe head injury (GCS score, 3–8 points after resuscitation) and an admission CT scan revealing hematoma, contusion, edema, or compressed basal cisterns. ICP monitoring may also be appropriate in the setting of severe head injury and a normal admission CT if two or more of the following features are present at admission: age >40 years, posturing, systolic blood pressure <90 mmHg.
- Deterioration in conscious level, developing neurological deficits, or focal signs (e.g., unilateral pupillary dilatation) should prompt urgent repeat CT scanning for late complications (e.g., subdural hematoma).
- An unstable neck fracture should be assumed until excluded by expert opinion and appropriate investigations.
- If a basal skull fracture is suspected (e.g., radiographs, rhinorrhea, otorrhea), avoid nasal insertion of feeding or endotracheal tubes.

Complications

- Actively manage increased ICP.
- Actively treat seizures with anticonvulsants to prevent further hypoxemic cerebral damage, and reduce cerebral oxygen requirements and ICP. All patients with severe closed head injury should be loaded with IV phenytoin and treated for 7 days as seizure prophylaxis. Consider additional causes such as hypoglycemia, development of a new space-occupying lesion, recreational drugs, and infection.
- Diabetes insipidus suggests hypothalamic injury and carries a poor prognosis. Desmopressin 1 to 4 µg IV should be given daily to maintain urine output of 100 to 150 mL/h.
- Actively manage hyperpyrexia. Some studies show long-term benefit from induced hypothermia, but this needs to be aggressively instituted as early as possible after the injury to be effective.
- Actively manage hyperglycemia with insulin, and avoid hypoglycemia.

Key papers

Clifton GL, Miller ER, Choi SC, *et al.* Lack of effect of induction of hypothermia after acute brain injury. *N Engl J Med* 2001; **344**:556–63.
Rovlias A, Kotsou S. The influence of hyperglycemia on neurological outcome in patients with severe head injury. *Neurosurgery* 2000; **46**:335–42.

See also

Analgesia and sedation

- Adequate analgesia (usually opiates) must be given to the head-injured patient because pain and agitation will increase ICP, thereby causing a secondary insult.
- Short-acting sedation should be used because this enables rapid assessment of the underlying level of consciousness and any focal neurological deficit.

Respiratory management

- Hyperventilation is no longer recommended apart from short-term management of increased ICP. If ventilated, aim to maintain $PaCO_2$ at 35 to 40 mmHg.
- Face or neck injuries may require emergency cricothyroidotomy or tracheostomy to obtain a patent airway. If orotracheally intubated, ensure local swelling has subsided (nasendoscopy, air leak around deflated cuff) before extubation.
- Severe agitation and confusion may last for several weeks; this will often delay weaning and extubation. Judicious sedation (e.g., with haloperidol) may be necessary. Early tracheostomy facilitates ventilator weaning while maintaining airway patency and pulmonary toileting in patients with head injury.

Circulatory management

- Hypotension should be avoided with adequate fluid resuscitation ± vasopressor therapy.
- Elevated blood pressures may be tolerated unless excessive.
- β-blockers may be useful in reducing the myocardial effects of excessive catecholamine levels.

Other drug therapy

- Antibiotic prophylaxis is not routinely recommended.
- High-dose steroid therapy is not beneficial.
- Trials of other neuroprotective agents (e.g., free radical scavengers) have also failed to show benefit.

See also

Ventilatory support—indications, p. 4; Endotracheal intubation, p. 36; ICP monitoring, p. 134; Jugular venous bulb saturation, p. 136; Hypotension, p. 310; Increased ICP, p. 384; Pain, p. 534

Spinal cord injury

Spinal injury, with or without damage to the cord, may be apparent soon after admission to the hospital; however, deterioration may occur, requiring a high index of suspicion and careful monitoring.

Immobilization

- The spine should be immobilized until a surgical opinion has confirmed that no unstable fracture is present, both radiologically and clinically.
- Place a hard cervical collar if a neck fracture is possible. This does not stabilize the spine; either skull traction or operative stabilization will be needed for an unstable fracture.
- Move the patient by 'log rolling' or straight lifting, using at least four staff members. Exercise care with neck manipulation. Intubation should be performed only by an experienced operator.

Circulatory instability

- So-called 'spinal shock' may occur with marked hypotension resulting from sympathetic outflow disturbance. Hypovolemia should be excluded first. Consider damage to other organs/vessels (e.g., spleen, aorta).
- Vasopressor therapy may be necessary if evidence of tissue hypoperfusion persists (e.g., oliguria, metabolic acidosis).
- Postural hypotension and circulatory instability (including symptomatic bradycardia) is commonplace for the first few weeks. Autonomic dysfunction affects 50% of cervical and high thoracic cord injuries.

Respiratory management

- High cervical cord injury above C5 results in loss of diaphragmatic function, whereas above C8 can result in loss of intercostal function. This may compromise or prevent breathing and weaning from IPPV.
- When able, the patient should be managed in an upright posture.
- Atelectasis is common and requires meticulous pulmonary toileting.
- Early tracheostomy may facilitate support and comfort.

General measures

- Carefully monitor neurological function to enable early detection of spinal cord compression and referral for urgent remedial surgery.
- Give low-molecular weight heparin SC for thromboembolism prophylaxis.
- The incidence of stress ulceration is high. Ideally, enteral nutrition should be instituted at an early stage. Drugs (e.g., sucralfate, H_2 blockers) may be needed.
- Enteral feeding may be difficult to institute initially because gastric distension and paralytic ileus is common after spinal cord injury. A nasogastric tube should be inserted for gastric decompression. An enterostomy may eventually be needed to enable long-term feeding.
- Bowel and bladder function may be deranged. Long-term bladder catheters, and regular laxative and enema therapy should be instituted at an early stage.

- Special care is needed to prevent pressure sores.
- Institute regular physical therapy to prevent contractures.
- Psychological support for patient and family is crucial, particularly if long-term disability is likely.
- High-dose steroid therapy may be beneficial if started within 8 h, although this still remains controversial.
- Hyperbaric oxygen therapy is of unproven benefit.
- After spinal injury, muscle relaxants may cause severe hyperkalemia.
- Steroids have been shown to be useful, but this remains controversial.

Key trial

Bracken MB, et al. Administration of methylprednisolone for 24 or 48 hours or tirilazad mesylate for 48 hours in the treatment of acute spinal cord injury. Results of the Third National Acute Spinal Cord Injury Randomized Controlled Trial. National Acute Spinal Cord Injury Study. JAMA 1997; **277**:1597–604.

See also

Burns—fluid management

Patients with major thermal injuries (i.e., >20% body surface area) are admitted to an ICU specializing in the management of burns for meticulous attention to fluid resuscitation, prevention of infection, and the frequent need for mechanical ventilation.

Monitoring

- The fluid loss from major burns requires careful assessment of intravascular volume status. The traditional markers of fluid resuscitation in burns of central venous pressure, urine output, and hematocrit are generally inadequate.
- Cardiac output monitoring may be needed for accurate titration of fluid. This is particularly applicable in the presence of a hyperdynamic, vasodilated circulation that often commences within 1 to 2 days. Although infection is not necessarily present, vasopressor therapy may be needed to maintain adequate systemic blood pressures.
- Pulmonary artery and central venous catheters should not be inserted through affected skin areas if at all possible.
- Insertion of intravascular catheters, urinary catheters and nasogastric tubes should be carried out soon after admission, because rapid-onset swelling within a few hours may make these procedures impossible.

Fluid management

- The extent of injury will have been estimated by burn surgeons who will also determine the proportion of full-thickness dermal injury to calculate the approximate fluid resuscitation required.
- Fluid management varies among centers. Many institutional protocols originated from the early work of Baxter at Parkland Hospital in the 1960s. Many formulas exist. These estimations are different in both the volumes of fluid per weight and the type of crystalloid ± colloid administered. No formula has been found to be superior. These formulas only provide an approximate guide and frequently underestimate losses both into the interstitial spaces and through the lost skin barrier. Evaporative losses are approximately 2 mL/kg/h. Water losses may be increased if wounds are not covered. Losses increase further with inhalation injury.
- Overzealous fluid infusion should be avoided to minimize edema.
- The increased permeability and fluid leak phase lasts approximately 1 to 2 days. After 2 to 5 days, a diuretic phase usually commences when excess tissue fluid is lost and body swelling reduces.
- Electrolyte levels (especially K^+ and Mg^{2+} can fluctuate widely during both periods, requiring monitoring and replacement as necessary.
- Although some hemolysis may occur, blood transfusion requirements are usually low, but debridement will result in major blood loss often requiring major transfusion (>8–10 U). Coagulopathy will often occur, in part as a result of a dilutional effect of the albumin infusion.

Fluid resuscitation regimen

Note: These regimens should be used as a guide only. With either of the following formulas, give blood as necessary to maintain Hb >10 g/dL. Reassess cardiorespiratory variables and urine output at frequent intervals to determine whether volume replacement is inadequate or excessive, and adjust fluid input accordingly.

Adapted from Parkland formula

- Total volume of Ringer's lactate for the first 24 hours = 4 mL Ringer's lactate solution × body weight (kg) × % burn.
- Half the volume is administered in the first 8 h; the rest is delivered over the next 16 h.

Adapted from Mount Vernon formula

- Divide first 36 h from the time of burn into six consecutive periods of 4, 4, 4, 6, 6, and 12 h.
- For each period give 0.5 mL 5% albumin × body wt (kg) × % burn.
- Give 1.5 to 2 mL/kg/h 5% glucose.

See also

Blood pressure monitoring, p. 112; Central venous catheter—use, p. 116; Colloid osmotic pressure, p. 172; Crystalloids, p. 176; Colloids, p. 180; Basic resuscitation, p. 268; Fluid challenge, p. 272; Hypotension, p. 310; Oliguria, p. 328; Burns—general management, p. 506

Burns—general management

Surgery

- Escharotomy may be needed on hospital admission to affected limbs, as well as to the neck and/or chest if a circumferential burn is present.
- Debridement of necrotic tissue is often begun within the first few days, because early grafting is associated with improved outcome. Coverage is obtained using either split skin grafts from the patient's own unaffected skin, donor skin grafts, or even experimental 'skin.' Blood loss may be rapid and massive (e.g., 100 mL per 1% of body surface grafted).

Wound care

- Early application of dressings and silver sulfadiazine cream, which has antibacterial properties against Gram-negative bacteria, may usefully prevent secondary infection.
- Early grafting often takes place within the first 2 to 3 days to provide a protective skin barrier.

Nutrition

- Enteral nutrition should be commenced soon after admission because studies have shown that early enteral nutrition improves outcome.
- Target intake is protein of 1 g/kg + 2 g per percent burn and a calorie intake of 20 Cal/kg + 50 Cal per percent burn.

Infection

- Prophylactic antibiotics are often not given to burn patients.
- Body temperature increases on days 1 to 2, as high as 40°C, may persist for several days and do not indicate secondary infection.
- Likely infecting agents include streptococci, staphylococci, and Gram-negative bacteria such as *Pseudomonas*. Appropriate antibiotic treatment should be given as indicated.

Other considerations

- Any suspected inhalation injury should be diagnosed and treated.
- Ensure adequate analgesia (opiates). Ketamine is a useful anesthetic because it has analgesic properties as well.
- Tetanus toxoid should be given soon after hospital admission.
- Reduce heat and fluid losses by placing the patient on a heated air-fluidized bed, and by early coverage of burned skin through application of occlusive dressings and placement of affected limbs in transparent plastic bags.
- Stress ulceration can usually be avoided through prompt resuscitation and early enteral nutrition.
- Pressure sores and contractures should be prevented by careful nursing and physiotherapy.
- Succinylcholine should be avoided from 5 to 150 days postburn because of the risk of rapid and severe hyperkalemia.
- Increasing resistance to nondepolarizing muscle relaxants may be seen.
- β-blockade has been associated with outcome improvement in children who sustain a burn injury.

See also

Physical disorders

Hypothermia

Clinical features
- >33°C—Shivering is usually marked in an attempt to correct body temperature.
- <33°C—Neurological signs of dysarthria and slowness appear.
- <31°C—Hypertonicity and sluggish reflexes with cardiovascular dysfunction become life threatening.
- <28°C—Arterial pulses often become impalpable. Hypothermic rigidity is difficult to distinguish from death.
- Prognosis depends on the degree and duration of hypothermia.

ECG changes
Sinus bradycardia is followed by atrial flutter and fibrillation with ventricular ectopics. The PR interval, QRS complex, and QT interval are prolonged. Atrial activity eventually ceases. The J wave is most often seen at <31°C, and ventricular fibrillation is common at <30°C, giving way to asystole at <28 °C.

Complications
Hypoxemia is common as a result of hypoventilation and ventilation–perfusion mismatch. Hypovolemia and metabolic acidosis are common. Renal tubular damage may result from renal blood flow reduction. Acute pancreatitis, rhabdomyolysis, and gastric erosions are common.

Management
1. Oxygen (FiO_2 0.6–1.0) to maintain SaO_2 >95%
2. Fluid replacement with careful monitoring
3. Rewarming—All hypothermic patients with no evidence of other fatal disease should be assumed fully recoverable. In the event of cardiac arrest full resuscitation should continue until the patient is normothermic (VF is resistant to defibrillation between 28°C and 30°C). The technique used for rewarming depends on the core temperature (measured with a low-reading rectal thermometer) and the clinical circumstance.

Rapid central rewarming
In cases when the temperature is <28°C (<33°C with acute-exposure hypothermia), or when there is cardiac arrest, rapid rewarming may be achieved by continuous AV rewarming circuits, peritoneal dialysis, and gastric or bladder lavage with warmed fluids. Cardiopulmonary bypass is an effective rewarming strategy for patients with cardiac arrest resistant to defibrillation. These techniques may achieve rewarming rates of 1 to 5°C/h. Active surface rewarming with a heated blanket or warm-air blanket can achieve rates of 1 to 7°C/h and is less invasive. Hemodynamic changes may be dramatic during active rewarming, requiring careful monitoring and support. If extracorporeal rewarming is available, rates of 3 to 15°C/h may be achieved with the addition of cardiovascular support.

Spontaneous rewarming

Spontaneous rewarming proceeds at a rate inversely proportional to the duration of hypothermia. With good insulation (space blanket), rewarming rates of 0.1 to 0.7°C/h can be achieved. Core temperature may decrease during spontaneous rewarming as cold blood is returned from the periphery to the central circulation.

Causes of hypothermia

- Coma and immobility
- Cold-water immersion
- Exposure
- Hypothyroidism
- Hypopituitarism
- Sepsis
- Erythroderma

See also

Ventilatory support—indications, p. 4; Endotracheal intubation, p. 36; Defibrillation, p. 45; Peritoneal dialysis, p. 68; ECG monitoring, p. 110; Basic resuscitation, p. 268; Cardiac arrest, p. 270; Fluid challenge, p. 272; Tachyarrhythmias, p. 314; Bradyarrhythmias, p. 316; Pancreatitis, p. 354; Thyroid emergencies, p. 448; Rhabdomyolysis, p. 530

Pyrexia (1)

Mechanisms underlying an increase in temperature are poorly understood. It reflects the balance between heat loss and heat production. There may be an inability to lose heat (e.g., high ambient temperature), 'thermostat' dysregulation within the hypothalamus, or increased heat generation (e.g., as a result of mitochondrial uncoupling). There is some laboratory evidence that a indicates that an increased temperature may be beneficial in terms of white cell response, heat shock protein activation, and mitochondrial protection. Septic patients presenting with a low temperature have a poorer prognosis.

An excessive temperature may be unpleasant to the patient (e.g., rigors), will increase metabolic rate and therefore oxygen demand, and may induce excessive vasodilatation and salt and water loss. At very high temperatures, biochemical function is disrupted with altered enzyme function and increased cell breakdown (e.g., rhabdomyolysis).

Causes

Infection

The most common cause of pyrexia in the ICU patient is infection, although it is overdiagnosed. The main sites are chest and intravascular catheter sites. Urinary tract infections are difficult to diagnose in the presence of a urethral catheter. Similarly, the respiratory tract is routinely colonized with bacteria within a few days of ICU admission, and differentiation between colonizing and pathogenic bacteria is difficult. Consider tropical illnesses (e.g., malaria) in patients who have visited endemic areas. Antibiotic therapy may itself be a cause of pyrexia.

Inflammation

Inflammation unrelated to infection will usually generate a pyrexic response; after cardiac surgery, burns, and MI; and with vasculitis, glomerulonephritis, hepatitis, and acalculous cholecystitis. Other than specific therapy (e.g., immunosuppression for vasculitis), management is generally symptom oriented to include cooling.

Adverse drug reaction

Numerous drugs may induce an idiosyncratic pyrexia, including antibiotics, sedatives, paralyzing agents, and amphetamines. Usually, removal of the offending drug is sufficient, but more active measures may have to be taken, including active cooling and dantrolene.

Adverse reaction to blood transfusion

An adverse reaction to a blood transfusion may be related to an immunological reaction to one of the cellular constituents, or to contamination with an organism, bacterial cell products, or other pyrogen.

Ambient heating

Excessive heating or prevention of heat loss may cause pyrexia. Consider strong sunlight, excess temperature control settings on specialized beds or mattresses, and heat-retaining bed clothing.

Miscellaneous

Other causes of pyrexia include neoplasm and postcerebral insult (e.g., head injury, CVA).

Key paper

Circiumaru B, *et al*. A prospective study of fever in the intensive care unit. *Intensive Care Med* 1999; **25**:668–73.

Pyrexia (2)

Currently, the optimal temperature to target in disease states is not known, other than cerebral insults, for which normo- or even hypothermia appears to offer neuroprotection by reducing cerebral metabolic rate. In other conditions it seems reasonable to accept pyrexia, provided it is tolerated by the patient.

Principles of management

1. Diagnose then remove or treat the offending cause. For example, seek and treat infection, stop blood infusion and send discontinued bag to laboratory for analysis, use anti-inflammatory ± immuno-suppressive agents for vasculitis.
2. Cooling aids symptomatic recovery, reduces metabolic rate, and lowers pressor requirements.
   - Increase evaporative losses (e.g., tepid sponging, wet sheets, ice packs).
   - Increase convective losses (e.g., fanning to improve air circulation).
   - Administer antipyretics (e.g., Tylenol, aspirin).
   - Attempt more aggressive cooling if temperature is >40°C.
   - Aim to lower temperature to <38.5°C, then reassess.

See also

Hyperthermia

Hyperthermia is defined as a core temperature >41°C.

Clinical features
- Delirium and seizures are associated with temperatures of 40 to 42°C.
- Coma is associated with temperatures >42°C.
- Tachycardia
- Tachypnea
- Salt water depletion
- Rhabdomyolysis
- DIC
- Heart failure with ST depression and T-wave flattening

Causes
- Hyperthermia may be an extreme form of pyrogen-induced fever associated with infection, inflammation, neoplasm, or CVA.
- Heat stroke is associated with severe exercise in high environmental temperatures and humidity. There may be excess clothing or hypovolemia reducing the body's ability to dissipate heat production.
- Malignant hyperthermia is a drug-induced myopathy associated with a hereditary calcium transfer defect in patients receiving volatile anesthetics or taking muscle relaxants, antidepressants, alcohol, or Ecstasy. Heat production is increased by muscle catabolism, spasm, and peripheral vasoconstriction.
- Neuroleptic malignant syndrome is a drug-induced hyperthermic syndrome secondary to phenothiazines or butyrophenones. It is associated with muscle rigidity, akinesia, impaired consciousness, and autonomic dysfunction, and continues for 1 to 2 weeks.

Management
1. Rapid cooling should be instituted when temperatures exceed 41°C.
2. Supportive treatment includes fluid replacement and seizure control.
3. Clothing should be removed and patients should be nursed in a cool environment.
4. Surface cooling may be achieved with a fan, tepid sponging, wet sheets, ice packs, or a cool bath.
5. Handling should be minimized and active cooling measures should be stopped when the core temperature is <39°C.
6. Internal cooling may be considered by gastric lavage or peritoneal lavage using cooled fluids.
7. Phenothiazines may be used to reduce temperature and prevent shivering (not in neuroleptic malignant syndrome).
8. Muscle relaxants should be used if the patient is ventilated.
9. For malignant hyperthermia, the offending drug should be stopped and dantrolene 1 mg/kg given IV every 5 min to a maximum dose of 10 mg/kg.
10. Mechanical ventilation with high FiO_2 and treatment of hyperkalemia are required.
11. Neuroleptic malignant syndrome is treated by stopping the offending drug, giving dantrolene as mentioned, and administering dopamine agonists (e.g., L-dopa or bromocriptine).

See also

Electrocution

The effects of electrocution are the result of the effects of the current and the conversion of electrical energy to heat energy on passage through the tissues. Important factors are the following:

- Energy delivered—heat = amperage^2 × resistance × time (i.e., the amperage is the most important determinant of heat production)
- Resistance to current flow—tissues are resistant to current flow in the following decreasing order: bone, fat, tendon, skin, muscle, blood vessels, nerves. A high skin resistance and short duration of contact concentrate the effects locally. However, skin contaminants, moisture, and burning reduce resistance.
- Type of current—alternating current is more dangerous than direct current. Tetanic muscle contractions may prevent the victim from releasing the current source whereas the single, strong muscle contraction with direct current often throws the victim clear. Alternating current is more likely to reach central tissues, with consequent sustained apnea and VF (with as little as 50–100 mA for 1–10 ms).
- Current pathway—cardiorespiratory arrest is more likely the closer the contact is with the chest and heart.

Lightening strike differs from contact electrocution in that high-intensity, ultrashort duration of current may produce cardiac arrest with little tissue destruction.

Clinical features

- Tachyarrhythmias including VI and VF
- Asystole—more likely with high current (>10 A)
- Myocardial injury—heat injury, coronary artery spasm, arrhythmias, myocardial spasm
- Respiratory arrest—tetanic contraction of the diaphragm, arrhythmias, cerebral medullary dysfunction
- Trauma—tetanic muscle contraction, falling, or being thrown clear
- Burns—skin and internal tissues

Management

Most severe electrical injuries require urgent field treatment prior to hospital admission.

1. The first priority is to ensure that the source of the electrical injury is not a hazard to rescuers.
2. Manage cardiorespiratory arrest.
3. Prevent further injury (e.g., spinal protection, removal of smoldering clothes).

After hospital admission and restoration of the circulation, management is directed toward the complications.

1. Maintain ventilatory support.
2. Manage hypovolemia associated with burn injury. Fluid requirements are usually greater than for victims of thermal burns and require close monitoring.
3. Check cardiac enzymes for degree of myocardial injury. Treat heart failure and/or arrhythmias as indicated.

4. Manage rhabdomyolysis and covert compartment syndrome.
5. Perform surgical debridement of necrotic tissue and fixation of bony injury.

See also

Near-drowning

After near-drowning, the major complications are lung injury, hypothermia, and the effects of prolonged hypoxia. Although hypothermia bestows protective effects against organ damage, rewarming carries particular hazards.

Pathophysiology

Prolonged immersion usually results in inhalation of fluid; however, 10% to 20% of patients develop intense laryngospasm, leading to so-called 'dry drowning'. Traditionally, freshwater drowning was considered to lead to rapid absorption of water into the circulation, with hemolysis, hypoosmolality, and possible electrolyte disturbance, whereas inhalation of hypertonic fluid from seawater drowning produced a marked flux of fluid into the alveoli. In practice, there seems to be little distinction between fresh water and sea water because both cause loss of surfactant and severe inflammatory disruption of the alveolar–capillary membrane, leading to an ARDS-type picture. Initially, hemodynamic instability is often minor. A similar picture often develops after 'dry drowning' and subsequent endotracheal intubation.

Acute hypothermia often accompanies near-drowning, with loss of consciousness and hemodynamic alterations.

Management

1. Oxygen (FiO_2, 0.6–1) should be given, either by face mask if the patient is spontaneously breathing, or via mechanical ventilation. Comatose patients should be intubated. Early CPAP or PEEP may be useful.
2. Bronchospasm is often present and may require nebulized β_2 agonists, and either nebulized or SC epinephrine.
3. Fluid replacement should be directed by appropriate monitoring. Inotrope therapy may be necessary if hypoperfusion persists after adequate fluid resuscitation. Intravascular fluid overload is uncommon, and the role of early diuretic therapy as a therapy to prevent intracranial hypertension is controversial. Hemolysis may occur and requires blood transfusion.
4. Arrhythmias may arise secondary to myocardial hypoxia, hypothermia, and electrolyte abnormalities. These should be treated conventionally.
5. Metabolic acidosis (lactate) may be profound, but sodium bicarbonate therapy is rarely indicated because the acidosis will usually correct on restoration of adequate tissue perfusion.
6. Electrolyte abnormalities are usually minor and should be managed conventionally.
7. Rewarming follows conventional practice; cardiopulmonary bypass may be considered if core temperature is <30°C. Cardiopulmonary resuscitation including cardiac massage should be continued until normothermia is achieved.
8. Cerebral protection usually follows increased ICP protocols, although, as mentioned earlier, the roles of diuretic therapy and fluid restriction are controversial. Signs of brain damage such as seizures may become apparent and should be treated as they arise.

9. Antibiotic therapy (e.g., clindamycin, or cefuroxime plus metronidazole) should be given if strong evidence of aspiration exists. Otherwise, take specimens and treat as indicated.
10. Decompress the stomach using a nasogastric tube to lessen any risk of aspiration. Enteral feeding can be initiated afterward.

See also

Ventilatory support—indications, p. 4; Endotracheal intubation, p. 36; Positive end expiratory pressure (1), p. 22; Positive end expiratory pressure (2), p. 24; Continuous positive airway pressure, p. 26; Bronchodilators, p. 186; Antiarrhythmics, p. 204; Antimicrobials, p. 258; Acute respiratory distress syndrome (1), p. 290; Acute respiratory distress syndrome (2), p. 292; Metabolic acidosis, p. 436; Hypothermia, p. 518

Rhabdomyolysis

Rhabdomyolysis is the breakdown of striated muscle, which may result in compartment syndrome, acute renal failure, and electrolyte abnormalities (hyperkalemia, hypocalcemia, hyperphosphatemia).

Causes
- Trauma, especially crush injury
- Prolonged immobilization (e.g., after fall, drug overdose)
- Drugs (e.g., opiates, cocaine, Ecstasy)
- Hyperpyrexia
- Vascular occlusion (including lengthy vascular surgery)
- Infection
- Burns/electrocution
- Severe hypophosphatemia
- Congenital myopathy (rare)

Diagnosis
- Suggested by disproportionately high serum creatinine level compared with urea (usual ratio is approximately 10 µmol:1 mmol)
- Inreased creatine kinase (usually >2000 IU/l)
- Myoglobinuria—this produces a positive urine dipstick to blood. Laboratory analysis is required to confirm myoglobin rather than blood or Hb. The urine is usually red or black, but may appear clear despite significant rhabdomyolysis.

General management
- Provide prompt fluid resuscitation.
- Hypocalcemia should not be treated unless the patient is symptomatic. Administered calcium may form crystals with the high circulating phosphate.
- Hyperkalemia may be resistant to medical management and may require urgent hemodialysis or hemofiltration.

Compartment syndrome
- Suspect compartment syndrome if limb is tender or painful and peripheries are cool. Loss of peripheral pulses and tense muscles are late signs.
- Manometry in muscle compartments reveal pressures >20 to 25 mmHg.
- Arm, leg, and buttock compartments may be affected.
- Management involves either prophylactic fasciotomies if at high risk or close monitoring (including regular manometry) with decompression if pressures exceed 20 to 25 mmHg.
- Fasciotomies may result in major blood loss.

Renal failure

- Renal failure is thought to be produced by a combination of free radical injury, hypovolemia, hypotension, and, possibly, myoglobin blocking the renal tubules.
- Renal failure may be prevented by prompt rehydration with 0.9% saline for 3 to 5 days. Alkalinization of the urine with sodium bicarbonate or diuresis with mannitol remain controversial. There is no evidence that these therapies offer any benefit over hydration alone and there may be complications to these approaches.
- Potassium, sodium, calcium, and magnesium levels should be regularly monitored and managed as appropriate.
- If renal failure is established, dialysis or filtration techniques will be required, usually for a period of 6 to 8 weeks.

Key paper

Better OS, Stein JH. Early management of shock and prophylaxis of acute renal failure in traumatic rhabdomyolysis. *N Engl J Med* 1990; **322**:825–9.

See also

Pain and postoperative intensive care

Pain

Pain results from many insults (e.g., trauma, invasive procedures, specific organ disease, and inflammatory processes). The relief of pain is one of the primary goals of medicine. Pain relief is necessary for physiological and psychological reasons:

- Anxiety and lack of sleep.
- Increased sympathetic activity contributing to an increased metabolic demand.
- The capacity of the circulation and respiratory system to meet the demands of metabolizing tissues may not be adequate.
- Myocardial ischemia is a significant risk.
- The endocrine response to injury is exaggerated with consequent salt and water retention.
- Physiological attempts to limit pain may include immobility and muscle splinting, and consequent reductions in ventilatory function and cough.

Pain perception

The degree of the pain stimulus is related to the magnitude of tissue damage. The site of injury is also important; thoracic and upper abdominal injury is more painful than injury elsewhere. However, the perception of pain is dependent on other factors (e.g., simultaneous sensory input, personality, cultural background, and previous experiences of pain).

Management of pain

Systemic analgesia

- Opioid analgesics form the mainstay of analgesic drug treatment in intensive care.
- Small, frequent IV doses or a continuous infusion provide the most stable blood levels. Because the degree of analgesia is dependent on blood levels, it is important that they are maintained.
- Higher doses are required to treat rather than prevent pain.
- The dose of drug required for a particular individual depends on his or her perception of pain and whether tolerance has built up to previous analgesic use.
- The use of nonopioid drugs may reduce the dose required of opioid drugs. This includes acetaminophen and NASIDs, ketamine, and dexmedetomidine.

Regional analgesia

- Regional techniques reduce respiratory depression but require experience to ensure procedures are performed safely.
- Epidural analgesia may be achieved with local anesthetic agents or opioids.
- Opioids avoid the vasodilatation and hypotension associated with local anesthetic agents, but do not produce as profound analgesia.
- The combination of opioid and local anesthetic is synergistic.
- IV opioids should be avoided, or close monitoring should continue for 24 h after cessation of epidural opioids because of the potential for late respiratory failure. Sample regimens are shown in Table 33.1.
- Local anesthetic agents may be used to block superficial nerves (e.g., intercostal nerve block with 3–5 mL 0.5% bupivacaine plus epinephrine).

Nonpharmacological techniques

Adequate explanation, positioning, and physical techniques may all reduce drug requirements.

Table 33.1 Regimens for epidural analgesia

Lumbar LA	10–15 mL 0.5% bupivacaine followed by an infusion of 5–20 mL/h 0.125% bupivacaine
Thoracic LA	4–6 mL 0.5% bupivacaine followed by an infusion of 6–10 mL/h 0.125% bupivacaine
Opioid Combined	5 mg morphine gives up to 12 h analgesia Infusion of 3–4 mL/h 0.125% bupivacaine with 0.3–0.4 mg/h morphine or 25–50 µg/h fentanyl

LA = local anesthetic

See also

Opioid analgesics, p. 232; Nonopioid analgesics, p. 234; Multiple trauma (1), p. 502; Multiple trauma (2), p. 504; Head injury (1), p. 506; Head injury (2), p. 508; Burns—general management, p. 514; Postoperative intensive care, p. 536

Post-operative intensive care

Patients may be admitted to the ICU after surgery, either electively (discussed later) or after unexpected perioperative complications.

General care
- Ensure surgical and anesthetic plan has been agreed to (e.g., overnight ventilation, special precautions (e.g., wire cutters if mandible wired), movement restrictions, hemodynamic targets).
- Provide adequate analgesia.
- Ensure adequate rewarming.
- Maintain euglycemia.
- Provide appropriate thrombosis and stress ulcer prophylaxis.
- Conduct blood gas, electrolyte, and Hb monitoring.

Postoperative respiratory problems
Postoperative respiratory problems are common in those with preexisting respiratory disease, especially with a reduced vital capacity or peak flow rate. Problems include
- Exacerbation of chronic chest disease
- Retained secretions
- Basal atelectasis
- Pneumonia
- Upper airway problems (e.g., laryngeal edema)

Anesthesia and surgery (especially upper abdominal surgery) reduce FRC, thoracic compliance, and cough. There is reduced macrophage function and systemic inflammatory activation, with infection, and acute lung injury as possible consequences.

Therapeutic aims
Preoperative preparation may help avoid some of the problems:
- Cessation of smoking for >1 week
- Bronchodilatation
- Respiratory muscle training
- Chest physiotherapy
- Avoidance of hypovolemia in the nil-by-mouth period

Postoperative clearance of secretions and maintenance of basal lung expansion are very important. These require effective analgesia and chest physiotherapy. Consider early use of noninvasive ventilation if spontaneously breathing but requiring high FiO_2. Mechanical ventilation assists basal expansion and secretion clearance when anesthetic recovery is expected to be prolonged or when surgery ± preexisting disease increases the risk of secretion retention and atelectasis. Ensure a patent airway prior to extubation when intubation was difficult or after upper airway surgery.

Postoperative circulatory problems
- Prevention of hypovolemia is crucial in avoiding inflammatory activation and, therefore, many postoperative complications.
- Hemorrhage is usually obvious and managed by resuscitation, correction of coagulation disturbance, and surgery.

- Subclinical hypovolemia is common postoperatively. Hypothermia and high catecholamine levels help to maintain central venous pressure and blood pressure despite continuing hypovolemia. Avoiding reduced stroke volume or metabolic acidosis are the best indicators of adequate resuscitation.
- Postoperative fluid management requires a high degree of suspicion of hypovolemia. Fluid challenges should be used to confirm and treat hypovolemia when there is any circulatory disturbance, metabolic acidosis, or oliguria.

Reasons for elective ICU admission

- Airway monitoring (e.g., major oral, head, and neck surgery)
- Respiratory monitoring (e.g., cardiothoracic surgery, upper abdominal surgery, prolonged anesthesia, previous respiratory disease)
- Cardiovascular monitoring (e.g., cardiac surgery, vascular surgery, major abdominal surgery, prolonged anesthesia, previous cardiovascular disease)
- Neurological monitoring (e.g., neurosurgery, cardiac surgery with circulatory arrest)
- Elective ventilation (e.g., cardiac surgery, major abdominal surgery, prolonged anesthesia, previous respiratory disease)

See also

Ventilatory support—indications, p. 4; Endotracheal intubation, p. 36; Noninvasive respiratory support, p. 32; Chest physiotherapy, p. 48; Pulse oximetry, p. 92; Blood gas analysis, p. 102; ECG monitoring, p. 110; Blood pressure monitoring, p. 112; Central venous catheter—use, p. 116; Central venous catheter—insertion, p. 118; Cardiac output—thermodilution, p. 124; Cardiac output—other invasive, p. 126; Cardiac output—noninvasive (1), p. 128; Cardiac output—non-invasive (2), p. 130; Electrolytes (Na^+, K^+, Cl^-, HCO_3^-), p. 146; Full blood count, p. 154; Coagulation monitoring, p. 156; Colloids, p. 180; Blood transfusion, p. 182; Bronchodilators, p. 186; Respiratory stimulants, p. 188; Opioid analgesics, p. 232; Nonopioid analgesics, p. 234; Sedatives, p. 236; Muscle relaxants, p. 238; Anticoagulants, p. 246; Coagulants and antifibrinolytics, p. 252; Fluid challenge, p. 272; Respiratory failure, p. 280; Atelectasis and pulmonary collapse, p. 282; Chronic airflow limitation, p. 284; Hypotension, p. 310; Oliguria, p. 328; Metabolic acidosis, p. 436; Hypothermia, p. 518; Pain, p. 534

Obstetric emergencies

Pre-eclampsia and eclampsia

Preeclampsia is defined as hypertension (systolic blood pressure >140 mmHg or diastolic blood pressure >90 mmHg) with proteinuria (>3 g/L in a 24-h specimen) in a previously normotensive woman. Eclampsia is the same condition associated with seizures. They are associated with cerebral edema and, in some cases, hemorrhage. A reduced plasma volume, increased peripheral resistance, and DIC all impair tissue perfusion, with possible renal and hepatic failure. Pulmonary edema may occur secondary to increased peripheral resistance and low COP.

Management

Hypertensive crises and seizures may continue for 48 h postpartum, during which time close monitoring in an intensive care area is essential.

Circulatory management

- High blood pressure resulting from arteriolar vasospasm may be controlled by plasma volume expansion with a fluid challenge regimen in the ICU.
- Oliguria may coexist with reduced plasma volume; controlled volume expansion is usually more appropriate than diuretic therapy.
- If plasma volume expansion fails to control hypertension, antihypertensives such as labetalol, nifedipine, or hydralazine may be used.

Seizures

- Seizures are best avoided by good blood pressure control.
- Initial seizure control may be achieved with small doses of benzodiazepines.
- Magnesium sulfate is the treatment of choice for eclamptic seizures. A clear threshold concentration for the prevention of seizures does not exist, although a range of 4.8 to 8.4 mg/dL has been recommended. Deep tendon reflexes are usually lost around 8 to 10 mg/dL, and respiratory depression can occur at levels >10 mg/dL.
- Prophylactic anticonvulsant therapy with magnesium may also be considered in preeclampsia.
- Excess sedation should be avoided because of the risk of aspiration, although continued seizures may require elective intubation, mechanical hyperventilation, and further anticonvulsant therapy.

Early fetal delivery

The definitive treatment for eclampsia is fetal delivery, but the needs of the fetus must be balanced against those of the mother. If fetal maturity has been reached, immediate delivery after control of seizures and hypertension is necessary. Antenatal corticosteroids accelerate fetal lung maturity and should be considered with an expert in maternal fetal medicine.

Table 34.1 Drug dosages

Labetalol	Start at 2 mg/min IV or quicker if a rapid response is required; labetalol is usually effective after 200 mg has been given, after which a maintenance infusion of 5–50 mg/h may be continued
Hydralazine	5–10 mg by slow IV bolus, repeat after 20–30 min; alternatively, by infusion starting at 200–300 µg/min and reducing to 50–150 µg/min
Magnesium	6 g over 15 min followed by 2–3 g/h by IV infusion until seizures have stopped for 24 h

Key papers

Magpie Trial Collaboration Group. Do women with pre-eclampsia, and their babies, benefit from magnesium sulphate? The Magpie Trial: A randomised placebo-controlled trial. *Lancet* 2002; **359**:1877–90.

Which anticonvulsant for women with eclampsia? Evidence from the Collaborative Eclampsia Trial. *Lancet* 1995; **345**:1455–63.

See also

Ventilatory support—indications, p. 4; Blood pressure monitoring, p. 112; Central venous catheter—use, p. 116; Central venous catheter—insertion, p. 118; EEG monitoring, p. 138; Coagulation monitoring, p. 156; Colloid osmotic pressure, p. 172; Colloids, p. 180; Hypotensive agents, p. 202; Anticonvulsants, p. 240; Fluid challenge, p. 272; Hypertension, p. 312; Generalized seizures, p. 372

HELLP syndrome

HELLP (hemolysis, elevated liver enzymes, and low platelets) syndrome is a pregnancy-related disorder associated with hemolysis, elevated liver function tests and low platelets. Criteria used for the diagnosis of HELLP are described later.

- Microangiopathic hemolysis results from destruction of red cells as they pass through damaged small vessels.
- Hepatic dysfunction is characterized by periportal necrosis and hyaline deposits in the sinusoids. In some cases, hepatic necrosis may proceed to hepatic hemorrhage or rupture.
- Thrombocytopenia results from increased platelet consumption, although PT and APTT are normal, unlike in DIC.

Clinical features

- Epigastric or right upper quadrant pain with malaise
- Nausea and vomiting
- Generalized edema
- Hypertension
- Proteinuria

Presentation may occur postpartum.

Criteria for diagnosis of HELLP syndrome

- Microangiopathic hemolytic anemia with schistocytes on a peripheral blood smear
- LDH >600 U/L or total bilirubin >1.2 mg/dL
- AST >70 U/L
- Platelets <100 × 10^9/L

Management

- Priorities for management include basic resuscitation and exclusion of hepatic hemorrhage or ruptured liver. In the latter case, an early cesarean section and definitive surgical repair are urgent.
- Prompt delivery is indicated if gestational age is ≥34 weeks, nonreassuring fetal heart rate, severe maternal disease (multisystem organ dysfunction, DIC, liver infarction, or hemorrhage), abruptio placenta are present.
- Microangiopathic hemolysis and thrombocytopenia may respond to plasma exchange and FFP infusion.
- Platelet transfusions should be avoided unless there is active bleeding.
- Magnesium sulfate is administered to prevent seizures.
- Blood pressure is managed similar to preeclampsia.
- Corticosteroids can be used to accelerate fetal lung maturity in pregnancies of <34 weeks' gestation.
- Consultation with an expert in maternal fetal medicine should be obtained.

See also

Postpartum hemorrhage

Postpartum hemorrhage is usually the result of incomplete uterine contraction after delivery, but may be the result of retained products. The magnitude of hemorrhage may be severe and life threatening. Postpartum hemorrhage occurs in about 3% of births.

Resuscitation

The principles of resuscitation are the same as those applying to any hemorrhagic condition. Blood transfusion requirements may be massive, and therefore there may be a need to replace coagulation factors. There may be significant retroplacental bleeding, which may lead to underestimation of blood volume loss. Rapidly establish large-bore IV access and consider managing fluid and blood replacement with hemodynamic monitoring.

Stimulated uterine contraction

Begin fundal massage and administer uterotonic drugs such as oxytocin (10–40 U in 1 L normal saline) or carboprost tromethamine (250 µg IM every 15–90 min for a total dose of 2 mg).

Aortic compression

Temporary reduction of hemorrhage may be achieved by compressing the aorta with a fist pushed firmly above the umbilicus, using the pressure between the fist and the vertebral column to achieve compression. This may buy time while definitive surgical repair is organized.

Arterial occlusion

Angiographic embolization or internal iliac artery ligation may avoid the need for hysterectomy in some cases. The disadvantages of these procedures include a significant delay in organization and, in the latter case, the high failure rate.

See also

Blood pressure monitoring, p. 112; Central venous catheter—use, p. 116; Central venous catheter—insertion, p. 118; Full blood count, p. 154; Coagulation monitoring, p. 156; Blood transfusion, p. 182

Amniotic fluid embolus

- Amniotic fluid embolus is an uncommon but dangerous complication of childbirth that presents with a precipitous onset of hypoxemic respiratory failure, DIC, and shock.
- There is a high early mortality associated with acute pulmonary hypertension.
- The initial response of the pulmonary vasculature to the presence of amniotic fluid is intense vasospasm resulting in severe pulmonary hypertension and hypoxemia.
- Right heart function is initially compromised severely, but returns to normal with a secondary phase, during which there is severe left heart failure and pulmonary edema.
- Amniotic fluid contains lipid-rich particulate material that stimulates a systemic inflammatory reaction. In this respect, the progress of the condition is similar to other causes of multiple-organ failure, with associated capillary leak and DIC.
- Diagnosis is supported by amniotic fluid and fetal cells in pulmonary artery blood and urine, although this finding is not specific for embolus.

Management

Management is entirely supportive. If amniotic fluid embolism occurs prior to delivery, urgent cesarean section must be performed to prevent further embolization.

Respiratory support

Oxygen (FiO$_2$, 0.6–1.0) must be provided. In many cases mechanical ventilation will be required.

Cardiovascular support

Standard resuscitation principles apply, with controlled fluid loading and inotropic support being started as required.

Hematological management

Management of the coagulopathy requires blood product therapy guided by laboratory assessment of coagulation times. In addition, some cases improve after treatment with cryoprecipitate, possibly the result of the effects of fibronectin replacement.

See also

Ventilatory support—indications, p. 4; Continuous positive airway pressure, p. 26; Pulmonary artery catheter—use, p. 120; Pulmonary artery catheter—insertion, p. 122; Fluid challenge, p. 272; Pulmonary embolus, p. 306; Heart failure—assessment, p. 322; Heart failure—management, p. 324; Systemic inflammation/multiorgan failure, p. 486

Death and the dying patient

Brain death

The ability to diagnose brain death correctly is an essential skill for any physician working in intensive care. The diagnosis of brain death allows pronouncement of death and closure for family members, and enables potential retrieval of organs for donation. Diagnosis of brain death is usually followed by asystole within a few days. Before brain stem function testing can be performed to confirm the diagnosis, the patient must have an underlying diagnosis compatible with brain death. There must be no hypothermia (temperature >35°C), evidence or suspicion of depressant drugs, significant metabolic abnormality, or muscle relaxant effect. There must be no spontaneous muscular movements, posturing, or seizures. Cessation of mechanical ventilation is seen by many laypeople as the final point of death. Clearly, this final step is easier if all are aware that it is to happen. If organ donation is considered, the transplant coordinator should be involved at an early stage.

Brain death testing

Procedures vary by institution. In most U.S. centers, clinical assessment of brain stem reflexes must be performed by two doctors who have experience in evaluating brain death (usually an intensivist, neurologist, or neurosurgeon). Some centers also require a confirmatory test (e.g., EEG, four-vessel angiogram).

Pupillary light reflex
Pupils should appear fixed in size and fail to respond to a light stimulus.

Corneal reflexes
Corneal reflexes should be absent bilaterally.

Pain response
There should be no cranial response to supraorbital pressure.

Vestibulo-ocular reflexes
After confirming that the tympanic membranes are clear and unobstructed, 20 mL iced water is syringed into the ear. The eyes would normally deviate toward the opposite direction. Absence of movement to bilateral cold stimulation confirms an absent reflex.

Oculocephalic reflexes
Oculocephalic reflexes are also called 'doll's eye' reflexes. With the eye lids held open, brisk lateral rotation of the head normally produces opposite rotation of the eyeball, as if to fix the gaze on an object. This rotation is lost in brain death.

Gag reflex
The gag reflex is absent in brain death. However, the gag reflex is also often lost in patients who are intubated.

Apnea test

While the reflex assessments are being performed, the patient should be preoxygenated with 100% oxygen. The ventilator can be disconnected and oxygen passed into the trachea via a catheter. Apneic oxygenation can sustain SaO_2 for prolonged periods, but there is an inevitable increase in $PaCO_2$ that should stimulate respiratory effort. After 3 to 5 min of disconnection, blood gas analyses are performed until $PaCO_2$ is >60 mmHg. Any respiratory effort negates the diagnosis of brain death.

Atropine test

There should be no increase in heart rate after 1 mg atropine is given IV.

See also

Blood gas analysis, p. 102; EEG monitoring, p. 138; Urea and creatinine, p. 144; Electrolytes (Na^+, K^+, Cl^-, HCO_3^-), p. 146; Toxicology, p. 162; Opioid analgesics, p. 232; Nonopioid analgesics, p. 234; Sedatives, p. 236; Muscle relaxants, p. 238; Cardiac arrest, p. 270; Hypoglycemia, p. 440; Hypothermia, p. 518; Care of the potential organ donor, p. 554

Withdrawal and withholding treatment

This (withdrawal and withholding treatment) is arguably the most difficult and stressful decision that has to be made for the critically ill patient. Withdrawal involves reduction or cessation of vasoactive drugs and/or respiratory support. In some ICUs the patient is heavily sedated and disconnected from the ventilator. Withholding involves noncommencement or nonescalation of treatment (e.g., applying an upper threshold dose for an inotrope and/or not starting renal replacement therapy).

Patients have the right to refuse any therapy, and this right is not relinquished when the patient lacks decision-making capacity because of critical illness. Surrogate decision makers (typically family or persons appointed by the patient) should be asked to speak on the patients' behalf in order that the health care team know the wishes of the patient. Furthermore, it is the duty of the physician to guide the patient and surrogate decision makers so that decisions that reflect the patient's goals are reached, rather than decisions that are simply easy. Simply asking surrogates questions like 'What do you want us to do?' or 'Does the patient want everything to be done?' does not further patient autonomy, and in fact is an abrogation of physician responsibility to explain options and consequences and to assist the patient in making difficult decisions.

It should be stressed to the patient and surrogate that the choice is never between care and lack of care, but that pain relief, comfort, and general nursing care will always be continued. Likewise, no decision is binding, but can be amended depending on the patient's progress (e.g., moving from withholding to withdrawal of therapy, or reinstitution of full treatment). A 'negotiated settlement' is often a useful interim compromise for families unable to accept a withdrawal decision, whereby limitation of treatment is instituted and subsequently reviewed.

Family members can sometimes be very distraught and, occasionally, irrational when discussing withdrawal/withholding of therapy. For many, this will be their first experience of the dying process in a loved one. A number of other factors including guilt, anger, and within-family disagreements may also surface. It should be stressed that the withdraw/withhold decision should not be left to the family alone, because this is an unfair burden for them to carry. Rather, it is their passive agreement with a medical recommendation that is being sought. Indeed the role of the surrogate is to speak for the patient, not for his or her own desires. Family members need to be dealt with both sensitively and honestly, and they should not feel pressured to make medical decisions.

Discussions should involve the patient's nurse and other involved caregivers as appropriate. It should be accurately documented in the progress notes to ensure good communication between caregivers.

See also

Communication, p. 566

Care of the potential organ donor

Patients with suspected brain death should be considered candidates for organ donation. The transplant coordinator should be contacted early (before the family is approached) to confirm likely suitability. If the family is amenable, the transplant coordinator will then initiate organ donation procedures. Medical criteria for organ donation are constantly evolving. For example potential donors with HIV or hepatitis B/C were once excluded but may now be considered by some transplant centers who may consider the organs for recipients with HIV or chronic hepatitis. Thus, local organ procurement agencies should be informed about all potential donors.

Management

1. Confirm brain death with appropriate testing and pronounce the patient.
2. Contact the coroner per local requirements.
3. Run laboratory tests for blood group, HIV, and hepatitis status, and electrolytes.
4. Maintain optimal cardiorespiratory status with fluid ± inotropes, optimal ventilation, and physiotherapy. Diabetes insipidus should be treated with replacement fluids and 1-deamino-8-D-arginine vasopressin.

See also

Blood gas analysis, p. 102; Urea and creatinine, p. 144; Electrolytes (Na$^+$, K$^+$, Cl$^-$, HCO$_3^-$), p. 146; Colloids, p. 180; Inotropes, p. 196; Vasopressors, p. 200; Fluid challenge, p. 272; Hypotension, p. 310

Chapter 36

ICU organization and management

ICU layout

The ICU should be easily accessible by departments from which patients are admitted and close to departments that share engineering services. It is desirable that critically ill patients are separated from those requiring coronary care or high-dependency care, for which a quieter environment is often needed. It is possible to provide intensive care and high-dependency care in the same unit, as long as patients can be separated within the unit. However, the differing requirements of these patients may limit such flexibility.

Size

Intensive care bed requirements depend on the activity of the hospital, with additional beds required for specialties such as cardiothoracic surgery or neurosurgery. Very small (less than six beds) or very large (>20 beds) units may be difficult to manage, although larger units may be divided operationally and allow better concentration of resources.

Patient areas

- Patient areas must provide unobstructed passage around the bed. Curtains or screens are required for privacy.
- Floors and ceilings must be constructed to support heavy equipment (some pieces may weigh 1000 kg).
- Doors must allow for passage of bulky equipment as well as wide beds.
- Every bed should have access to a wash sink.
- Air-conditioning should allow for positive and negative pressure control in cubicles, and temperature and humidity control.
- Services must include adequate electricity supply (at least 28 sockets per bed) with emergency backup supply. Oxygen, medical air, and suction outlets must be available for every bed.
- Some rooms for reverse isolation (negative pressure) are necessary, and rooms plumbed for dialysis are also recommended.
- The bed areas should have natural daylight, and patients and staff should ideally have an outside view.
- Communications systems include an adequate number of telephones to avoid all telephones being in use at once, intercom systems to allow bed-to-bed communication, and a system to control entry to the department.
- Computer networks should enable communication with central hospital administration and laboratory systems.

Other areas

Other areas include adequate storage space, dirty utility, clean utility, offices, laboratory, conference room, custodian room, staff rest room, locker room, toilets, and visitors' area.

ICU staffing (medical)

Intensive care has evolved from the early success in simple mechanical ventilation of the lungs of polio victims to the present day, when patients admitted to intensive care will usually have failure or dysfunction of one or more organ systems requiring mechanical support and monitoring. The ICU should have dedicated intensivists who can provide 24-h-per-day coverage on a rotating basis.

Required skills of intensive care medical staff

Management

Senior intensive care medical staff, assisted by senior nursing and pharmacy colleagues, command the primary responsibility for the financial management of the ICU. It is through their actions that treatment of the critically ill is initiated and perpetuated; they are ultimately responsible for the activity of the unit and patient outcome.

Decision making

In the ICU most decisions are ultimately made by team consensus. Clinical decisions in the ICU can be thought of under three categories: (1) decisions relating to common or routine problems for which a unit policy exists, (2) decisions relating to uncommon problems requiring discussion with all ICU and non-ICU staff currently involved, and (3) decisions of an urgent nature taken by intensive care staff without delay.

Practical skills

Expertise in the management of complex equipment, monitoring procedures, and performance of invasive procedures is required.

Clinical experience

Medical staff require experience in the recognition, prevention, and management of critical illness, infection control, anesthesia, and organ support.

Technical knowledge

The intensive care specialist has an important role in the choice of equipment used in the ICU.

Pharmacological knowledge

Drug therapy regimens are clearly open to the problems of drug interactions and, in addition, pharmacokinetics are often severely altered by the effects of major organ system dysfunction, particularly involving the liver and kidneys.

Teaching and training

The modern intensive care specialist has acquired a number of skills that cannot be gained outside the ICU. It is therefore necessary to be able to provide this education to junior doctors in training for intensive care.

Open versus closed units

Unlike in many other countries, many ICUs in the United States lack sufficient numbers of intensive care specialists to provide full and exclusive coverage of critically ill patients. Thus, a common model is an 'open ICU' where primary specialties (e.g., medicine, surgery) admit patients to the ICU and function as part of the extended ICU medical staff for their own patients. These physicians often receive considerable ICU training and experience as it pertains to the care of critically ill patients of the sort for whom they are caring as primary specialists. For example, most general surgeons receive training in the surgical ICU and acquire experience related to routine care of surgical patients in the ICU. Most general internists have the same type of training for medical patients in the medical ICU. Under this model, consultants are usually called in to manage more complex or unusual problems. Some units involve consultants to manage mechanical ventilation or renal replacement therapy or even to manage blood glucose or select antibiotics.

The downside to the open ICU model is that very complicated cases can result in numerous physicians attempting to manage individual problems without a clear 'team captain' who orchestrates the total care plan. Physicians who lack sufficient expertise in intensive care such that consultants are routinely needed also lack sufficient ability to manage the team effectively. As a result, confusion regarding who is responsible for what often arises, leading to frustration among staff and families.

The 'closed ICU' model, by contrast, restricts activities of physicians who are not part of the ICU team. These physicians may not write orders or do bedside procedures without approval, and often oversight, by the ICU medical staff. Consultants are called in to provide advice or to perform procedures, but do so only under the authority of the ICU team.

At the University of Pittsburgh, the ICUs are organized along subspecialty service lines (e.g., cardiac surgery, liver transplantation, trauma) and operate under a closed model in which physicians outside the service line or ICU staff have limited authority and generally may not write orders.

ICU staffing (nursing)

Critically ill patients require close nursing supervision. Some will require high-intensity nursing throughout a 24-h period whereas others are of a lower dependency and can share nurses. In addition to the bedside nurses, the department needs additional staff to manage the day-to-day operation of the unit, to assist in lifting and handling of patients, to relieve bedside nurses for rest periods, and to collect drugs and equipment. These additional nurses (or nurse assistants), by the nature of their duties, will usually include more senior-level nurses. The number of bedside nurses is dependent on activity, more patients require more nurses.

Communication

Good communication is essential to the smooth running of the ICU. This includes communication between the ICU staff, patients, visiting professionals, and relatives of the patient.

Patient communication

Critically ill patients may still be able to hear conversation despite sedation or apparent unconsciousness. Bedside discussions should take this into account and all procedures should be explained to the patient in simple terms before starting. The patient who lacks capacity to consent to treatment will nonetheless appreciate verbal discussion or explanation.

Doctor–nurse communication

It is essential that the multidisciplinary approach to intensive care involves medical and nursing staff in decision making. Ward rounds are a forum for such interdisciplinary communication, and the attending physician leading rounds should ensure that all present are truly involved. The plan for the day can be set on rounds, but is more likely to succeed if all involved in effecting the plan are involved in setting it. Similarly, all changes from the plan, whether the result of unforeseen emergencies or failure of the patient to respond, should be fully discussed—even if after the fact, in the case of emergencies.

Communication with visiting teams

The intensive care staff should be responsible for the day-to-day care of critically ill patients, including coordinating the input from various non-ICU professionals involved in the management of patients and affecting the treatment plan. The admitting team should be involved in major decisions. Visiting medical staff should not see patients without being accompanied by a member of the intensive care medical staff.

Communication with families

Family members are often overwhelmed by the environment of an ICU, are worried about the patient, and are easily confused by the information they are given about critically ill patients. Most communication should be face to face, avoiding lengthy discussions on the telephone. When several people are imparting information, differences in emphasis or content destroy any chance of effective communication. It is essential that the bedside nurse be present when family members are spoken to, because there are often questions and concerns that crop up later and are directed to the nurse. It is worth remembering that the family has greater contact with the nurses and often develops a relationship with them. When admitting teams need to communicate with families about a specific aspect of the illness, the bedside nurse and, ideally, a member of the intensive care medical staff, should be present. Most interviews with relatives should be away from the bedside, although it is often helpful to impart simple information at the bedside, particularly to demonstrate particular issues. Again, it must be remembered that the patient may hear the conversation. Although it is helpful to interview all relatives together, this is not always practical, either because they cannot all be present at the same time or because they do not relate to each other well. Information often changes when delivered second hand, so it is better to communicate directly with various family members separately in these circumstances.

Medicolegal aspects

The ICU is a source of many medicolegal problems. Patients often lack the capacity to consent to treatment. They may be admitted after trauma, violence, or poisoning, all of which may involve a legal process. Admission may also follow complications of treatment or medical mishaps occurring elsewhere in the hospital. The nature of critical illness is such that complications are common and litigation may follow.

Consent and agreement

Many procedures in intensive care are invasive or involve significant risk. The patient is often not able to provide informed consent for such treatment. It is important that the risks and benefits of the procedure are explained to the next of kin, and that this discussion is documented in the patient's chart. For major decisions, particularly those involving withdrawal or withholding of life support, the patient should ideally be involved in discussions. If not feasible, the patient's surrogate should be asked to give his or her view of what the patient would want in this situation.

Record keeping

It is impossible to record everything that happens in intensive care in the progress notes. The electronic medical record provides the most detailed record of what has happened, but summary notes are essential. Such notes must be factual, without unsubstantiated opinions about the patient or about previous treatment. All entries must be timed and signed. It must be remembered that the notes may be used later in legal proceedings. They may be used against you, but, if well kept, will usually form the best defense. In the event of a medical mishap, the episode should be clearly documented after witnessed explanation occure to the patient and/or family.

Dealing with the police

Most police inquiries relate to patients who are admitted after suspicious circumstances. Although there is a duty to patient confidentiality, it may be in the patient's interests to impart information about him or her. This may be with the consent of the patient or the next of kin. Written statements or verbal information may be requested. Any information given should avoid opinion and should be strictly factual.

Dealing with the coroner

Regulations pertaining to the role of the coroner for in-hospital deaths vary by state. In general, the coroner or medical examiner must be informed of any death for which a death certificate cannot be issued. Death certificates can be issued when the death is the result of a 'natural cause'. Some jurisdictions require that all deaths be reported to the coroner, whereas others have specific guidelines. When there is any doubt, the coroner should be informed.

Clinical governance

Clinical governance is a framework through which health care organizations are accountable for continuously improving the quality of their services and safeguarding high standards of care by creating an environment in which excellence in clinical care will flourish. For the ICU, clinical governance requires the culture, the systems, and the support mechanisms to achieve good clinical performance and to ensure that quality improvement is embedded into the unit's routine. This includes action to ensure risks are managed, adverse effects are rapidly detected, openly investigated and lessons learned, good practice is rapidly disseminated and systems are in place to ensure continuous improvements in clinical care. There must be systems to ensure all clinicians have the right education, training, skills and competencies to deliver the care needed by patients. There must be systems in place to recognize and act on poor performance.

Essential components of clinical governance

Clear management arrangements

Everyone must know to whom they are accountable, the limits of their decision making, and whom must be informed in the decision-making process.

Quality improvement

Through the process of clinical case review, the standard of practice is monitored and changes are effected to improve quality.

Clinical effectiveness

Evidence-based practice is essential when evidence exists to support clinical decisions. Protocols and guidelines standardize practice.

Risk assessment and management

An ongoing assessment of clinical risks should be performed. An action plan should be developed for managing each risk.

Staff and organizational development

Including continued professional education, clinical supervision, and professional regulation.

Patient input

Complaint monitoring should be used to learn lessons and improve practice within the ICU. Patient and family surveys can be used to adapt quality initiatives to the needs of patients.

See also

Quality Improvement, p. 572

Quality improvement

Quality improvement has become an essential part of medical practice. The main purpose is to improve quality of care that, in the ICU, must involve all members of the multidisciplinary team. Change in practice in one discipline will inevitably have an effect on others. Quality improvementl may involve a review of activity, performance against predetermined indicators, or an assessment of cost-effectiveness. Quality improvement may focus on specific topics or may encompass the performance of several ICUs. Successful quality improvement requires commitment from senior staff to ensure practice is defined, data are collected, and change is effected when necessary. When change is suggested by quality improvement, a further review is required to ensure that the change has occurred.

Data collection

Ideally, a basic data set should be common to all ICUs nationally to allow meaningful comparisons to be made. This requires the data set to be detailed enough to answer questions posed but not so detailed that collection becomes unsustainable. Resources must be provided in terms of computer databases and staff to collect and analyze data. Those collecting the data should be provided with regular summary reviews to ensure that enthusiasm continues and quality control is maintained. Methods of data entry should consider the time involved and the fact that most of those collecting data are not keyboard experts. Typographical mistakes destroy the value of collected data such that error trapping and data validation must form part of the housekeeping in any database used. Some quality improvement topics require data collection that is not part of the basic data set. Collecting appropriate data requires clarity in posing the question to be answered and care in choosing data items that will truly answer the question.

Quality improvement meetings

Regular quality improvement meetings should follow a predefined timetable. This helps to ensure maximum staff attendance and also sets target dates for data collection and analysis. Audit meetings should be chaired and have defined aims. Discussion of the topic being audited must lead to recommended changes in practice, and these must be followed through after the meeting. It is clear that all staff cannot attend all meetings. Dissemination of information prior to implementing proposed changes improves the likelihood of the proposed changes becoming successfully implemented.

See also
Clinical governance, p. 570

ICU scoring systems

Various ICU scoring systems have evolved to provide
- An index of disease severity (e.g., APACHE, Simplified Acute Physiology Score [SAPS])
- An index of workload and consumption of resources (e.g., Therapeutic Intervention Scoring System [TISS])
- A means of comparison for:
  1. Auditing performance—either in the same ICU or between ICUs
  2. Research (e.g., evaluation of new products or treatment regimens)
- Patient management objectives (e.g. sedation, pressure area care)

Other than the GCS, there is no universal system practiced by every ICU. Although APACHE is the predominant system used in the United States and the United Kingdom for scoring disease severity, SAPS is more popular in mainland Europe. Interpretation of the same system can also be highly variable.

TISS
- This system attaches a score to procedures and techniques performed on an individual patient (e.g., use and number of vasoactive drug infusions, renal replacement therapy, administration of enteral nutrition).
- It has been used by some ICUs to develop a means of costing individual patients by attaching a monetary value to each TISS point scored.
- It is also used as an index of workload activity.
- A discharge TISS score can be used to estimate the amount of nursing interventions required for a patient in step-down facilities or on the general ward.
- TISS does not accurately measure nursing workload activity because it fails to account for tasks and duties such as coping with the irritable or confused patient, dealing with grieving relatives, and so forth.

GCS
First described by Teasdale and Jennett in 1974, the GCS utilizes eye opening, best motor response and best verbal response to categorize neurological status. It is the only system used universally in ICUs, although limitations exist in mechanically ventilated, sedated patients. It can be used for prognostication and is also frequently used for therapeutic decision making (e.g., elective ventilation in patients presenting with a GCS scored <8 points).

Sedation
A variety of systems gauge and record the level of sedation in a mechanically ventilated patient. This assists the staff in titrating the dose of sedative agents to avoid either over- or undersedation. Developed in 1974, the Ramsay Sedation Scale consists of a 6-point scoring system separated into three awake and three asleep levels in which the patient responds to a tap or loud auditory stimulus with either brisk, sluggish, or no response at all. The main problem lies in achieving reproducibility of the tap or loud auditory stimulus. A 'modified Ramsay' scale is currently in use in many units.

Table 36.1 Glasgow coma scale

Score (pt)	Eyes open	Best motor response	Best verbal response
6	—	Obeys commands	—
5	—	Localizes pain	Orientated
4	Spontaneously	Flexion withdrawal	Confused
3	To speech	Decerebrate flexion	Inappropriate words
2	To pain	Decerebrate extension	Incomprehensible sounds
1	Never	No response	Silent

Modified Ramsay Sedation Scale

1 Anxious, agitated, or restless
2 Cooperative, oriented, and tranquil
3 Sedated but responds to commands
4 Asleep but easily roused
5 Asleep, sluggish response to stimuli
6 No response to noxious stimuli

ICU scoring systems—APACHE II

- Devised by Knaus and colleagues, this system uses a point score derived from the degree of abnormality of readily obtainable physiological and laboratory variables in the first 24 h of ICU admission, plus extra points for age and chronic ill health.
- The summated score provides a measure of severity whereas the percentage risk of subsequent death can be computed from specific coefficients applied to a wide range of admission disorders (excluding burns and cardiac surgery).
- APACHE I, first described in 1981, utilized 34 physiological and biochemical variables.
- A simplified version, APACHE II, utilizing just 12 variables was published in 1985 and has been extensively validated in a number of countries.
- A further refinement published in 1990, APACHE III, claims to improve on the statistical predictive power by adding five new physiological variables (albumin, bilirubin, glucose, urea, urine output).
  - Changing thresholds and weighting of existing variables
  - Comparing both admission and 24 h scores
  - Incorporating the admission source (e.g., ward, operating room)
  - Reassessing effects of age, chronic health, and specific disease category. Wide acceptance of APACHE III may be limited because its risk stratification system is proprietary and has to be purchased.

Chronic health points

Two points for elective postoperative admission or 5 points if emergency operation or nonoperative admission, if patient has either

- Biopsy-proved cirrhosis, portal hypertension, or previous hepatic failure
- Chronic heart failure (NYHA grade 4)
- Chronic hypoxia, hypercapnia, severe exercise limitation, 2 second-degree polycythaemia, or pulmonary hypertension
- Dialysis-dependent renal disease
- Immunosuppression by disease or drugs

Table 36.2 APACHE II

	+4	+3	+2	+1	0	+1	+2	+3	+4
Core temperature (°C)	≥41	39–40.9		38.2–38.9	36–38.4	34–35.9	32–33.9	30–31	≤29.9
Mean BP (mmHg)	≥160	130–159	110–129		70–109		50–69		≤49
Heart rate (bpm)	≥180	140–179	110–139		70–109		55–69	40–54	≤39
Respiratory rate (breaths/min)	≥50	35–49		25–34	12–24	10–11	6–9		≤5
If FO$_2$ ≥0.5, A-aDO$_2$ (mmHg)	≥500	350–499	200–349	<200					
If FO$_2$ <0.5, PO$_2$ (mmHg)					>70	61–70		55–60	
Arterial pH	≥7.7	7.6–7.69		7.5–7.59	7.33–7.49		7.25–7.32	7.15–7.24	≤7.15
Serum Na$^+$ (mmol/L)	≥180	160–179	155–159	150–154	130–149		120–129	111–119	≤110
Serum K$^+$ (mmol/L)	≥7	6–6.9		5.5–5.9	3.5–5.4		3–3.4	2.5–2.9	≤2.5
Serum creatinine (mg/dL)*									
	≥3.4	1.9–3.4	1.4–1.8		0.6–1.4	<0.6			
Hematocrit (%)	≥60		50–59.9	46–49.9	30–45.9		20–29.9		≤20
Leukocytes (/mm^3)	≥40		20–39.9	15–19.9	3–14.9		1–2.9		≤1

* Double points if acute renal failure.
Neurological points =15 (GCS)
A-aDO$_2$; FO$_2$BP, blood pressure.

Key paper

Knaus WA, et al. APACHE II: A severity of disease classification system. *Crit Care Med* 1985; **13**:818–29.

ICU scoring systems—SAPS II

- SAPS II has a similar role to APACHE II, but is more widely used in mainland Europe. SAPS was devised by Le Gall and colleagues in 1984 (SAPS I) and with modified by the same group in 1993 (SAPS II). SAPS III is in development.
- Similar to APACHE II, burns and cardiac surgical patients are excluded from analysis.
- The original version used 14 readily measured clinical and biochemical variables whereas the updated version, SAPS II, comprises 12 physiology variables, age, type of admission (medical, scheduled or unscheduled surgical), and three underlying disease variables.
- A point score is based on the degree and prognostic importance of derangement of these variables in the first 24 h after ICU admission. The point scoring was assigned based on logistic regression modeling of data obtained from 8369 patients in 137 adult ICUs in both Europe and North America, and was validated in an additional 4628 patients.
- The claimed advantage of this system is that it estimates the risk of death without having to specify a primary diagnosis.

Table 36.3 SAPS II

Age	<40 (0); 40–59 (7); 60–69 (12); 70–74 (15); 75–79 (16); ≥80 (18)
Heart rate (bpm)	<40 (11); 40–69 (2); 70–119 (0); 120–159 (4); ≥160 (7)
Systolic BP (mmHg)	<70 (13); 70–99 (5); 100–199 (0); ≥200 (2)
Body temperature (°C)	<39 (0); ≥39 (3)
PaO$_2$/FO$_2$ (mmHg) only if ventilated or on CPAP	<1.77 (11); 1.77–3.52 (9); ≥3.53 (6)
Urine output (L/day)	<0.5 (11); 0.5–0.999 (4); ≥1 (0)
BUN (mmol/L)	<28 (0); 28–83 (6); ≥84 (10)
White cell count (/mm^3)	<1 (12); 1–19.9 (0); ≥20 (3)
Serum K (mmol/L)	<3 (3); 3–4.9 (0); ≥5 (3)
Serum Na$^+$ (mmol/L)	<125 (5); 125–144 (0); ≥145 (1)
Serum HCO$_3^-$ (mmol/L)	<15 (6); 15–19 (3); ≥20 (0)
Serum bilirubin (mg/dL)	<4 (0); 4–5.99 (4); ≥6 (9)
GCS score	<6 (26); 6–8 (13); 9–10 (7); 11–13 (5); 14–15 (0)
Chronic disease	Metastatic cancer (9), hematological malignancy (10), AIDS (17)
Type of admission	Scheduled surgical (0), medical (6), unscheduled surgical (8)

Scores (points) are included parentheses. BP, blood pressure.

Key paper

Le Gall JR, *et al.* A new Simplified Acute Physiology Score (SAPS II) based on a European/North American multicenter study. *JAMA* 1993; **270**:2957–63.

ICU scoring systems—SOFA

A limitation of the APACHE and SAPS scoring systems is that they were designed and validated on data obtained during the first 24 h of intensive care admission. Various systems have been developed to enable daily scoring (e.g., Sequential Organ Failure Assessment [SOFA], Riyadh Intensive Care Program score, Multiple Organ Dysfunction Score) to allow a better assessment of change in the patient's condition.

Because the physiological and biochemical status of the patient is determined in part by disease severity, but also by the degree of medical intervention, these sequential scoring systems incorporate the use of various therapies and procedures.

The SOFA system was initially designed to improve patient characterization for multicenter drug trials in sepsis (SOFA initially stood for Sepsis Organ Failure Assessment) but has subsequently been applied to intensive care patients in general, with 'Sequential' being substituted for 'Sepsis'.

Although it has not been validated in the sense that a point score denoting severity of dysfunction in one organ system does not translate directly to an equivalent severity in another organ, it has been used successfully to prognosticate and to follow changes in patient status throughout their intensive care stay.

Table 36.4 SOFA

	0	1	2	3	4
Respiratory PaO_2-ot-FO_2 ratio (mmHg)	>400	>400	≤300	≤200*	<100*
Renal Creatinine (mg/dL) or Urine output (mL/d)	<1.2	1.2–1.9	2.0–3.4	3.5–4.9 <500 mL/da	≤5.0 <200 mL/da
Hepatic Bilirubin (mg/dL)	<1.2	1.2–1.9	2.0–5.9	6.0–11.9	12.0
Cardiovascular MAP (mmHg)	No hypotension	MAP >70	Dopamine ≤5 or, dobutamine (any dose)†	Dopamine >5 or, epinephrine ≤0.1 epinephrine ≤0.1†	Dopamine >15 or epinephrine >0.1 epinephrine >0.1†
Hematological Platelet count (x10^3/mm^3)	>150	≤150	≤100	≤50	≤20
Neurological GCS	15	13–14	10–12	6–9	<6

*With ventilatory support
†Adrenergic agents administered for at least 1 h (doses in micrograms per kilograms per minute).

Key paper

Moreno R, Vincent JL, Matos R, et al. The use of maximum SOFA score to quantify organ dysfunction/failure in intensive care. Results of a prospective, multicentre study. Working Group on Sepsis Related Problems of the ESICM. *Intensive Care Med* 1999; **25**:686–96.

ICU scoring systems—trauma

Scoring systems have been developed in trauma for
- Rapid field triage to direct the patient to appropriate levels of care
- Quality assurance
- Developing and improving trauma care systems by categorizing patients and identifying problems within the systems
- Making comparisons between groups from different hospitals, in the same hospital over time, and/or undergoing different treatments

The Injury Severity Score (ISS) is a severity scoring system for patients based on the anatomic injuries sustained. The Revised Trauma Score (RTS) utilizes measures of physiological abnormality to predict survival. A combination of ISS and RTS—(TRISS)—was developed to overcome the shortcomings of anatomic or physiological scoring alone. The TRISS methodology uses ISS, RTS, patient age, and whether the injury was blunt or penetrating to provide a measure of the probability of survival.

Injury Severity Score

1. Use theAbbreviated Injury Score 1990 dictionary to score. injury
2. Identify highest abbreviated injury scale score for each of the following:
   - Head and neck
   - Abdomen and pelvic contents
   - Bony pelvis and limbs
   - Face
   - Chest
   - Body surface
3. Add the squares of the three highest area scores.

Table 36.5 Revised trauma score

	Measure	Coded value	x = Score weighting
Respiratory rate (breaths/min)	10–29	4	
	>29	3	
	6–9	2	0.2908
	1–5	1	
	0	0	
Systolic blood pressure (mmHg)	>89	4	
	76–89	3	
	50–75	2	0.7326
	1–49	1	
	0	0	
GCS score (pt)	13–15	4	
	9–12	3	
	6–8	2	0.9368
	4–5	1	
	3	0	

Total = revised trauma score.

Sedation scale—RASS

The RASS uses the duration of eye contact after verbal stimulation as the principal means of titrating sedation. The RASS has good interrater reliability in a broad range of adult ICU patients and validity when compared with a visual analogue scale and other sedation scales.

Richmond Agitation Sedation Scale (RASS)

+4	Combative	Overtly combative, violent, immediate danger to staff
+3	Very agitated	Pulls or removes tubes or catheters aggressive
+2	Agitated	Frequent nonpurposeful movement, fights ventilator
+1	Restless	Anxious, but movements not aggressive or vigorous
0	Alert/calm	
−1	Drowsy	Not fully alert, but has sustained awakening (eyeopening/eye contact) to voice (>10 s)
−2	Light sedation	Briefly awakens with eye contact to voice (<10 s)
−3	Moderate sedation	Movement or eye opening to voice (but no eye contact)
−4	Deep sedation	No response to voice, but movement or eye opening to physical stimulation
−5	Unable to be roused	No response to voice or physical stimulation

Procedure for RASS Assessment

1. Observe patient.
   a. Patient is alert, restless, or agitated (score, 0 to +4).
2. If not alert, state patient's name and tell patient to open eyes and look at speaker.
   b. Patient awakens with sustained eye opening and eye contact. (score, −1)
   c. Patient awakens with eye opening and eye contact, but not sustained (score, −2).
   d. Patient has any movement in response to voice but no eye contact. (score, −3).
3. When no response to verbal stimulation, physically stimulate patient by shaking shoulder and/or rubbing sternum.
   e. Patient has any movement to physical stimulation (score, −4).
   f. Patient has no response to any stimulation. (score, −5).

Key trial

Ely EW, *et al.* Monitoring sedation status over time in ICU patients: The reliability and validity of the Richmond Agitation Sedation Scale (RASS). *JAMA* 2003; **289**:2983–91.

See also

Sedatives, p. 236

Index

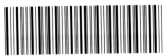
DATE DUE

Normal hemodynamic parameters–adults